Short and Sweet

In my teenage years, I read a novel by H. G. Wells called *The Island of Dr. Moreau*. The strength of the book lay in its vivid descriptions of the eponymous doctor's shocking treatment of wild animals during his attempts, by means of vivisection, to change them into human beings. In the book, the House of Pain referred to the laboratory in which Moreau conducted his hideous experiments, without any regard for the extraordinary pain that the animals endured under his scalpel. These medical monstrosities were called the Beast Folk.

In my book, the House of Pain refers to the hospitals and medical centers which the Veterans Administration owns and mismanages. The modern day Moreaus are the indifferent people that the VA employs: administrators, doctors, and medical so-called professionals.

I was seriously wounded in Vietnam by three bullets and an enemy grenade. I spent thirteen months recuperating in Army hospitals; three of those months I was held firmly in place by traction bars. After I was discharged with a 60% disability rating, I suffered a lifetime of strong discomfort that culminated in severe chronic pain due largely to a sciatic nerve which had been damaged when an enemy bullet shattered my left femur.

Every bit of this pain could have been eliminated if the VA medical personnel wanted to help me. None did.

When I mentioned this chronic pain, the doctor who was assigned to treat me threw me out of his office - on two occasions - and on another occasion he had a tantrum, screamed in my ear and called me a dope addict, and fled the office in the middle of the examination, never to return, leaving me all alone in his office. I swear these incidents happened exactly the way I described them in this book.

The hospital director supported this behavior and denied my numerous requests to be transferred to a different doctor.

The chronic pain clinic prescribed over-the-counter skin cream to treat my chronic sciatic pain. When I complained that the cream did not help, I was kicked out of the clinic.

Hard to believe? Welcome to VA medical (dis)service.

This modern version of the House of Pain is found in the Veterans Administration's medical centers, in which veterans – chiefly those who suffer from long-time aftereffects of their time spent in Vietnam – are mistreated, misunderstood., and disregarded as yesteryear's forgotten soldiers from a misguided and forgotten war. The inhuman Beast Folk are the VA's medical staff. Most of them, anyway.

I have had the misfortune to have experienced firsthand the dire machinations of the VA's apathetic medical system.

This book tells it all: from my personal combat actions as a rifleman in the 25th Infantryman Division in Vietnam, to a long-time patient in various Army hospitals, through a lifetime of anguish as a disabled civilian, to my ultimate confrontation with today's Veterans Administration, whose modern banner reads like a quote from W. C. Fields, "Go away kid, ya bother me."

Here is my story about modern VA medical mistreatment. This is the kind of treatment that today's soldiers can expect to receive if they are ever wounded in combat.

Caveat emptor, as the Romans used to say. Let the buyer beware . . . if you enlist.

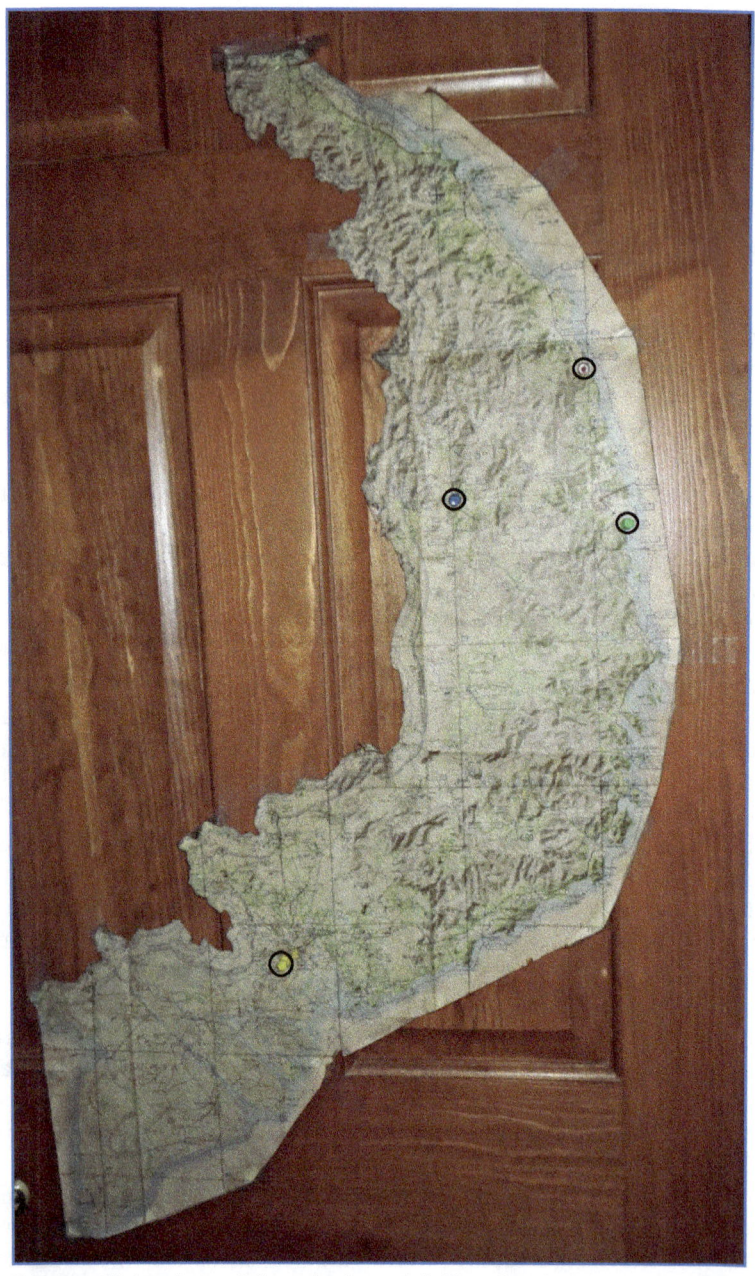

This map of Vietnam is mounted on a door in my study. The yellow pin designates Saigon. The blue pin designates Pleiku. The red pin designates Duc Pho. The green pin designates Qui Nhon.

Note the colophon at the bottom of the opposite page. I designed the colophon. Cheryl drew the volcano. I drew the lightning bolt by copying it from the insignia of the 25th Infantry Division.

The House of Pain

Veterans Administration's Mistreatment of Wounded Vietnam Veterans

by Gary Gentile

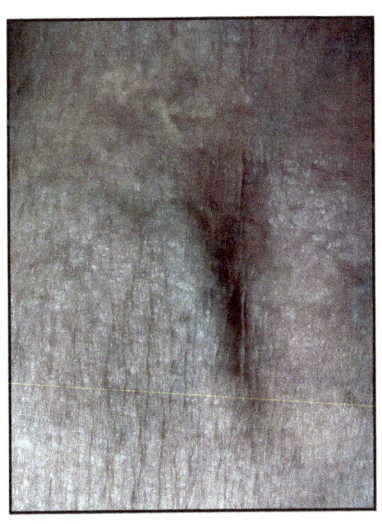

Note the white horizontal scar above the vertical blood vessel on the inside of my elbow. This is called a cut-down. Had it not been for this emergency procedure, you would not be reading this book today. Read on.

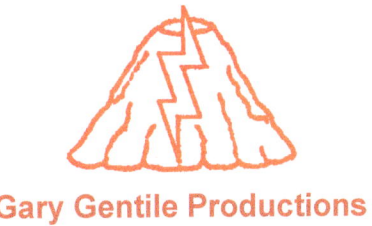

Gary Gentile Productions

Copyright 2024 by Gary Gentile

All rights reserved. Except for the use of brief quotations embodied in critical articles and reviews, this book may not be reproduced in part or in whole, in any manner (including mechanical, electronic, photographic, and photocopy means), transmitted in any form, or recorded by any data storage and/or retrieval device, without express written permission from the author. Address all queries to:

Bellerophon Bookworks
500 Lehigh Gorge Drive
Jim Thorpe, PA 18229

Additional copies of this book may be purchased from the same address by sending a check or money order in the amount of $20 U.S. for each copy (plus $4 postage per order, not per book, in the U.S. Inquire for shipping cost to foreign countries). Alternatively, copies may be ordered from the author's website and paid by credit card:

http://www.ggentile.com

Picture Credits

All uncredited photographs were taken by the author. Photographs that are credited as "Archival photo" are those that were obtained from archival sources, either directly or indirectly. The front cover bottom photo and the three rear cover photos are Archival photos.

> This book is dedicated to
> all the soldiers and civilians,
> and especially to the medical personnel,
> who served in Vietnam, plus to
> those people who served in any capacity
> in stateside military hospitals during the
> Vietnam Conflict.

International Standard Book Numbers (ISBN)
1-883056-60-8
978-1-883056-60-5

First Edition

Printed in U.S.A.

Introduction

During the height of the American Civil War, the person who was the largest and most powerful slaveowner in the country – in the world – was President Abraham Lincoln.

You were not taught this in school.

You were taught instead about Lincoln's Emancipation Proclamation. Most graduates today believe that January 1, 1863 put an end to slavery in the United States of America. In fact, the Emancipation Proclamation did not free a single solitary slave. People who were slaves before the Proclamation remained slaves after the Proclamation. The reason that the Proclamation was as worthless as the paper it was printed on was because all the slaveowners and their slaves lived in the Confederate States of America, where, by means of Southern cessation, Lincoln did not have jurisdiction.

Three months later – on March 3, 1863 – Lincoln enacted the Civil War Military Draft Act. The first response to this Act was a series of riots in New York City, where more than a hundred people were killed, most by gunfire. This act was so repulsive to the public that after the Civil War ended, the Thirteenth Amendment was added to the Constitution of the United States. It states in full:

>Section 1. Neither slavery nor involuntary servitude, except for punishment for crime whereof the party shall have been duly convicted, shall exist within the United States, or any place subject to their jurisdiction.
>
>Section 2. Congress shall have power to enforce this article by appropriate legislation.

The bard of Avon wrote in *Romeo and Juliet*, Act 2, Scene 2: "A rose by any other name would smell as sweet." By analogy, the terms "slavery" and involuntary servitude go by many names: deprivation of freedom, bondage, peonage, tyranny, feudalism, indentureship, compulsory service, servility, conscription, and the draft, just to name a few.

All these words possess the same meaning in different forms: the military draft was, is, and always will be not only unconstitutional, but patently wrong. Yet Lincoln embraced slavery in order to get what he really wanted: not freedom for slaves but a country united. Not that there was anything wrong with a United States of American, but people need to understand that Lincoln's primary goal was winning the war, not freeing slaves.

Freeing slaves was only an afterthought, a political move to justify the war. Had Lincoln truly cared about the slavery issue, he would have proposed the Emancipation Proclamation at the beginning of the war, not in the middle.

It is ironic that the only way he could win the war was by creating a system of slavery that he called the draft. It is also ironic that the Emancipation Proclamation that set black slaves free, should also have freed Caucasian draftees. Think about that.

In the United States Declaration of Independence, the freedom sentiment is written thus: "We hold these truths to be self-evident, that all men are created equal, that they are endowed by their Creator with certain unalienable Rights, that among these are Life, Liberty and the pursuit of Happiness." To add another irony, half of the signatories of the Declaration of Independence owned slaves; slaves which they did not free after they signed the Declaration. Thomas Jefferson, an otherwise paragon of virtue, even went so far as to have children by his slaves. More food for thought.

It is as if the primary U.S. government rule is "do as I say, not as I do." Or as Arline Rosenfeld once said to me, "Don't listen to what I say, understand what I mean." (Whatever that means. I thought it best not to argue with her.)

Imagine my horror when I learned that the federal government of the United States habitually disregarded both the Constitution and the Declaration of Independence, as if the law against slavery was arbitrary and capricious; and that the federal government could dispense with my freedom and make me a slave any time it wished to do so. In 1966, it wished to do so. And it continued to do so for a decade.

Millions of male citizens between the ages of 18 and 26 were wrested from their homes, their jobs, their schools, their lives, and sent to the other side of the world to fight a war that they knew nothing about; while the politicians who were responsible for uprooting them from their lives sat comfortably on their seats in office.

The irony of the Vietnam draft was that I was old enough to die for my country, but not old enough to vote for it.

At that time, I was a geology major at Temple University, in Philadelphia, Pennsylvania. I was also taking courses in archaeology, anthropology, mineralogy, and chemistry. My goal was to eventually earn a degree in paleontology.

But the government had different plans. There was a war – sorry, a conflict – in Vietnam, and cannon fodder was in short demand. So short that the government decided by fiat that it had the right to violate my Constitutional rights of life, liberty, and the pursuit of happiness, to draft me between semesters.

I was given two choices: two years in the U.S. Army or five years in a federal penitentiary.

I made the wrong choice.

I've been paying for that choice ever since.

The House of Pain demonstrates explicitly how much I have paid for making that wrong choice.

Another irony of the Vietnam conflict was that the U.S. government forced me to fight for another country's freedom, when I did not possess that freedom in my own country. Perhaps the Vietnamese army should have sent soldiers to fight for my rights instead.

To give you an idea of what it was like to be drafted, look at it this way (or ways).

You're 32 years old and have just been promoted to a higher position in the company that employs you. Now you earn enough money to purchase that larger house that you need so that you and your wife can afford to have children. You put a downpayment on your dream house and move in two months later. You receive a letter from the government. The letter tells you that you have 30 days to settle your affairs, and to inform your family that you will be going away for two years.

You are a mother of two children. You also run a business from home. You have just learned that you are pregnant again. You and your husband move one child into the other child's bedroom. You repaint the walls in the vacated bedroom in anticipation of the blessed event. An FBI agent knocks on your door. He or she informs you that you have skill sets that the government needs. Prepare to leave your family for the next couple of years.

Certainly, these are extreme examples. I have created them purposely to demonstrate that unwanted interference in a person's life is just as disruptive and horrible for those imaginary families as it is for a single male who has recently graduated from high school, and whose life is just as important to him as your life is to you.

Try to imagine how you would feel if your life were interrupted by government interference. Try hard. Then you may – just *may* – be able to feel how a draftee felt when his life was suddenly turned upside down. Think about it. Think hard. Think harder.

This book is partly about how much I paid for my non-existent rights. It is also about how an invasive government that once betrayed my life, now willingly keeps me in physical pain, through an unjust and corrupt government agency called the Veterans Administration: a sinecure for disgraceful administrators who have a history of letting veterans die rather than treating their needs.

Mine is an ugly story, not fit for underage children. Parts of it are not even fit for adults. But every word is true. Nor is the story unique. This is not only my story. It is the story of every man who was drafted in order to fight an overseas war, then had to pick up the pieces that were left of his life, all the while ducking the hatred of an unappreciative band of citizens.

Read it and weep, as the saying goes in the book business. Read it and weep – for the dead, for the wounded, and for the emotionally challenged. For those men who went to war, then returned to America only to have to fight a civilian war.

My story is more than just my story; it is an example of every draftee's story. Some of their stories are worse than mine. Some of their stories are worse than I can imagine. Yet, whenever the VA pulled another trick on me, or refused to treat my wounds, or flagrantly appeared not to care about me the way I thought that a national medical system should respond to me, I think of what my Baptist minister once said to me:

"I wept because I had no shoes, till I met a man who had no feet."

This book is about one soldier whose shoes were stolen by the Veterans Administration.

Now that I've given my rebuke, read on for my supporting evidence.

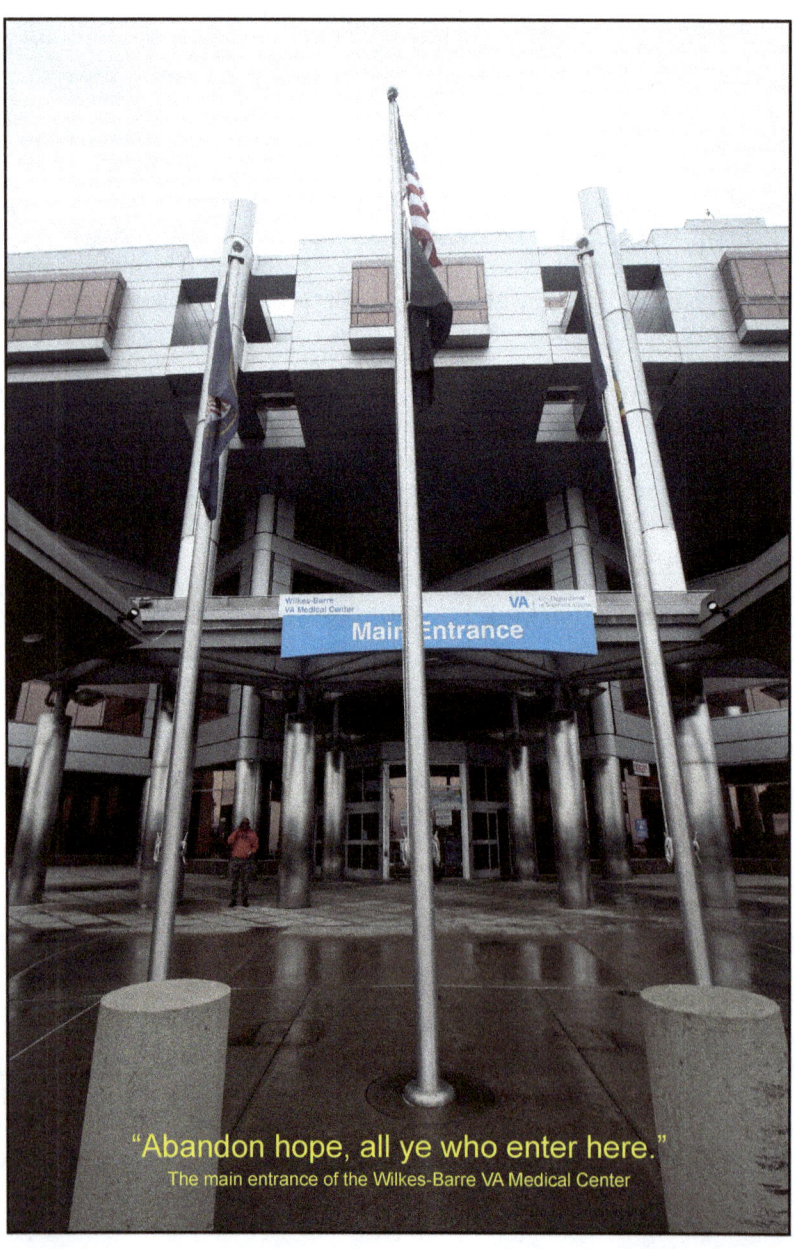

"Abandon hope, all ye who enter here."
The main entrance of the Wilkes-Barre VA Medical Center

Part 1 – Combat

Civilian Life

I was an early saver. I did odd jobs for my grandfather and kept my earnings in a piggy bank. I also saved money that I received as Christmas presents and birthday gifts. My parents couldn't afford to buy a bicycle for me, but by the age of 9, I had saved enough money to buy a bike for myself. It cost $25. I became a voracious bike rider. I rode my bike everywhere, even into the woods where paths were unknown. Yet when I rode along the sidewalks and saw anthills in the cracks between the squares, I swerved to avoid running over the hill and any nearby scurrying ants.

Once I found a baby opossum at the base of a tree in the woods. It was so weak that it could hardly drag itself by using its front paws; its hind legs were paralyzed. I looked all around for its mother or father or siblings. I even climbed the tree, thinking that the parents might have dropped the joey accidentally. When I could not find any adult opossums or joeys on or around the tree, I carried it home in the palm of my hand.

Not knowing what to feed it or how to take care of it, I called the Philadelphia Zoo. A zookeeper told me to feed it milk with an eyedropper, and to keep it warm. He thought that the paralysis of the hind legs was due to malnutrition. By the end of the week the opossum was walking naturally. When I placed it inside by pajama top, it scampered along my body and out through the neck opening; its tiny claws tickled.

The zookeeper called me a week later to ask about the opossum's health. When I told him how well it was doing, he suggested that instead of releasing it in the woods where I had found it, as I expected to do, I should donate it to the petting zoo: a children's zoo within the zoo where children could touch and pet animals that had been raised in captivity and had become tame. So that is what I did.

As an early teen I worked for my great-uncle Joe picking watermelons in August. Sometimes when I picked up a melon and rolled it over in my arms, I spotted a black widow spider on the underside. I didn't squash it under my palm. I brushed it off gently and continued on my way.

My cousin Michael – Uncle Joe's grandson and three months younger than I – taught me how to shoot a BB gun (actually a rifle). He took me to a pond where terrapins sunned themselves on logs. Target practice consisted of "plinking" the shell – which did not hurt the terrapin – until it got annoyed enough to slide off the log and into the water. I was an instant marksman. Nearly every time I pulled the trigger, I plinked a terrapin's shell.

I got so excited that when a bird landed on a nearby tree limb, I spun around and aimed at it, and without thinking, I pulled the trigger. The result was that I shot the bird in the neck and killed it. When I realized what I had done, I burst into tears. I cried and cried and cried. All I could think about was the baby birds whose mommy or daddy would not be returning to the nest to take care of them. I was inconsolable. I never fired the BB gun again.

I didn't know it at the time, but I was a natural.

My point in relating these incidents is to demonstrate how sensitive I was as a child. I have maintained that sensitivity throughout my life. Just a week ago – as I write these words in 2022 – I saw a squirrel struck by a car. After the car passed, I saw the tail stand up straight and wave like a flag in the wind. Then the tail flopped over. The body lay in the middle of the road. I picked up the squirrel and carried its body into the adjacent forest. Tears rolled down my cheeks as I petted the inanimate body, and thought about the bird that I had shot so long ago with my cousin's BB gun.

Soon my petting turned into a first-aid check, which I had done several times with car crash victims. The squirrel's body was not crushed, nor was there any sign of blood. I gently palpated the body, then did the same for the limbs. I thought that I could detect a faint heartbeat, although I couldn't be certain. I decided that the squirrel had bumped its head on the rolling tire and knocked itself unconscious. I placed it in a safe location adjacent to a tree. When I returned a few hours later, the squirrel was gone.

None of these attributes compares with those that were found in a soldier or a warrior. I had hopes of becoming a scientist. At Temple University, I took courses in geology, chemistry, calculus, anthropology, and similar scientific courses. My primary goal was to become a paleontologist, although I was flexible enough to consider specializing in a related earth science. That goal was terminated when I was drafted between semesters. Uncle Sam decided that the country needed cannon fodder more than it needed another paleontologist.

I was taught to be an infantryman.

Basic Training, or Learning through Torture

Fast forward to basic training. At the semi-automatic M-14 rifle proficiency assessment, each participant fired at 84-four targets. The closest targets were head silhouettes placed at a distance of 25 meters (82 feet); the farthest targets were full-body silhouettes placed at 450 meters (1,476 feet; for urbanites that's nearly 3 blocks; for rural folks it's more than a quarter mile). In between those distances were silhouettes whose size was graduated in accordance with the distance between the shooter and the target.

I knocked down 69 out of 84 targets. A kid from Winston-Salem, North Carolina flattened 70. Both of us qualified as experts, but he got the trophy.

Shooting a Colt-45 semi-automatic pistol from a distance of 25 meters (82 feet), I hit a man-sized target in the chest, neck, or head, 23 times out of 28 shots. And this was in combat posture.

If you watch YouTube videos of police shootouts, you'll see that cops habitually shoot unarmed civilians in the back, so they can afford to face the target and hold the gun with two hands. In combat, the targets return fire. Therefore, infantrymen use the single arm stance, with the body turned perpendicular to the enemy, and with the shooting arm stretched out straight, so as to present the smallest possible target to return fire.

The rifle posture is similar: the rifle is tucked against the chest, the shooting side faces the target with the body perpendicular to the target, and the trigger arm is held down and tucked close against the body so that the elbow pressed hard against the abdomen – not stuck out like a wing the way actors portrayed soldiers in the movies, because the wing stance increased the shooter's silhouette to enemy fire.

I also trained in the Mk 2 fragmentation grenade. When you see one of these being used in a movie, the result is nearly always a gigantic ball of yellow flame as large as a two-story house, which the grenade completely demolishes. I refer to these grenades as Hollywood grenades, or Stallone grenades. The effect in real life is less dramatic: a sphere of white light about the size of a soccer ball. There is no flame, no roar, just a loud whump that lasts a second or so. If a grenade detonates over loose dirt, there may be a large puff of dust that makes the explosion appear larger than it is.

I once saw a ball of flame like those that Hollywood hand grenades produce; it took the detonation of two 55-gallon drum that were filled with gasoline and iron filings. Remember this the next time you see Rambo shoot an arrow with an explosive pellet the size of a cigarette filter.

The outer shell of a fragmentation grenade is made of cast iron that has been scored so that upon detonation the shell breaks into small pieces that are dispersed in a 360-degree pattern that is designed to kill anyone within a radius of 15 feet (called the kill zone), and to severely wound anyone within 25 feet. It does not destroy multi-story buildings made of brick.

In kids' sports I never played pitcher or quarterback. I did not have a good throwing arm. In grenade training we threw a dummy grenade at a post that was surrounded by rings on the ground, much like a horizontal dart board. The closer the grenade landed to the post, the higher number of points the thrower received. In the qualification test I managed to score 92 points out of a 100: pretty good considering my weak background. As the army saying goes, " 'Almost' only counts in horseshoes and hand grenades," where a close call can still be a winner, or fatal.

I also had acquaintance with rifle combat by using pugil sticks to represent rifles. A pugil stick looks like a gigantic cotton swab about 5 feet in length, with each bushy swab being nearly a foot in diameter. The idea was to punch the opponent on the side of the head with either end; one end represented the steel barrel while the other end represented the wooden stock. We wore padded helmets when we engaged each other. Some punches were so hard that they knocked off the helmet. More than one person was sent to the infirmary.

The plastic stock an M-16 was likely to shatter on contact.

We also practiced use of the bayonet. For this exercise we fought against dummies (cadre excepted) so that no one would get hurt or killed. The specific motions were easy to learn. We also learned how to avoid those motions from enemy soldiers. But we didn't spend enough practice time for such combat forms to become instinctive in a pinch. Everything we were taught was like that. Basic Training was more like a familiarization course than long-term proficiency semester. More time was spent on bed making, shoe shining, and parading in step than was spent on combat training.

One item that I did not learn until I reached Vietnam was *proper* use of the bayonet. If you have ever watched Civil War movies, you might recall that soldiers carried rifles with very long bayonets whose blades were mounted parallel to the ground. That kind of bayonet was not practical in a jungle where it would get snagged on tree limbs and other entangling foliage. But although the bayonets that were designed to mount on the M-14 and the M-16 were shorter, they were not necessarily effective in hand-to-hand combat, because the blade was mounted vertically. That meant that the blade would not slide between the ribs, but would jam between them with only an inch or so of penetration: enough to hurt but not enough to kill. That might be okay when fighting only one soldier, but not so good when being overrun by hundreds of approaching enemy soldiers, because the blade might get stuck in the bone.

(This same situation arises in murder mysteries in which a murderer stabs a victim (usually in the back) with the blade striking the body perpendicular to the ribs. The blade would not penetrate enough to kill if the victim was left for dead. A knife should be held with the blade held parallel with the ground if the victim is standing, so it can slide between the ribs. These descriptions sound gruesome, but combat *is* gruesome.

Picture the human skeleton. The ribs have slight curves to them but are fixed predominantly parallel to the plane of the ground. Yet the bayonets for the M-14 and the M-16 were mounted vertically with respect to the surface plane. I figured this out one night while I was on guard duty. Later, I practiced rotating my rifle 90 degrees during a practice lunge. Thankfully, I never had to perform this maneuver in combat.

As the subject of this book is pain, I must not forget to mention the Army's standard teaching methodology. Any time a recruit made a mistake during training, he got knocked to the ground by the fist of a screaming lieutenant or punched in the head by a sergeant with a long-handled paddle. I don't know why the Army thought that these cruel acts of brutality increased memory retention, but there it is. The Army seemed to believe that the more pain that a recruit was made to suffer, the more knowledge that recruit could absorb.

I have a friend who is a jet plane pilot instructor. He once told me that people don't learn by being yelled at. When a trainee makes a mistake, he repeats instructions in a soft and calm voice. If that method works in civilian life, I don't understand why it shouldn't work equally as well in military training.

I preferred the scholastic method, but the Army relied on pain, fear, torture, and intimidation as learning incentives. Whether a recruit learned anything was irrelevant. There were no written exams, and everyone graduated. If you were assigned to KP (Kitchen Police), you missed whatever subject was being taught that day. There were no make-up days.

At the end of eight weeks, I was an expert at spit-shining boots, making my bed, and marching in step across the parade ground: skills that were decidedly unnecessary for a combat soldier.

Learning through Greater Torture
AIT (Advanced Infantry Training)

I attended Jungle Warfare School in Fort Polk, Louisiana, in an area that was known as Tiger Land. Weapons training was extended to include the M-16 automatic rifle, M-60 machine gun, M-79 grenade launcher, claymore antipersonnel mine, and the light antitank weapon (whose acronym was LAW).

The LAW was like the World War 2 bazooka in that it launched a rocket through a tube that was held on the shoulder. The tube of the LAW was shorter than that of the bazooka, and it was made of cardboard instead of steel. The LAW was disposable, for one-time use only. After firing, the tube was crushed out of shape so that it could not be re-used by the enemy, and the plastic sight was stomped to pieces.

The rockets that I was trained to fire could hit a tank on the other side of a tree or a revetment's blast wall. Standard rocket vanes were straight, whereas the vanes on the rockets that I fired were curved or slanted like stripes on a barber's pole. In flight, the angled vanes caused the rocket to spin in ever-widening circles. The shooter had to estimate not only the distance to the target, but the elevation of the tube so that as the circular trajectory enabled the rocket to approach the target, the rocket did not hit the tree but passed around the side of it. At the end of the flight pattern, the rocket had to be

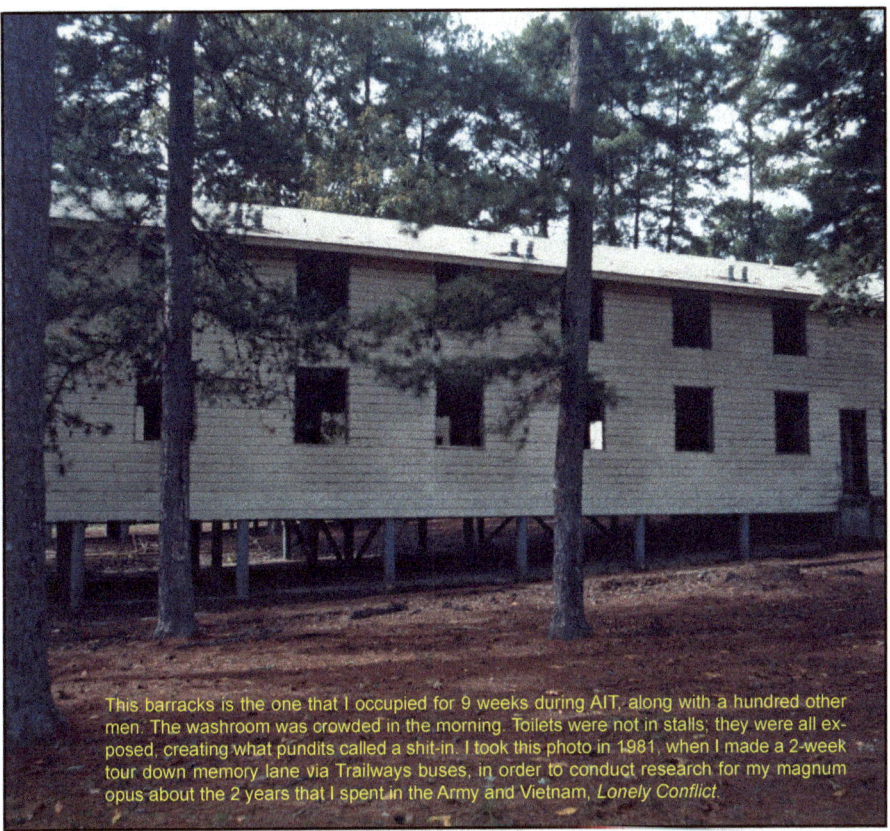

This barracks is the one that I occupied for 9 weeks during AIT, along with a hundred other men. The washroom was crowded in the morning. Toilets were not in stalls; they were all exposed, creating what pundits called a shit-in. I took this photo in 1981, when I made a 2-week tour down memory lane via Trailways buses, in order to conduct research for my magnum opus about the 2 years that I spent in the Army and Vietnam, *Lonely Conflict*.

close enough to the ground to hit the target, without passing before, beyond, or over the target, or slamming into the ground before reaching the target.

I was trained for familiarization only, not enough to become proficient in use.

(I must mention that my description of the LAW's rocket contradicts a description that I read online while conducting research for this book. No mention was made of the rocket's ability to circle around objects during flight. Yet I distinctly remember watching the expanding flight path as the rocket swooped around a tree (although there was no tank in evidence). Am I misremembering, or did I train in an alternate Universe?

There was also training in small-arms tactics, escape and evasion, hand-to-hand combat, survival, and use of a compass.

I was part of a squad of California hopheads (as they called themselves). They had marijuana mailed to them in envelopes that had no return address. In case the letter was lost or opened for inspection, it could not be traced back to the sender. The hopheads used to leave the barracks after dark and smoke joints in the adjoining forest. They got so wasted that I had to go after them before lights out (10 o'clock bed check) and lead them by the hand to the barracks. This led me to the conclusion that soldiers did not get hooked on marijuana after landing in Vietnam, as the press would have us believe, but took the habit with them, after which it spread to other units because the weed was so readily available. Food for thought.

Fort Polk was located in the middle of nowhere. One night the company was broken into squads and taken to a vast swamp that was situated twenty miles farther into nowhere. At midnight, my squad of hopheads was driven to the swamp where we were dropped off at a predetermined location. We each carried a rifle but were not issued bullets, so no one would accidentally shoot himself or anyone else, including the cadre. Neither did we have flashlights. We were given one lensatic compass (alias sighting compass) and a heading in degrees.

Because I neither drank alcohol nor smoked cigarettes or marijuana, my fellow trainees automatically elected me as the squad leader. I was proficient with the compass because I had been taught how to use it in the Boy Scouts. We had run compass courses (now called orienteering) to earn a merit badge. Army training was just as good, the only difference being the removal of the steel pot when taking a reading because the proximity of steel to the compass when held before the eyes caused deflection of the needle.

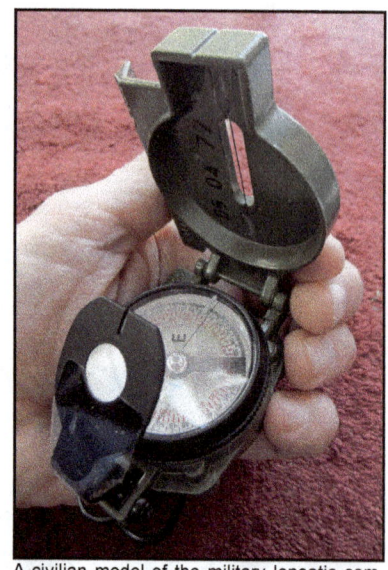

A civilian model of the military lensatic compass. The sighting lens is located at the lower left, where one can look down at the compass bearing and ahead past the sighting wire, at upper right.

I took the compass. According to the driver, a truck would be waiting for us five miles away, with the headlights switched on so we could find it in the dark. Upon arrival at our destination, several jeeps would be waiting to transport squads to the barracks upon safe arrival.

I rotated the bezel of the lensatic compass to set the declination, which I had memorized from class. The compass face glowed a faint luminescent green from a thin veneer of radium paint, the kind that was used on wristwatch hands. Despite the absence of the Moon, faint starlight forced its way through the clouds, and enabled me to read the cardinal numbers that designated degrees. While peering through the folding magnifying lens at the proper heading, I also looked through the notch where a thin vertical wire aligned on a tall tree at the far side of an open field. There were no trails through the swamp; our trek was conducted strictly by bushwhacking from one compass point to the next.

When I started walking, the hopheads followed me in line like a brood of scared ducklings.

Perhaps I exaggerated. They were not scared, just uncertain . . . until a rabbit dashed from under a bush and darted in front of a soldier. He squealed out loud. The soldier, not the rabbit. And I do mean squealed. Geez! These were the kind of men who were being sent into combat. What chance did they have against professional soldiers who were born and raised in the jungle?

We were negotiating a huge swamp that consisted of large tussocks and ankle-deep water when we reached a stream that measured ten feet in width. I crossed first. The crotch-deep water was cold but tolerable. (This was in November.) I held my rifle high. After scrambling up the opposite bank, I told the next man in line to wade to me.

A few minutes later, as I was taking another compass heading, I heard a splash and a curse. Someone had stumbled and dropped his rifle in the stream. I stepped back into the water. Four of us waltzed back and forth until someone stepped on the rifle, reached down to recover it, and handed it to the owner. I shook my head in the darkness, hoping that when these guys reached Vietnam, they were not assigned to frontline duty.

Then we entered a forest so thick that I couldn't see the face of the man standing next to me, much less anything to sight on the compass. I couldn't even see the compass in my hand. I led the way. I used the sashay method: after I passed around a tree on the left, I passed around the next tree on the right. This approximated a relatively straight course. Some of the men held onto the pistol belt of the man in front of him. We chattered as a way to establish the location of the man in front and the man behind. There were some grumbles of disgust, but no one was unduly frightened by the darkness. Better yet, no one got lost.

As soon as we got out of the dense woods, I stopped long enough to remove my steel pot and take a sighting. The terrain got easier after the swamp and the black forest. We were able to maintain a steady pace over undulating ground. We took no water breaks; each person drank from his canteen as we hiked. I kept taking sightings: not always on trees, but sometimes on the space between trees, if that was the correct heading.

The ground ascending gently. Soon we were rustling through dry dead leaves. The forest thinned out but I had no trouble taking sightings. Our clothes were still soaked so we walked fast as a way to keep warm. Because we were training for jungle warfare, we were not allowed to wear jackets, because jackets were not part of the jungle fatigue outfit, even though the temperature was in the mid-40 degrees Fahrenheit. This system was called military intelligence.

We encountered a steep rise that was in the open where trees were sparse and the undergrowth was moderate. We climbed to the top of a bushy knoll. In the near distance directly in front of us glowed the beam of a pair of headlights that pointed directly at us through a thin mist. We heard music in the air. The squad let out a series of whoops.

No longer did I need to take a sighting. We climbed down the other side of the knoll and rushed toward the headlights, half a mile away. Low bushes and occasional trees did not beget a formidable barrier.

Ten minutes later, I stepped out of the brush and announced my arrival: "Hello!"

Three men wearing fatigues were lounging in chairs around a small campfire. They all jumped to a standing position as if I had just fired a rifle. One of them stammered, "Who, who are you?"

I gave him our identification in the form of company, platoon, and squad. At this remove I don't remember the ID, but in that strange and misunderstood entity that is called the mind, I can somehow recall my basic training ID: D-6-2.

After some stammering, one of the men muttered, "When did you start?"

"Twelve o'clock."

He glanced at his watch.

"It's two thirty. That's two and a half hours. No one has ever made it that fast."

I shrugged.

After exchanging glances with the other two men, he said something like, "Well, come on in. We'll drive you to the barracks." By "we" he meant one of his two subordinates.

We (my squad) climbed into the back of a small truck which sported neither a cab nor a roof. We each took a place on the floor behind the two front seats. The dirt roads were lumpy and uneven. An hour later the truck stopped in front of our barracks. We disembarked, thanked the PFC (private first class) for the ride, entered the empty building, and went straight to bed.

I slept until 0830. (The military used the 24-hour clock.) The barracks was mostly empty. We had the day off to do as we wished. Some men were still asleep, some were sitting on the edge of their bunks, a few stood groggily. I took a shower, donned a clean set of fatigues, and moseyed to the mess hall. Like the barracks, the mess hall was largely empty. I could have as much food as I wanted. The specialty was steak and eggs, which I promptly ordered, medium rare. I drank orange juice and lingered over numerous cups of coffee. None of the handful of men was from my squad.

Squads dribbled into the compound throughout the day. They all appeared the way my fellow squad members and I must have appeared when we arrived: weak and dirty, wet and muddy, exhausted. We were not given food for the compass course; only one canteen filled with water. Most men staggered straight to the mess hall in their grubby fatigues.

By lunchtime, half the company had arrived at the compound. Men continued to trickle in all afternoon. Some squads were missing one or more of their members. Arrivals became mixed with men from different squads. They were both tired and famished. They had had no sleep the night before, hadn't eaten since the previous day's dinner, and unless they had drunk out of streams, they were badly dehydrated and not thinking clearly.

By the end of the day, three men were still missing in action: separated from their squads in the dark, lost in the endless wilderness, possibly hurt and unable to move or call for help. Neither search parties nor rescue teams were dispatched.

About mid-morning of day two, one man showed up when he stepped off the base bus. He had made it out of the woods to a tarred road, hitched a ride from a long-distance truck driver who took him to Leesville, where he caught the public bus to Fort Polk.

Late afternoon, just before chow call, another man showed up in a taxicab.

On day three, the last missing man was dropped at the compound by a local farmer. He was much the worse for wear.

All three men had horrible stories to tell about how they wandered "over the hills and through the woods" but never found grandmothers house, then shivered throughout the night (or nights) awaiting daybreak (or dawns).

There were no tests or make-up exams. No one failed the course. Diplomas were worthless because there was an endless line of expendables to take the place of the KIA's. Simply raise the draft numbers or remove the exemptions.

Our fates were sealed the moment we received a draft notice in the mail. This was a gentler way of procuring victims than employing press gangs, but the result was still the same. American soldiers no longer needed names; they had been replaced by serial numbers that were stamped on the dog tags that they wore around their necks. They were the generation of expendables.

Trainees were expected to have every bit of jungle warfare tactics pounded into their heads by paddles or punches. Everyone was shipped to Vietnam: the good, the bad, and the ugly. I have often wondered how many of my fellow trainees returned from the 'Nam alive. How many individuals lost civilian opportunities. How many families were torn apart by their absence. How many "summer soldiers and sunshine patriots" lost arms and legs. They all lost years of their lives; many lost their lives.

And as I was fated to learn, few people in the civilian world really gave a wit (or some other word.)

Vietnam – Descent into Horror

The day I landed in-country, I was ordered to place my personal belongings in a locker. I was issued jungle fatigues, jungle boots, jungle underwear (olive drab), web gear, and an M-16 automatic rifle (a pistol-grip assault rifle) and spare magazines. I left the underwear in the locker. T-shirts were too warm and boxer shorts were a nuisance: the legs tended to cling to sweat-covered thighs and ride up toward the crack between the buttocks with every step, until they bunched and had to be pulled down by the bottom hem.

The next day, I was transported by cargo plane to join my outfit in Pleiku, home of the Montagnards, who lived in the Central Highlands. Without having the opportunity to sight my rifle, I was dispatched on jungle patrol with elements of the 25th Infantry Division. I was totally unprepared for combat. But then, no one was ever prepared for combat until it happened.

And even then . . .

After traipsing through the jungle and climbing mountainous terrain all day, I spent the night in a foxhole. I have always said that there are no racists in foxholes. I was paired with a Negro (as Blacks were called before the latter word became capitalized). The color of a partner was irrelevant because he was there to have my back, just as I was there to have his. Anyway, once the sun set, neither of us could see the color of the other.

(As information, I went to an integrated grade school where all the kids played together and didn't recognize any distinctions such as skin color. The only difference between Blacks and Whites occurred when the nurse came to our homeroom to perform a lice inspection. The school was located in a low-income area. The Caucasian kids lined up so the nurse could run a pencil through our hair in a search for lice or their eggs (nits). The Negro kids were excused from this head search because, as we were told, black kids didn't get lice. None of us thought anything about it; that was just the way it was.)

With our entrenching tools, we dug a rectangular two-person foxhole with a sloped bottom that led to a sump hole in the middle, in case an enemy soldier tossed a grenade into our hole. In that case, the shrapnel would be directed upward while we would turn away from the blast and press our faces against the dirt.

I don't remember my partner's name. We took turns standing guard: one slept behind the mound of dirt that we extracted from the foxhole, while the other stood guard from inside the foxhole. Unlike the first sentence in old-time mystery books, it was a dark and quiet night.

The next day, the newbies (new recruits) stayed dug in while the others went on patrol. We mingled with Montagnards in a nearby village, where we traded C-rations for fresh pineapples and coconuts. Montagnards were friendly because they were on the side of the U.S. in the conflict, and they were glad to have us nearby for protection.

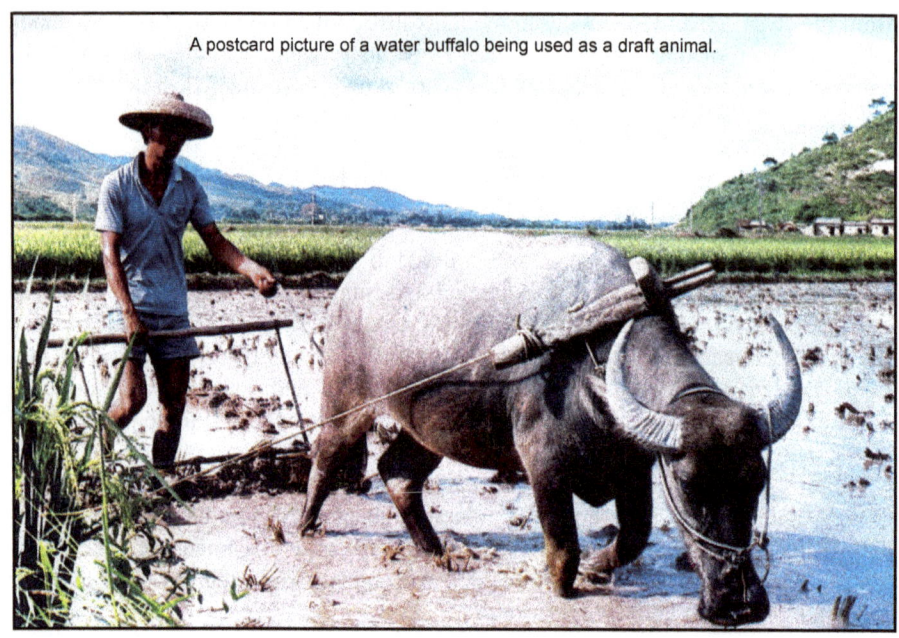
A postcard picture of a water buffalo being used as a draft animal.

    The only incident of the day occurred with the approach of an aged mamasan (a nonpejorative word that U.S. troops used to call Vietnamese women). She stood about five feet high, weighed about eighty pounds, and looked to be a hundred years old; even her wrinkles had wrinkles. Her sole attire was a pair of short-shorts. Her sagging breasts hung down like ancient prunes. She was tugging a thousand-pound water buffalo by means of a short length of twine that was connected to a ring in the mammal's nose; she yanked the twine and cursed in the local lingo whenever her stubborn pet walked too slowly to suit her fancy.
    The absurdity of the scene was uproarious to all of us except to the pair of newbies in the next foxhole to our left. They had unknowingly dug their foxhole next to a sandy pathway. They leaped out of their foxhole and scrambled clear of the approaching couple in time to avoid being trod by the beast. Barefoot mamasan ignored them.
    The rest of us laughed. It was the only laugh that I ever heard or had in Vietnam; and it was the only time I even smiled, much less laughed. Constant combat is not a laughing matter.
    A week later, after I had been transferred to the lowlands, I encountered another water buffalo; this one was on the rampage. When we emerged from the jungle, it was grazing on a patch of grass along the edge of a rice paddy that seemed to extend over the far horizon. I was third in line of a two-column patrol across the dry rice paddy when the water buffalo spotted us and charged between the point man and the next man in the opposite column, and headed straight for me. I jumped aside in time to avoid being gored; the left horn missed me by inches. Then it turned and charged through the rest of the squad, scattering soldiers as if they were pins on a bowling alley in the middle of a strike. No one got hurt. The water buffalo stopped running a few feet away, stared at us, then ignored us and calmly resumed grazing.
    No one even lifted his rifle, much less fired a shot. We were not allowed to shoot

water buffaloes. They were personal property of the people we were sent ten thousand miles to protect.

There wasn't much action in the Central Highlands. I never even flipped my rifle's safety switch off "safe," much less touched the trigger. After a while spent "humping the boonies" on fruitless patrols, a bunch of us was flown in a cargo plane to the rice paddy lowlands near the coastal village of Duc Pho, where the Army had built a forward firebase that was occupied by several hundred soldiers and a number of artillery guns. This area was under the command of the 4th Infantry Division, to which we were temporarily attached. Duc Pho was located midway between Qui Nhon and the DMZ (Demilitarized Zone). This was where the charging water buffalo incident occurred.

After landing and checking in with the top sergeant, I had the afternoon to sight my rifle, eat a hot meal, and sleep on a cot in a tent. This was the only time in-country when I did not sleep on the ground or on the floor of a cargo plane. The next morning, a Huey gunship flew me and two other soldiers to a company that occupied a sandbagged entrenchment in a dry rice paddy adjacent to thick coarse jungle.

Like every Huey that I ever saw, it had no doors or seats, just a flat cargo bay. The removal of these components saved weight so that the Huey could carry more men or supplies, or so it could take-off faster in an emergency, such as when enemy soldiers were trying to shoot it down.

Both of my fellow travelers belonged to the company. One was returning from R&R (rest and recuperation: a week-long vacation when soldiers were sent to places such as Australia or Japan, where they could rest and recuperate from non-stop combat). The other was returning from the hospital. He had gone outside the perimeter to take a crap in the dark. He was on his way back when the rustling noise he made as he walked through dry grass alerted a guard who was half asleep, and thought that an enemy soldier was sneaking toward the compound. The guard tripped the switch for the claymore anti-personnel mine. The returning soldier had already passed the location where the

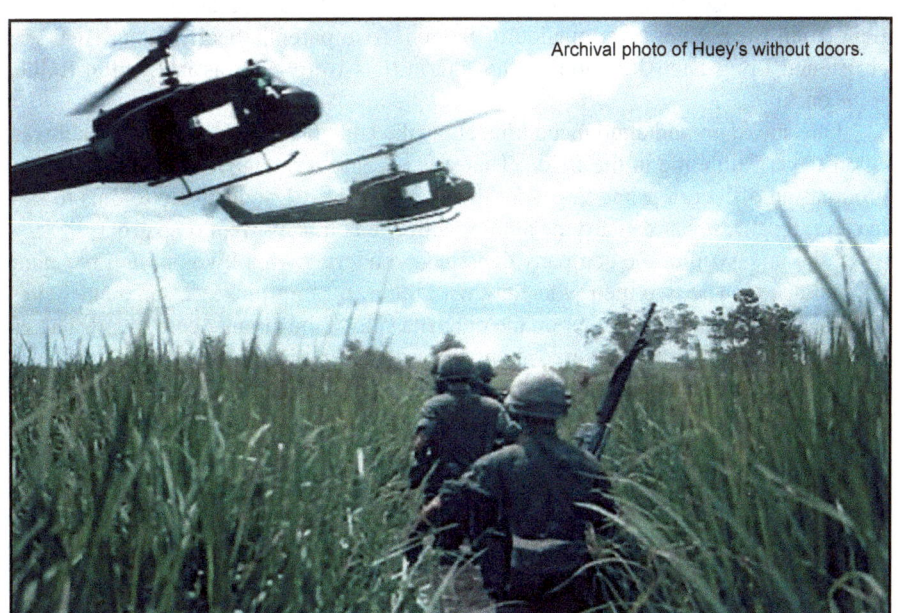
Archival photo of Huey's without doors.

claymore was planted, but the backscatter sent a flurry of pellets into the sole of his boot and through his foot.

It was the returning soldier's fault for not announcing to the guard while passing his station that he was going outside the perimeter.

An interesting fact that the men told me was that when they were in the forward firing base, resting between patrols, they smoked marijuana. But once they were out in the bush, the tune changed. To put it in their approximate words and accent, "Ain't nobody smokin' no shit in the bush. Charlie everywhere. You got to be alert or you be dead." They were dead serious. Bad allusion. Not "dead" serious, but you know what I mean. They spoke softly – as softly as a person could speak above the noise of the Huey's blades as they swished through the humid air – but I heard it loudly. These two men were experienced soldiers who had a vast amount of knowledge about combat, and, to put it in literary words, they knew whereof they spoke.

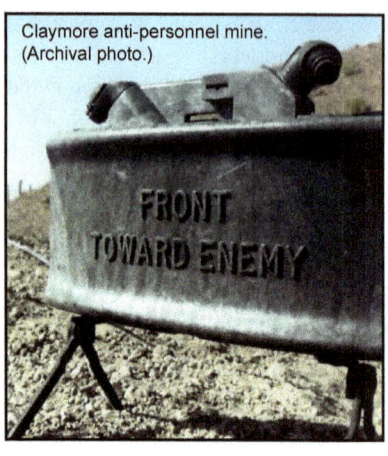
Claymore anti-personnel mine. (Archival photo.)

Their dry tone and relaxed composure gave me shudders.

As we landed, the downwash from the helicopter's rotating blades created a minor sandstorm. After the sand settled, we three checked in with the captain while "volunteers" unloaded a resupply of ammunition, cases of C-rations, and a hot breakfast for the troops. Even in the morning heat, the men found a hot meal refreshing.

We approached a group of men who were gathered close together. I presumed that they were officers but did not know which one was the company commander. No one wore insignia of any kind: no name tags, no signs of rank, just dirty jungle fatigues like everyone else. (I was still wearing the same outfit that had been issued to me at Long Bien (near Bien Hoa, outside of Saigon. Also parenthetically, Long Bien was christened Long Bien Junction so that the initials were LBJ, as in Lyndon Baines Johnson.)

One spoke up and announced himself as the captain. The first thing he said was, "Don't ever salute me in the field." That was because a salute singled him out of the group as an officer: a prime target for a watching sniper. I nodded. He told us to stay in camp for the day and guard the ammo while the company went on patrol.

I felt uneasy after the company departed, wondering what I would do if the camp were attacked. The two men who flew with me into camp picked a sandbag shelter. They told me to stay in a shelter on the opposite side of the circular compound. The diameter of the compound measured about 50 yards. The perimeter was dotted with cube-shaped shelters that stood four feet high and measured four feet square. The overhead planks were covered with two layers of sandbags, plus an extra row facing outward as protection for nighttime guards. Inside, a narrow slit enabled me to gaze across a vast rice paddy that was currently left fallow. The paddy seemed to extend forever.

The air was unbearably hot: about 110 degrees in the shade. I spent most of the day inside a shelter, staring alternately through the slit or through the doorway across the camp at the jungle. I had my choice of C-rations for lunch. The day dragged on quietly until an armed soldier emerged from the jungle. I leaped into a crouched position with my rifle pointing toward the lone soldier. Then more men followed him as he waved his rifle at me. He was the point man of my company. I started breathing again.

After the company settled down, I was assigned to a squad that was shorter in personnel than most. Company strength was supposed to be 120 men; recent casualties were so high that the company was down to 90. My squad should have had eight soldiers but was down to five; I made six: one corporal and five PFC's. I remember three names: squad leader Corporal Yawn, PFC Tye, and PFC White (who was Black).

By Hollywood standards, we made the perfect representative squad: four Caucasians, one Negro, and one Hispanic. Yawn and Tye were rifleman. One Caucasian was the M-60 machine gunner: he carried the 23-pound machinegun plus one belt of ammo that was locked and loaded. White was the machine gunner's assistant; he carried two belts of linked cartridges crisscrossed over his shoulders and chest, the tripod on his back, and two spare barrels in his fanny pack. (In the literal heat of battle, the machinegun barrel could turn cherry red; if the barrel was not exchanged, the steel would get soft and cause the barrel to sag.) The Hispanic carried an M-79 grenade launcher that was secured below the barrel of his M-16. Back at base camp we had a dedicated M-79 grenade launcher for nighttime use against an attack on the compound.

The M-16 weighed seven pounds. Because the M-16 was an automatic rifle, there were three switch positions: safe, single, and automatic (like a machinegun: the weapon would continue to fire as long as the trigger was depressed.). During my entire time in Vietnam, I fired my M-16 on automatic only once: and that was not at a target but because the captain wanted us to provide covering fire while the other platoons engaged the enemy. I even fired the machine gunner's M-16: one rifle in each hand, like a later day Rambo.

Movies always showed riflemen firing on full automatic, generally from the waist, and spraying bullets from side to side like water from a garden hose, I suppose because it appeared macho and dramatic. In reality, firing on automatic was a waste of ammu-

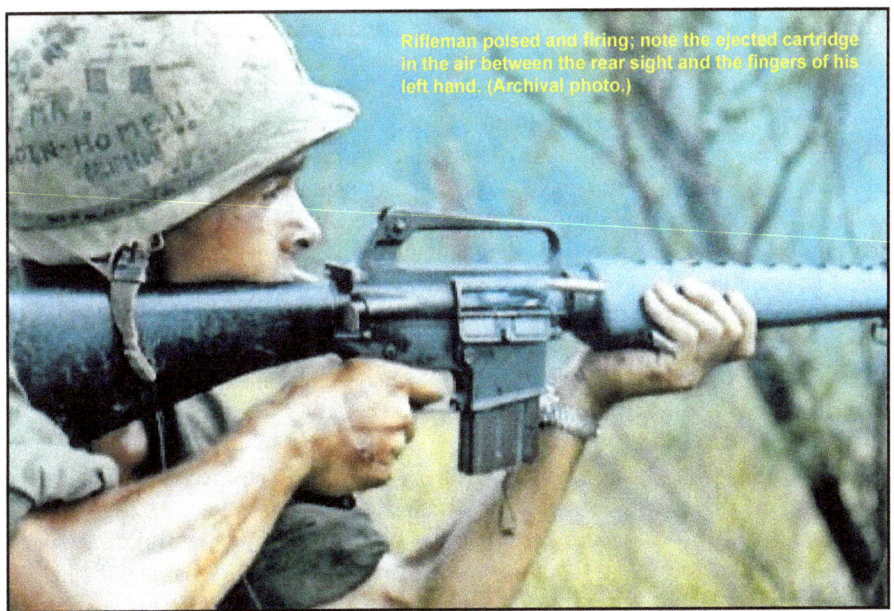

Rifleman poised and firing; note the ejected cartridge in the air between the rear sight and the fingers of his left hand. (Archival photo.)

nition. By holding down the trigger while the selector switch was positioned on auto, the M-16 could empty a 20-round magazine in less than 5 seconds. It takes longer than that to change magazines. It is more efficient to aim at a target and fire. I generally fired 3 single shots: grouping my bullets, not spraying them into the air.

What the movie makers don't realize is that, due to the rifling inside the barrel (which imparts spin on the bullet so it shoots straight, in the manner of a quarterback throwing a football), the spin on the bullet caused the barrel to track up and to the right. On a compass this would be equivalent to 45 degrees. In order to hit a target, the shooter firing on full automatic must aim left of the target's kneecap so that the barrel would track diagonally across the target's abdomen or chest.

Yawn made me the grenadier. This was ironic in that I scored only 92 points out of a hundred in the hand grenade accuracy test. (I was never chosen as pitcher in school baseball games.) Each day I carried half a dozen Mark 2 fragmentation grenades: 3 clipped to each front strap of my web gear suspenders. On my pistol belt I clipped a fanny pack in which were stuffed two C-ration meals plus incidentals; tied to the pack was a poncho and an entrenching tool. Also clipped to the belt were 2 canteens and 4 ammo pouches. The ammo pouches were World War Two leftovers that were designed to fit a magazine of twenty 7.62-millimeter bullets for the M-14 rifle. Because the size of M-16 bullets measured 5.56 millimeters, two of its 20-round magazines fit into each ammo pouch. This gave me a capacity for 181 rounds: 8 magazines in pouches, 1 magazine locked onto the rifle, and 1 bullet loaded in the chamber: in other words, locked and loaded. The safety switch remained in the "safe" position.

After introductions were made, I stood guard while the rest of the squad cleaned their rifles after a hard day of combat. We ate C-rations for dinner (and for breakfast and lunch). Yawn assigned times for nighttime guard duty. Night fell quickly. After dark, the men brushed their teeth with water from a puddle in the middle of the compound.

Yawn ordered me to deploy the claymore anti-personnel mine. The M18A1 measured about 7 inches across, and weighed about 2 and a half pounds. With the claymore in hand, I low-crawled over the low dune that had been built around the compound, into a thicket of tall grass where an enemy observer (hopefully) could not see me. I low-crawled (on my belly) for a hundred feet while changing direction stealthily. I placed the claymore behind a clump of grass, pushed the thin legs into the ground, then uprooted tufts of nearby grass which I pressed against the convex front of the mine. I connected the electrical blasting cap by feel. I sighted the mine from the rear, and tilted it a tiny bit upward. I unrolled the detonation cord as I crawled back to the sandbag hut. I attached the cord to the command detonator. A press of the button would now trigger the C-4 explosive that would spray some 700 steel balls the size of buckshot or BB's into the enemy's face.

Claymore deployment became my permanent job. The claymore was retrieved by the last person on guard duty before first light.

I picked a place on the ground to sleep. We all slept fully clothed and booted and with rifle in hand. I lay on my right side with my legs bent at the knees so I could wedge the butt of my rifle between my thighs. I wrapped my fingers around the trigger guard and slept like a child clutching a teddy bear. I used my steel pot as a pillow. When it rained, I couldn't sleep with raindrops pelting my eyelids, so I separated the helmet liner from the steel pot, lay my head on the steel pot, and balanced the helmet liner on the side of my face in such a way that my eyes were protected from the raindrops. Many mornings I awoke soaking set. We did not have tarps, tents, sleeping bags, or spare clothes (except for an extra pair of socks).

Just as I was about to close my eyes, I saw lightning bugs zipping across the compound. A second or two later I heard the chatter of machine gun fire. I leaped off the ground and made a mad dash to the sandbag shelter. Yawn was there before I was. Then the other four men crowded in behind me. We were crammed together like a bunch of college students in a phone booth. Yawn and I were nose to nose, crouched together due to the low height of the ceiling. White's knee was between my legs, and one on my legs was between Yawn's legs. The barrel of my rifle was pressed against my ear. How all of us fit in that four-by-four compartment I cannot now imagine. It's amazing what you can do when someone is trying to kill you.

Yawn peered through the narrow slit in the front of the hut; the slit was high enough to fit a rifle or a grenade launcher (one that was not mounted to the bottom of the barrel of an M-16). Each squad had an M-79 grenade launcher in the hut. We heard retaliatory fire from the opposite side of the compound. The machine gun fire ceased. The sniper quit shooting and melted into the jungle. Return fire withered, then stopped. All was quiet. This kind of harassment happened every night. Every night. Sometimes more than once.

We searched for Charlie during the day, and Charlie sniped at us at night. Even if Charlie didn't hit anyone, the sniping depleted our energy by keeping us awake.

Yawn turned his head toward me. In the darkness I could see only his silhouette. "Congratulations, Gentile. You just earned your C.I.B." (Combat Infantryman Badge.)

I was too happy to be alive to care about the badge that I could now wear on my dress uniform (which was back at Long Bien). Such was my introduction to combat.

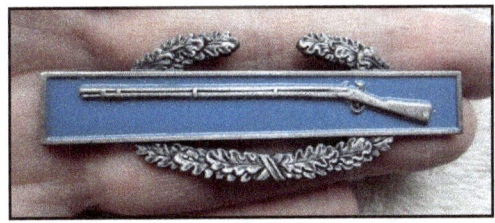

Although I earned the C.I.B. by dint of having fought in action - and have the scars to prove it - I was never awarded the paperwork that allowed me to wear the badge. Ironically, the U.S. Army does not *give* the badge to recipients; they must buy it from the PX (Post Exchange). I bought mine 57 years later, just so I could picture it in this book. It cost $6.95 plus sales tax online. The shipping was free.

The Daily Grind

Not a day went by without a firefight, or at the very least a skirmish. Sometimes it was short, such as when we found an enemy soldier in a grass-covered spider hole, in which case we overpowered him with rifle fire or hand grenades. Sometimes it was long, such as when the company met an enemy force that attacked us or defended a position. Every day there were bodies. My company was lucky in that, so far during my attachment, the body count was numbered strictly on Charlie's side.

Why was an enemy soldier called Charlie? In casual conversation, Vietcong was shortened to VC. In the radio alphabet, VC was pronounced Victor Charlie. An enemy soldier was not called Victor because of the connotation of the word's dictionary definition: "one who defeats or vanquishes an adversary; the winner in a fight, battle, or war." Thus Charlie.

We wore the same uniform for a week or so, day and night. Whenever an American soldier died in the bush, he died with his boots on. That's because, as noted above, we slept with our boots on, and with rifle in hand.

Whenever it was convenient, such as when our ammunition was low and a Huey was dispatched to resupply our company reserves, we received a clean change of clothing (and hopefully hot food that was kept warm in insulated canisters). As noted, we wore only pants, shirts, socks, and boots; no underwear. Clean clothing was packed and compressed in bundles whose strings were cut free after the Huey landed inside the compound. The helicopter crew tossed the clothes out of the cargo bay onto the ground, then spread them over a convenient dry spot. We were called one squad at a time, with rifles but without web gear.

We stripped down at the apparel pile, tossed our dirty laundry into the hamper pile, then (wearing only socks and boots) rummaged through the clean clothing to find a shirt and a pair of pants that came somewhat close to fitting. After donning the fatigues, we grabbed two pairs of fresh dry socks, sat on the ground, removed our boots and dirty stinky socks, pulled on a pair of clean socks, donned our dirty, muddy boots, left two pairs of socks in the hamper pile, and returned to our squad's area.

The helicopter crew stowed all the dirty clothes in the cabin, then flew them to the forward fire base for laundering.

We also had a bath on unscheduled days. At a hopefully safe spot between firefight locations, we established a guard detail on the side of a river, along with an APC or two. (APC is short for armored personnel carrier: a steel-plated vehicle that was treaded like a tank, and that could also drive on water, albeit slowly.) One squad at a time (with firearms nearby on the bank), stripped down naked and waded into the water with a small bar of soap. Hurriedly, each soldier rubbed his body with soap and then rinsed as quickly as possible. There was no time for water fights.

Laundry day and bathing day never coincided. After the bath, we donned our dirty, sweaty clothes and returned to combat.

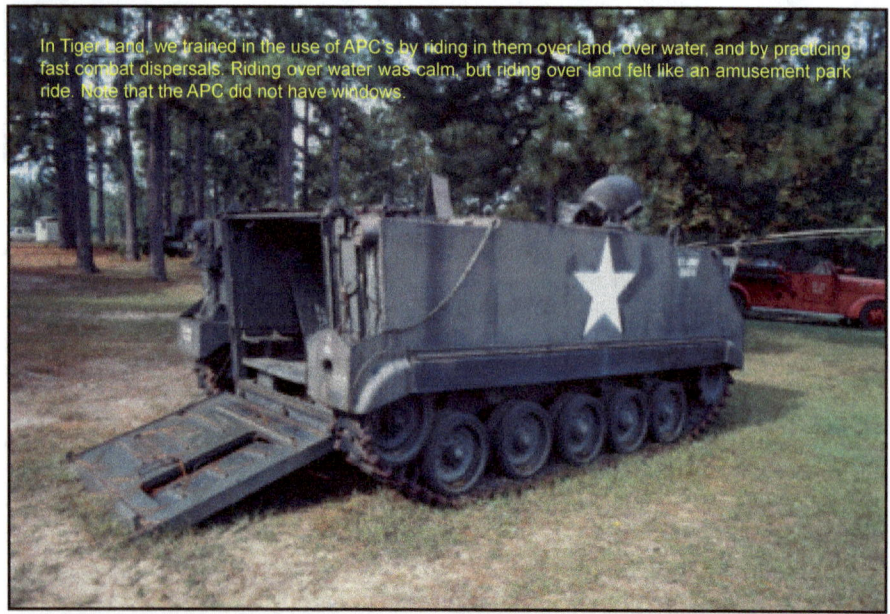

In Tiger Land, we trained in the use of APC's by riding in them over land, over water, and by practicing fast combat dispersals. Riding over water was calm, but riding over land felt like an amusement park ride. Note that the APC did not have windows.

No one shaved. There was neither time nor energy nor inclination.

Every night we did field maintenance on our weapons – one person at a time while the rest of the squad stood guard. The first thing I did was swab the inside of the barrel with a small cotton patch on the end of a metal cleaning rod (which was stowed inside the stock). This removed gunpowder residue. Then I did some light lubrication with gun oil. Finally, I cleaned the magazines and ammunition.

I dripped gun oil on the spring of the empty magazines, then refilled them with cartridges that were fresh out of a watertight ammo can. For each magazine that still held cartridges, I removed the bullets and laid them on a dry sock. One by one, I wiped each bullet clean with the other dry sock, then reinserted bullet into the freshly oiled magazine. If it had been a slow day, I might have as many as a hundred bullets to clean. The more combat action, the more bullets were expended, and the fewer bullets had to be cleaned. Uncleaned bullets were coated with dust and dirt, which tended to jam in the breach while firing, and had to be removed manually under fire before the rifle was usable again.

After the last bullet was wiped and all nine magazines were lubricated and filled, I donned dry socks (those that I had worn the day before) and tucked the damp socks under a strap on the fanny pack to dry.

Our rifles were not equipped with slings. We had to carry our rifles by hand all day, either by the rear sight if conditions warranted, or by closing the hand around the hand grip and trigger guard if action was anticipated. Whipping a slung rifle off the shoulder and bringing it to bear added a second or so to the shooting time. This amount of time delay was unacceptable because many of our combat actions started when the enemy fired at us in ambush from the jungle. Immediate return fire was crucially important.

Local Lingo

American soldiers in Vietnam developed their own language. It consisted of a mixture of abbreviations, expressions, shortcuts (such as "Charlie," as previously noted), corruptions, and quasi-Vietnamese and English words linked together. Here are the most common words and phrases that I heard in the bush:

Ao dai: a long dress worn by Vietnamese women
Didi: hurry or run
Didi mau: run fast
Frag: to kill an unpopular officer with a hand grenade
Hooch: a hut or house, generally made with bamboo walls, a thatched roof, and a dirt floor
Ville: a village (larger than a hamlet)
Hamlet: a small village, sometimes consisting of only a handful of hooches
Ho Chi Min racing slicks: sandals made by cutting lasts from a rubber tire, and attaching straps
Klick: a kilometer (about five-eighths of a mile)
NVA: North Vietnamese Army (regulars engaged in coordinated offensive operations)
VC: Vietcong (guerrillas who fought individually by using snipe and run techniques)

Into the Jungle

No one flunked jungle warfare school. Nine weeks of accelerated training was all the preparation I received in order to engage a military force whose soldiers had been born in the jungle, raised in the jungle, and taught since childhood to fight in the jungle. In this unequal contest of amateurs opposing professionals, the amateurs had the advantages of unlimited resources and absolute control of the air against the stealth and concealment of the professionals.

There was no front line in the accepted meaning of the term. The entire Republic of South Vietnam was a vast battleground on which two great armies intermingled like grains of salt and pepper on a jungle salad. Saturation bombing, napalm strikes, and defoliation offensives were large scale American tactics that seemed inappropriate under ordinary rules of engagement. To the uninitiated, these tactics might seem like burning down a house in order to exterminate a nest of wasps that was clinging to the eave, or using a chainsaw to excise a pea-sized cancerous tumor.

On the other hand, the problem that the American military faced in the bush was that, for the most part, the Vietcong and the North Vietnamese Army declined to fight full-scale battles. They fought only when the odds were in their favor; otherwise, they stayed hidden until the odds changed.

The primary practice of the VC and the NVA was to nip at the heels of the U.S. Army, like a bunch of angry chihuahuas that were too fast to catch or kick in the snout. Vietcong guerrillas and regulars of the North Vietnam Army played a deadly game of snipe and run that was difficult to combat.

America politicians should have been fully aware of such frustrating strategies, because American colonists practiced the same tricks against the British army in the American Revolution. As philosopher George Santayana wrote, "Those who cannot remember the past are condemned to repeat it."

This was why American small unit actions of company strength were more effective in fighting the enemy than large sweeping assaults.

I was part of what I call a canary campaign. In coal mines with long tunnels where deadly gases accumulated, miners used canaries that keeled over in their cages to warn the miners of poisonous vapors. In the jungle, we scouted hamlets and villages in order to sniff out the enemy. If we made contact with a large force of defenders, reserves were choppered in to join the firefight.

We were the sacrificial canaries.

My First Huey Assault

The Hueys flew low over the jungle that bordered our tight perimeter, barely cropping the trees in their effort to avoid enemy fire. Snipers had picked us apart throughout the night, and we were anxious to get out of there even if our next assignment was a search and destroy mission against a suspected Vietcong village. Dawn was half an hour away.

My belly was full of cold C-rations: ham and eggs chopped, because I was the only one in the company, perhaps in the whole army, who liked them.

Clipped to the front straps of my web suspenders were six fragmentation grenades. The ammo pouches on my pistol belt held one-hundred-sixty 5.56-millimeter rounds for the fully loaded M-16 assault rifle that I held tightly by the rear sight. A pair of can-

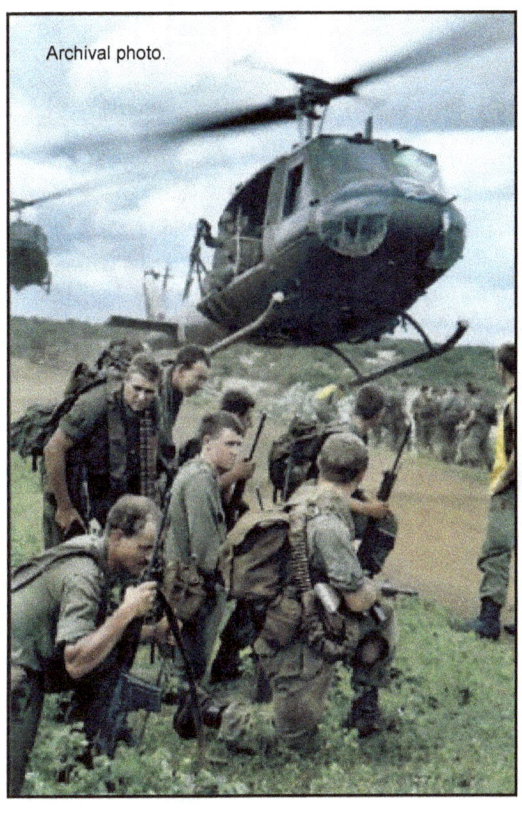

Archival photo.

teens, rain gear, sundries, extra socks, and "C's" completed my accoutrements. My raiment was a pair of dirty jungle fatigues, well-worn boots, and a steel pot on my head. We traveled light, depending upon resupply if we got into a major firefight.

The distinctive whup-whup-whup of rotating blades sent a chill along my spine, for I equated the raucous resonance with incipient fear and danger. Eight gunships touched down in the pre-dawn dust of the dry rice paddy where ninety-some armed men crouched in wait. As soon as the landing skids hit the dirt, we ran hunched over for the doorless and seatless cargo compartment. I was the last one to board. There was no more space inside, so I had to sit on the outer edge of the platform with my legs dangling over the side, next to the door gunner who glanced at me over the barrel of his machine gun. No one spoke. No one grinned or smiled. This was serious business.

We flew away instantly – if in fact the Huey had ever landed. Usually they maintained a hover with very little weight of the machine feeling the ground. The operation was more like a touch-and-go than an actual landing and take-off. We zoomed away and gained altitude simultaneously.

From my position half-out of the cargo compartment, I had a perfect view of the lush jungle below. Vietnam was a beautiful country when seen from the air: a patchwork quilt of wet and dry paddies whose symmetry was artistically rendered by alternating hues of green and brown. Great curved swaths of untamed jungle separated concentrations of paddies as if a painter's brush had made broad verdant strokes across a living canvas.

Randomly placed mounts like giant gumdrops rose hundreds of feet vertically from the rice paddy plains. In the mountainous regions called the Highlands, I had seen both in the air and on the dirt the undulating triple-canopy jungle, which presented a picture of living radiance that merely hinted at the profusion of lifeforms that lay hidden beneath the towering treetops.

Only from the level of the ground did the illusion of innocent splendor disappear. The dry rice paddies were barren and lifeless, the wet ones were covered with scum. The jungle was often impenetrable by man and was crawling with tigers and boars and snakes and monstrous poisonous insects. Disease and squalor inhabited the hamlets,

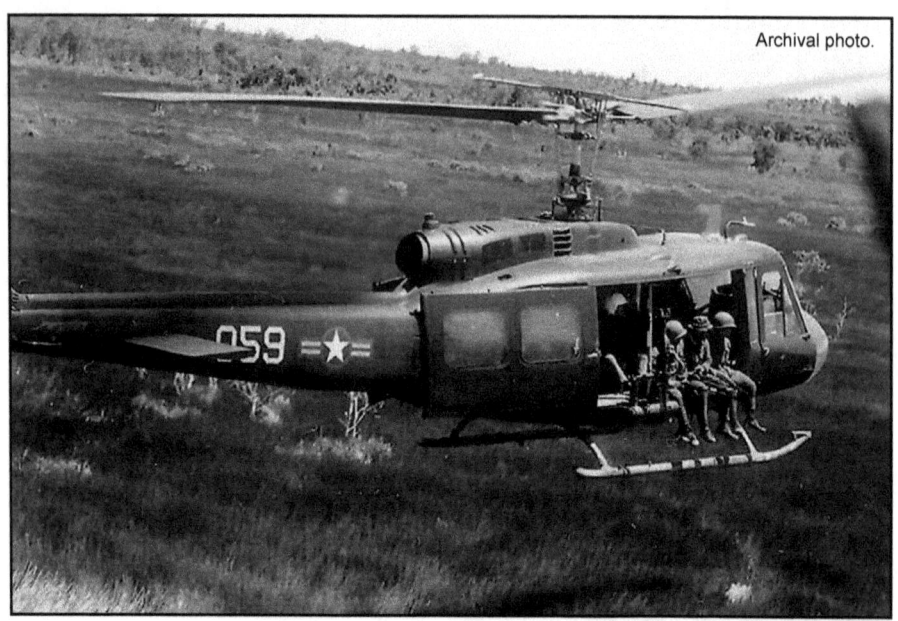
Archival photo.

poverty was the watchword. And worst of all, spread across the land was the ugliness of war.

The flight of Hueys swung north along the coast in the suffused early morning light. From an altitude of five thousand feet, I watched tumultuous waves of the turquoise water of the South China Sea crash against the white sandy beach. All below appeared calm.

We were flying over the surf line – albeit a mile high – when the Huey banked sharply for a turn to the west. So pronounced was the list of the aircraft that the deck I was perched on tilted instantly to a near vertical attitude. I gulped. My left hand gripped the bulkhead fiercely while my right hand squeezed my rifle, which lay across my lap. No longer was I looking out over placid pleasant scenery. Now I stared straight down into the jaws of death at the end of an accelerating descent, with no restraints against my body to prevent me from sliding off the deck. I teetered over the fathomless abyss, unable to do anything but hold on tight. Fortunately, inertia pinned me to the metal deck with the same principle of physics that prevents water from spilling out of a bucket that is swung horizontally in a circle. The Huey leveled out, and none but I knew of my moment of supreme terror.

The flight spiraled downward at a more moderate pace that was timed to reach our destination at sunrise. The Hueys gathered into formation like a flock of Canada geese. We dropped down close to the surface of the sea, then flew toward land out of the rising sun – just like in the future movie scene in *Apocalypse Now*, except that we had no speakers playing Wagner's *Ride of the Valkyries*.

When the beachside village hove into view, the Hueys pealed off to the left and right and announced our presence with machine-gun fire from multiple strafing runs. We swooped up to get a better view of the so-called enemy village and to allow the door gunners to sight targets who were trying to escape. We encountered no resistance, so the door gunners took out their frustrations on water buffalo that were wallowing helter-skelter in the paddies. American soldiers were not allowed to shoot water buffalo because Vietnamese peasants were so dependent upon them, but the door gunners did not seem to care about the rules of engagement.

We circled the landing zone once, then a voice behind me shouted over the noise of the screaming engine, "Get ready!"

There was no time to recover from my earlier fright – a greater one was coming. I swallowed my heart as I slid off the platform and planted my boots on the port landing skid; I steadied myself with my left hand, and with my right thumb I flipped the selector lever from safe to semi, and gripped my rifle by the hand grip and trigger guard.

We were still several hundred feet in the air and racing forward at nearly a hundred miles per hour. The wind whipped tears from my eyes. The village was ensconced within patches of jungle and stands of thick bamboo, all of which was surrounded by fields and paddies in which grew the simple staples on which the peasants managed to survive.

The Huey settled down over a dry paddy. The downdraft from the rotor blades churned loose dirt into a turbulent cloud of dust that temporarily blinded me. Then our forward motion ceased as we plummeted sickeningly toward the earth.

"*Go*"

Quick deployment and a rapid dispersal were necessary lest the Huey get shot down by enemy guns or rockets, or lest small arms fire decimate the troops before they even left the cabin. When I looked down past my boots, I saw nothing but a beige swirling miasma with no sign of the ground. We could be ten feet from the dirt – or a hundred. Above the roar of the engine, I heard automatic weapons fire and the whump of grenades detonating nearby.

I hesitated a split second too long. A hand smacked hard against my shoulder and shoved. I fell overboard. I braced my legs for a long drop from an indeterminate height. When I hit the ground after a fall but a foot, my stiffened muscles could not absorb the

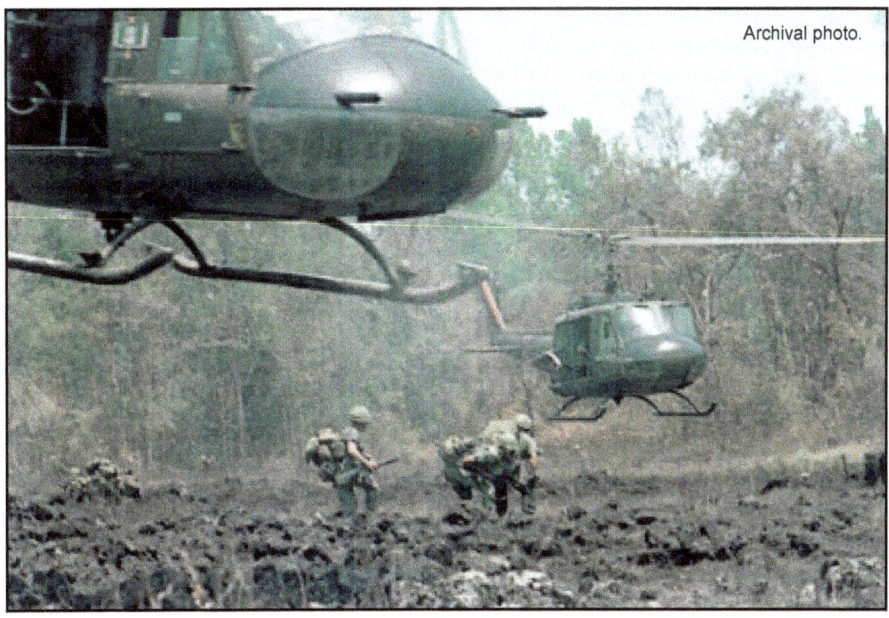

Archival photo.

shock. I tumbled onto my knees. Only my outthrust left hand prevented me from crashing flat onto my face. An instant later a pair of boots scraped my shoulder as someone stumbled over me. I scrambled forward on all threes – I clutched my rifle with my finger on the trigger, prepared to fire at a moment's notice – to avoid being trampled by the squad members behind me. Then I struggled to my feet and advanced in a low crouch through the swirling, blinding dust.

Gunfire surrounded me. I envisioned bullets whizzing by from all directions. I did not return fire because I saw nothing but airborne dust and dirt, now made worse by the revving of the engines of departing Hueys. A stark feeling of abandonment welled up inside me when the firepower of the gunships no longer backed up the ground troops. Now we were on our own.

Corporal Yawn indicated a direction and yelled in my ear, "Keep moving."

I did what the squad leader ordered. I glanced around and saw only two or three men through the haze. As I got farther away from the turbulence, the visibility in front of me increased. Conducting reconnaissance by fire, I sent a few rounds low into the tree line that demarcated the side of the paddy that bordered the 'ville. I crouched lower and scurried quicker, thankful when I saw a dike that rose about fifteen inches above the dry paddy bottom. I hit the ground ten feet before I reached the dike, then low-crawled frantically to the meager protection that was provided by the short rise.

The cacophony that was created by bursting grenades and the steady but sporadic rifle and machine-gun fire produced an atmosphere of frenzy. I poked my head above the dike, but only high enough to enable me to see ahead. A dense tangle of brush protected a bamboo thicket that acted as a natural rampart for the village. The bamboo had been cultivated for just that purpose. I could see nothing beyond – and certainly no targets at which to launch an offensive.

Seeking guidance in what course of action to take, I looked left and right – then left and right again. Then over my shoulder. Not a soul was in sight.

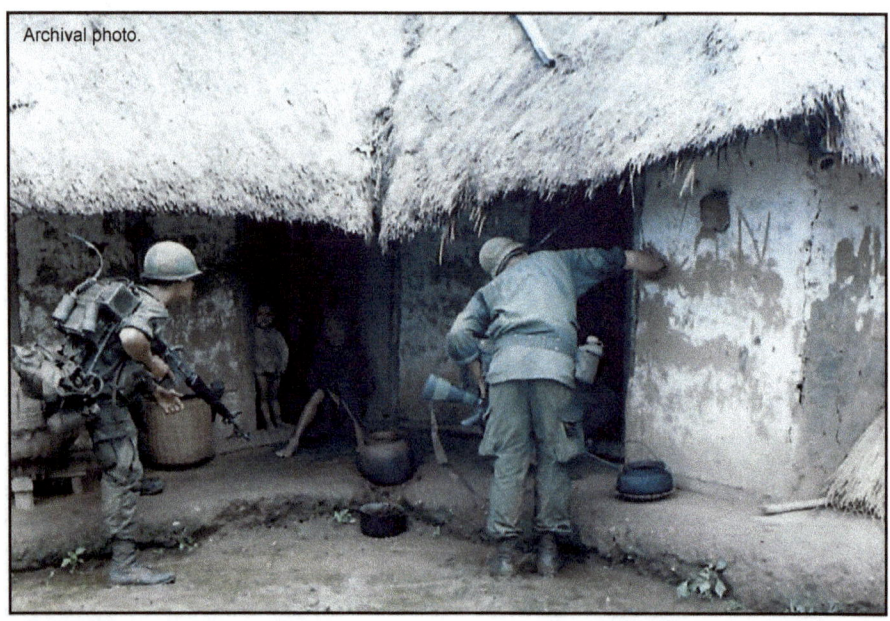
Archival photo.

I was alone.

I had advanced so fast and so far that I had outdistanced the entire company. Instinctively I wanted to jump up and dash back to the perception of safety in the numbers of my outfit. But then I envisioned what my mates might behold: a soldier looming out of the haze, olive drab in color, and running toward them bearing a rifle. Would they mistake me for an enemy soldier?

My heart thumped wildly. What was I to do in order to avoid being gunned down by friendly fire? The dust began to settle. Shapes coalesced. I turned away from the oncoming troops, placed my rifle on top of the dike, and fired into the bamboo thicket – not at anything, but in the direction which would illustrate whose side I was on.

Yawn stooped down beside me. "Good work, Gentile."

If he only knew.

I changed magazines and resumed firing, one bullet at a time. The rest of the squad plumped down on either side of me, as did the men from the other platoons that were forming a single rank. Several men hurled grenades high enough to clear the tops of the stalks, so the grenades did not bounce back at us. Machine guns shredded the dense foliage to confetti. Then, using entrenching tools, we chopped our way through the splintered barrier and into the outskirts of the village. We stayed off the paths because they might be booby-trapped.

By the time we reached the deserted hooches, I thought that the enemy had broken off the engagement and had melted into the jungle on the far side of the 'ville. We found no bodies, discovered no abandoned weapons, and saw not a single enemy soldier in the flesh – either dead or alive. I figured that the phantom army of Vietcong guerrillas fought on its own terms, much the same as the ragtag continental soldiers of the American Revolution played cat and mouse with British redcoats. History was repeating itself with the tables turned and with previous lessons forgotten by U.S. Army tacticians.

By day's end, when the tunnel vision of combat had worn off, I wondered how much of what I had seen and thought and felt that day was real, and how much was imaginary. Five decades years later, I still don't know.

However, when I think back on it, I cannot honesty say (or write) that I heard any enemy gunfire. We may have attacked an abandoned village which Army Intelligence *believed* was an enemy stronghold, or one that had been reactivated.

A lot of jet fuel and ammunition were wasted, but at least no one got hurt.

The Hearts and the Minds

The primary occupation of my company was to investigate 'villes and hamlets for signs of the enemy. Every day we tramped through the jungle or followed well-worn paths until we found a secluded 'ville. The 'villes were occupied by women, children, and old men. We seldom saw young or middle-aged males. The villagers were powerless against ninety armed men. They squatted on the ground or stood by their hooches as we approached. We never knew whether the people were friendly toward us or not. The routine was to enter each hooch and conduct a search the way we had been taught in jungle warfare school – in a place called Tiger Land, which was located outside of Fort Polk, Louisiana.

My pockets were always stuffed with sundries that we received from the Red

Cross. The sundry pack contained everyday necessities such as toothbrushes, toothpaste, shaving cream, aftershave lotion, razors, cookies, chocolate bars, cigarettes, beer and so on. Because I neither smoked nor drank alcoholic beverages, I gave my cigarettes and beer to the members of my squad. I drank hot Coca-Cola.

Because the temperature was 110 degrees, half the soda exploded into the air as soon as I popped the can open. The same thing happened with the beer. We were lucky if half a can of liquid reached our mouths.

We were not allowed to smoke on patrol because the scent would give away our position as we strode softly and slowly along the jungle trails. For the same reason, those who bothered to shave were not allowed to use aftershave lotion.

Because we had more sundries than we could use, eat, or drink, I stuffed my pockets with the leftovers. I distributed cookies and melted chocolate bars to the children whenever we walked into a 'ville. When they realized what I was doing, I was soon surrounded by beggars with their hands in my face.

Afterward, when it was time for business, I stepped into a hooch and conducted a close but careful search of the premises. The average hooch had little more than a handmade table and some chairs, and perhaps a bureau or chest. I looked for weapons that might be secreted in the bamboo walls. The sharp eyes of the occupants watched me closely as I rummaged through drawers. Most of them owned little more than the clothes they were wearing. I was careful not to break anything. These people had so few possessions that a broken item might be irreplaceable. On my way outside, I left two cans of C-rations on the table.

Small Unit Tactics

Movie portrayals of soldiers on combat patrol differ markedly from reality. Many times, I've seen on film that when the patrol leader raises his fist in the air, everyone

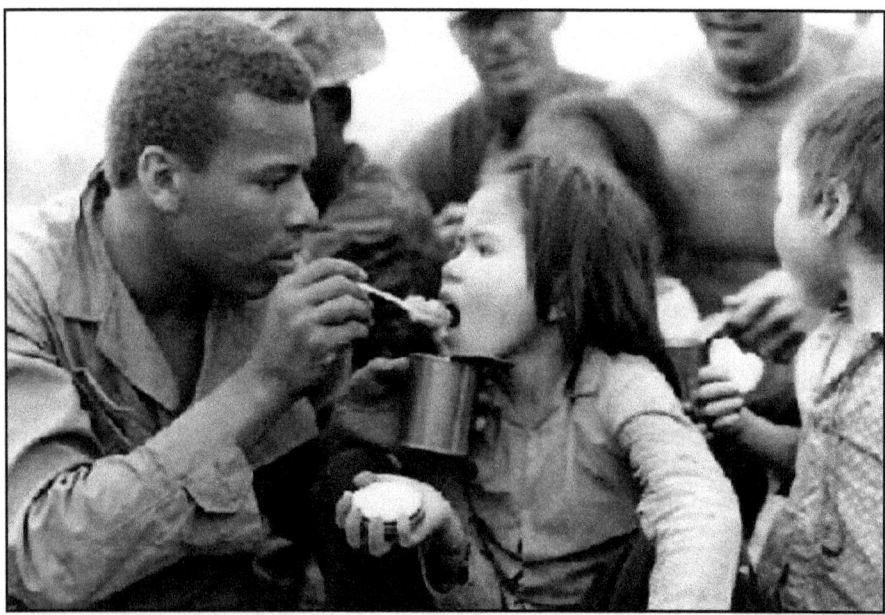

else immediately comes to a halt. That never happens in actual combat, and for several good reasons.

In order to get all the actors in the shot, so that dialogue can pass among them, movies often show soldiers bunched together like grapes on a stem. On real combat patrols, soldiers spread out and keep their distance from each other so that an antipersonnel mine or a hand grenade or machine gun fire or a mortar shell or an artillery shell would not kill everyone at once.

For the same reasons, soldiers advancing across a rice paddy spread sideways in order to maintain lateral distance. On a jungle trail, soldiers walked in a straight line and spread front to back. The prescribed distance in both circumstances was 15 feet. This distance was based on the kill zone of a fragmentation grenade.

The kill zone is the area that was defined by the length of the radius from the point of detonation, within which everyone was killed when a grenade detonated. The wound zone was the area that was defined by the length of the radius of 25 feet; in other words, anyone standing 25 feet from the point of detonation was likely to be wounded, but not killed.

Another reason for maintaining a safe distance from adjacent soldiers was the possibility of the presence of a booby trap, or antipersonnel mine. (A booby trap is now called an IED, for improvised explosive device.) If a soldier stepped on and triggered a booby trap, or tripped the wire of a booby trap, it was likely that adjacent soldiers who were fifteen feet away would *not* be killed, but only wounded. This was because the explosive charge in such a device was small: just enough to blow off a soldier's leg. That kind of wound was enough to take the soldier out of service, permanently. In addition, the presence of such mines had a strong psychological effect on surviving soldiers.

The possibility of the presence of antipersonnel mines was the reason that soldiers walked in a straight line on jungle trails, instead of in a staggered formation: there was less opportunity of triggering a mine where a preceding soldier had already placed his foot.

When it comes to tactics, every soldier on patrol – in either a sideways spread or in a front-to-back line – was responsible for observing his field of view. He was not just strolling along and daydreaming. In the paddy spread, each soldier was not simply staring ahead at the horizon, but was glancing at the ground for mines and trip wires. On a jungle trail, each soldier was assigned to watch a side: soldier one to the right side, soldier two to the left side, soldier three to the right side, and so on.

If the point man or platoon leader were to signal a halt under these circumstances, no one who was doing his job would have seen the raised fist. The raised fist signal to halt was a movie myth. It worked only if every soldier was constantly looking at the point man or platoon leader, which was never done in practice.

Death can still occur even when soldiers adhere to these precautions.

Close Call

To confuse the enemy, every morning we left the compound in a different direction. On one patrol, I was peering into the jungle on my right when I felt a puff of air against my ear, and almost simultaneously heard the clap of air rushing into the vacuum behind a passing bullet, before I heard the report of a rifle to my left. In a single fluid motion,

I spun leftward in a semicircle as I dropped to one knee as I flipped the safety switch to semi as I moved my finger from the guard to the trigger as I raised the rifle to my eye as the sniper broke from cover as I fired five rounds into his back. The entire action occurred in less than 3 seconds. Neither the man in front of me nor the one behind me had time to so much as raise their rifles.

I have extremely fast reflexes, plus the ability to assess a situation instantly and intuitively, as well as the sense to act appropriately. I don't know how I do it. I just do it. I don't take time to think; I just react instinctively. This inborn ability has never let me down.

As experienced troops, every soldier in the company dropped to one knee and aimed his rifle at the jungle, each alternate man facing in the opposite direction. No other targets presented themselves, no enemy fire ensued. This was not an ambush but a lone sniper who had waited for a target of opportunity. His shot to the back of my head had been slightly misaimed; or perhaps I swiveled my head at the fortuitous moment.

The company commander raced back along the path in a crouch. We were on a stealth patrol in which silence was a prerequisite. In a fierce hush he demanded, "Who fired those shots?"

I raised my hand. He squatted next to me. In a few curt sentences I explained that the sniper had fired the first shot – which announced our presence and position – and that I had returned fire. I pointed to the tree where the sniper had hidden before he broke cover and tried to run. Yawn and Tye nodded in confirmation. They saw the sniper break cover as I fired. In my ignorance, I asked, "Shall I go after him?"

For a long moment the experienced captain stared thoughtfully into the jungle, and thirty feet of clearing that afforded the sniper his shot. "No. That's just what they want us to do."

I realized then that the clearing could have been filled with hidden punji stakes that were smeared with feces, or the jungle floor could have been sown with pressure actuated booby-traps, or the trees could be strung with trip wires connected to explosive charges, or a full-scale ambush could be waiting for us just inside the tree line.

The captain slapped me on the shoulder. "Good work, soldier."

We continued the march along the jungle path, more alert than ever. Back at camp at the end of the patrol, I did not have time to dwell on the fact that my life had been only a fraction of an inch from death. My rifle had to be cleaned. My magazines needed to be oiled. My leftover bullets had to be wiped. I had to gulp down some C-rations. I had to deploy the claymore after dark. I had to stand guard duty during the night. I had to snatch a few winks of sleep before the morning routine started over again.

No one said anything to me about the sniper. There were no high fives, no handshakes, no fist bumps, no thumbs up, no jubilation, no congratulations. There was nothing special about my shooting an enemy soldier than there was about anyone else's shooting an enemy soldier. As much as I hate to write this – and I don't mean to sound smug or satirical – but in accordance with my job description it was just another day at the office: no different from fixing a paper jam in a copy machine.

It was my first kill.

Bullets and Water

The temperature was 110 degrees in the shade but we were in the sun. Sporadic gunfire erupted from the jungle thicket a few feet in front of my face. I ducked low behind the 18-inch-high berm and conserved my ammunition.

I didn't dare to throw a grenade for fear of hitting a tree and having the grenade ricochet back at me or someone else in my squad. Whenever I heard an enemy bullet whiz inches over my head, I fired at the origin of the sound: a three-bullet spread close to the ground. The ambushers were well hidden in the jungle, while we lay in the hot sand of a dry rice paddy.

We had been pinned down for two hours without being able to retreat or advance. I rolled over with my shoulders scrunched together, to take a quick swig from my canteen. It was only ten o'clock in the morning yet both canteens had been empty for an hour. I tried hopefully to find another drop to wet my tongue. The canteen was still empty. I was parched.

Corporal Yawn low-crawled behind the squad, hugging the ground like a frying griddle cake. He bumped into my shoulder. "Gentile, get everyone's canteens and go find water." This seemed like an impossible order to fulfill.

At a normal drink stop, we stood in a circle facing each other. This enabled all of us to see past the opposing man. One man removed his canteen from its pouch, gulped barely enough water to slake some of his thirst, then passed the canteen to the man standing next to him. That man took a drink and passed the canteen onward. Whoever was holding the canteen when it became empty, removed his canteen from its pouch, put the empty canteen into the vacated pouch, took another drink, then passed the canteen onward in a continuous round robin until we all had had our fill or until all the canteens were empty. In this game of musical canteens, no one possessed a personal canteen. And for a good reason.

A canteen had only two conditions: it was either full or empty; there was no in-between. This was because water in a partially filled canteen sloshed noisily, which could give away our position to listening enemy soldiers. This system was always followed on stealth patrols, when absolute silence was essential. No one took a drink whenever he was thirsty; he had to wait until the platoon or company stopped for that specific purpose.

I used to hike with a knapsack but hated the sweat that accumulated on my back. So I bought web gear from I. Goldberg, an Army surplus store in downtown Philly. I rigged it the way I wore it in Vietnam: fanny pack in the middle and canteens on either side. No grenades. Note the cap holder, and the metal cup with folding handle, both of which are contoured to fit the canteen. These items are not as grubby as they were in the bush. The splattered mud comes from riding my mountain bike through puddles.

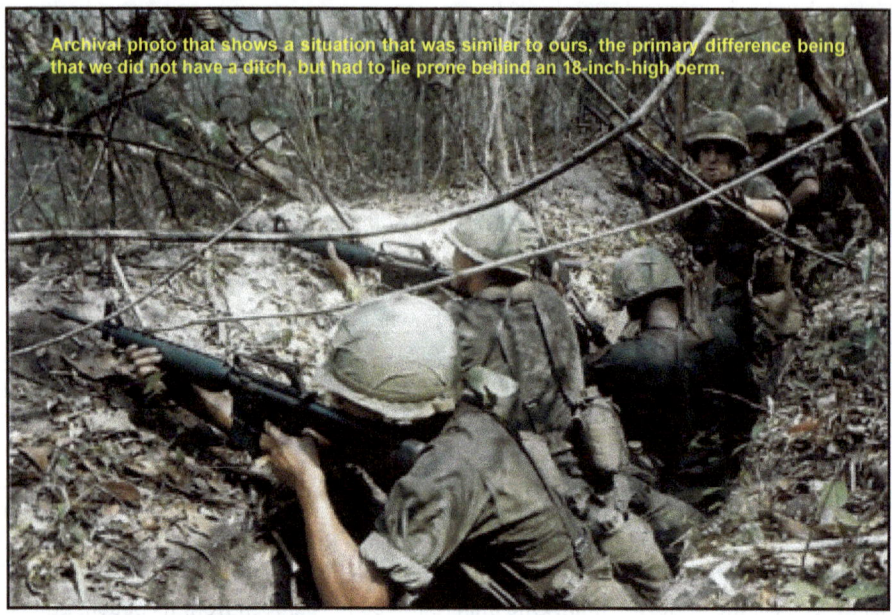

Archival photo that shows a situation that was similar to ours, the primary difference being that we did not have a ditch, but had to lie prone behind an 18-inch-high berm.

You must fully understand the importance of these precautions. Charlie could be anywhere – or everywhere – in the jungle, because the jungle was his home. All of Vietnam was enemy territory. Every day, American soldiers were killed in downtown Saigon.

I rolled onto my side with my back facing Yawn. "Get a spare boot lace out of my fanny pack."

Yawn undid the straps, pulled out the C-ration boxes, felt around inside the pack, retrieved a boot lace, returned the C-rations, and tightened the straps. Yawn handed his canteens to me. I ran the lace through the cap keeper of the canteens, then tied a knot that would keep the canteens in place.

I looked over the dry paddy. "I'll head for that grove of trees."

Yawn nodded. "Signal when you're ready. I'll give you cover fire."

There was a great deal of unspoken language in that short exchange. Each of us knew exactly what I planned to do, even though we had not discussed it. Combat soldiers exchanged information without articulating every word. We all thought alike. I simply pointed to a grove of trees about a quarter mile away from our position where the paddy and the jungle met, and that was not in the line of fire from the enemy.

I low-crawled along the berm in the direction that was away from the grove, explained the situation to my squad members, gathered canteens, then turned back and low-crawled in the direction toward the grove – all while shots were being fired by both opponents and while enemy bullets zinged by inches over my head. Again, I hate to sound macho, but bullets passing so close as the enemy bullets were passing were so common an occurrence that I hardly took notice of them unless I was in real danger of stopping one of them. A two-inch miss was the same as a mile. This firefight was no different from any other firefight.

After I had the last canteen on my string, I tied a knot through the ultimate cap keeper. I dragged the empty canteens about a hundred feet as I slithered along the berm.

When I felt that I was clear of the line of fire, I looked at Yawn and waved my hand. He gave the order to commence cover fire.

The first sound I heard was the chatter of the machine gun. It was followed immediately by the M-16's firing on spaced single shots. I did not run for it, as you might think. I low-crawled as fast as I could while keeping my body flat, more like a sinuous sidewinder than a baby crawling after a toy. I kept looking all around for enemy soldiers who may have heard the plastic canteens clattering together: a noise that was distinctly different from gunshots. To me the bouncing canteens sounded like church bells.

As I keep reiterating, everything around me was enemy territory. The very ground that I was crawling over could have been boobytrapped.

After a quarter-mile low-crawl, I reached the grove without incident. When I waved at Yawn, he ordered the men to cease cover fire. There could have been enemy soldiers hiding in the grove, so I stayed alert and kept my finger on the trigger. The grove was shaped like a lozenge that measured 50 feet in width. I was exceptionally cautious of boobytraps as I crawled through the dense understory to the opposite end, less than 50 feet away. I peeked out of the foliage.

The vast paddy seemed more than a mile in length in one direction, half a mile in the other. The patchwork of dikes separated squares of fields. Near me the paddies were dry. In the distance the paddies were flooded, yet I saw no peasants working in the fields.

I opted to head toward the jungle that lay half a mile away. First I studied the fringe for signs of movement or enemy emplacements; I saw neither. I stretched my body into low-crawl position, proceeded slowly. I continued to scan the jungle fringe. Halfway to the green jungle I chanced upon a paddy square that held a large puddle in the middle: about 30 feet in length and 10 feet at its widest.

Hastily I untied my string of canteens, all the while facing the jungle. I remained close to the ground so as to present the smallest possible target to the greenery.

I didn't like the appearance of the puddle. The top was covered with dark brownish scum that had the look of a mold culture – which in fact it was. I used both hands to part the scum. The water was clear underneath the scum, and about a foot deep. I unscrewed the cap of one canteen, covered the opening with my hand, submerged the canteen to the bottom of the puddle, tilted it slightly upward, and removed my hand. This was a Boy Scout trick for siphoning the cleanest water through the mouth of the canteen; the surface scum did not get sucked into the opening.

The normal procedure for filling a canteen with "wild" water was to tighten the cap, remove the canteen from the water, unscrew the cap, drop an iodine tablet into the opening, replace the cap and screw it down partway but not tight, shake the canteen so that water splashed out and over the canteen's threads, tighten the cap, and wait 20 minutes before drinking.

I couldn't wait that long. My throat was parched. I don't think many people have a true appreciation for the power of thirst. I put the pill in my mouth and washed it down with water from the canteen. I chugged down a quart of water on a single breath without stopping. I followed the same procedure with the second quart of water, except that I stopped halfway to take a breath. Thus, I swallowed half a gallon of water in less than a minute. Try it sometime.

I continually glanced around the paddy and especially toward the jungle, where enemy soldiers were apt to appear. I was filling the canteen for the third time when in my peripheral vision I spotted movement in the water. At first I thought it was a slug that was crawling across the bottom of the puddle. It was about the size of my thumb. As I watched, its body elongated toward my hand: growing longer but becoming thinner. Then it bunched its body to its original corpulence, grew fatter and shorter, and stretched again in my direction.

I spotted two more, heading toward my hand from different directions.

Leaches!

Shades of *The African Queen*. No one told me that Vietnam harbored giant leaches. They were never mentioned in training, and they did not emerge in casual conversation. I had never seen one in real life. But I had seen pictures of them in biology books. I have seen slugs in my back yard, but unlike leeches, slugs did not change their size or shape; those that I had seen in the woods near my house were permanently rotund.

Leaches had the ability to sense heat. That was how they detected my hand in the water. That was why they converged not on the canteen but on the hand that held it.

The canteen was nearly full. The leaches were less than a foot away. They were stretching forward when I yanked my hand and the canteen out of the puddle, leaving the blood suckers without a victim.

I dropped an iodine tablet into the canteen, screwed the lid partway on, shook the canteen, tightened the lid, then picked up another canteen. I moved to a different part of the puddle, parted the scum, and resumed the filling process. The three leaches – plus additional culprits – followed me. I had to move three more times before I filled all the canteens.

Two canteens went into the pouches on my pistol belt. The other 10 I retied onto the boot lace. I drank and refilled one more canteen before I started my retreat. Instead of dragging 10 empty canteens, I now had to drag 20 pounds of water. (As my grandmother used to say, "A pint's a pound the world around." Each canteen held one quart, or two pints.) It was a lot of work, but nothing was going to make me stand up and

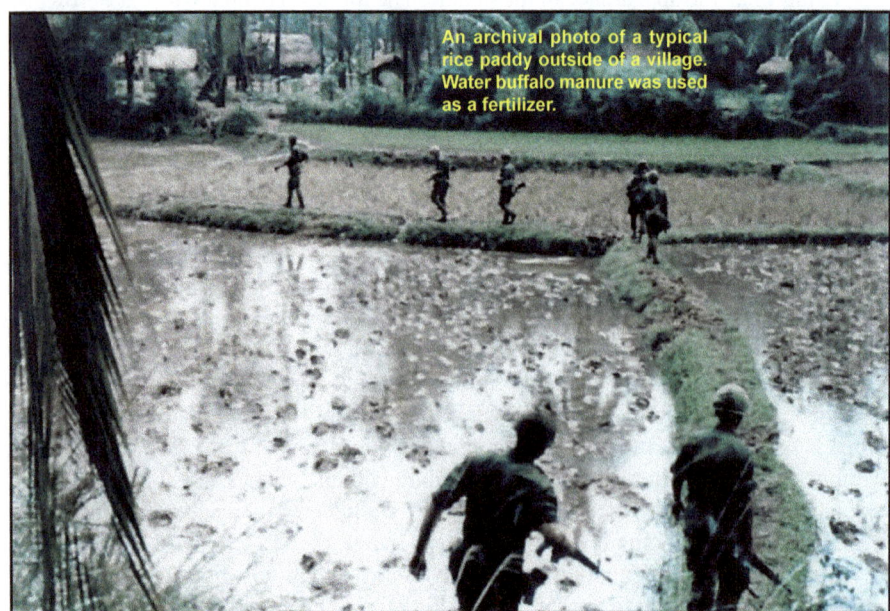

An archival photo of a typical rice paddy outside of a village. Water buffalo manure was used as a fertilizer.

carry them over my shoulders like machine gun belts. I kept low-crawling and looking over my shoulder for signs of the enemy.

I could still hear gunshots from the firefight in which my platoon was engaged. I crawled as fast as I could but the bouncing canteens slowed me down. After a long haul I reached the grove of trees. This was where I breathed a sigh of relief. My companions were fighting only a quarter mile away. I waited until I saw Yawn look in my direction, then I waved, all the while glancing at the jungle in front of me.

As soon as I heard the covering fire, I did a low-crawl dash across the open paddy to the berm. The covering fire ceased. I crawled along the berm and when I reached the first man on my team, I handed him two canteens. He paused long enough to empty one of them. Two bullets passed overhead, followed immediately by burps from an AK-47. My teammate started shooting at a presumed target. I moved on and made the rest of my deliveries, then rejoined the fracas.

I never told anyone about the scum-covered puddle. No one asked. The firefight continued.

This day was not yet over. Enemy fire gradually faded. Eventually, there seemed to be no more resistance. The lieutenant gave the order for the other squad to move forward. I slipped my finger off the trigger but did not put my safety switch to safe. The squad disappeared into the jungle. A couple of minutes later, my squad received the order to move forward.

We had taken only half a dozen steps when someone yelled, "Live grenade!" My platoon sergeant ran out of the jungle, bobbling an enemy grenade in his hands. My squad split and scattered like a flock of chickens getting away from a fox, of which I was one. As the sarge passed me, I saw him toss the grenade into a bomb hole and drop flat on his face as I leaped over a bush, landed on my feet, buckled my knees, and went flat onto my belly.

I squirmed back to my position behind the berm, rested my rifle on the hardpacked earth, and prepared to fire. I heard some M-16 chatter in the jungle.

There was no explosion. Either the grenade was a dud or the pin hadn't been pulled.

After a while, the sergeant raised his head a hair. He then crawled over the berm onto the paddy. There we lay. Five minutes later, the other squad's leader appeared and gave us the "all clear" sign.

When I stood up, I felt a stab of pain in my left ankle and fell back onto the ground. I didn't know what was wrong, only that I was in pain. Someone called the medic who happened to be nearby. I unlaced my boot. By the time the medic arrived, my ankle had swollen to twice its normal size. The medic felt it gently, but even gently gave pain.

The medic thought that I must have twisted it when I crash-landed during my avoidance of the grenade. He figured that the ankle was nothing more than a minor strain. He searched through his first-aid kit only to discover that he had not brought any Ace bandages with him. He instructed me to don another sock and tie my boot laces extra tight.

I did as he said. Not only did it hurt when I tightened the lace, but I felt a stabbing pain whenever I put my weight on the ankle. Every step felt as if I were being stabbed with an icepick.

Little did I know that this damaged ankle was going to plague me for the rest of my life.

The platoon regrouped, spread out wide, then proceeded through the jungle oh so slo-oo-owly, preceding every step with a hard visual examination of the ground in the search for booby traps and trip wires. Half an hour later we broke out of the jungle onto another dry rice paddy.

We found no blood, no bodies, no wounded enemy soldiers, no spider holes, not even a gun shell. It was as if no all-morning firefight had ever occurred. We stopped for lunch in the open. Afterward, we hiked 5 miles along flat dikes and jungle trails, back to our company's bivouac site. My ankle throbbed with every step.

It was another fruitless day in the fight for . . . whatever we were supposed to be fighting for.

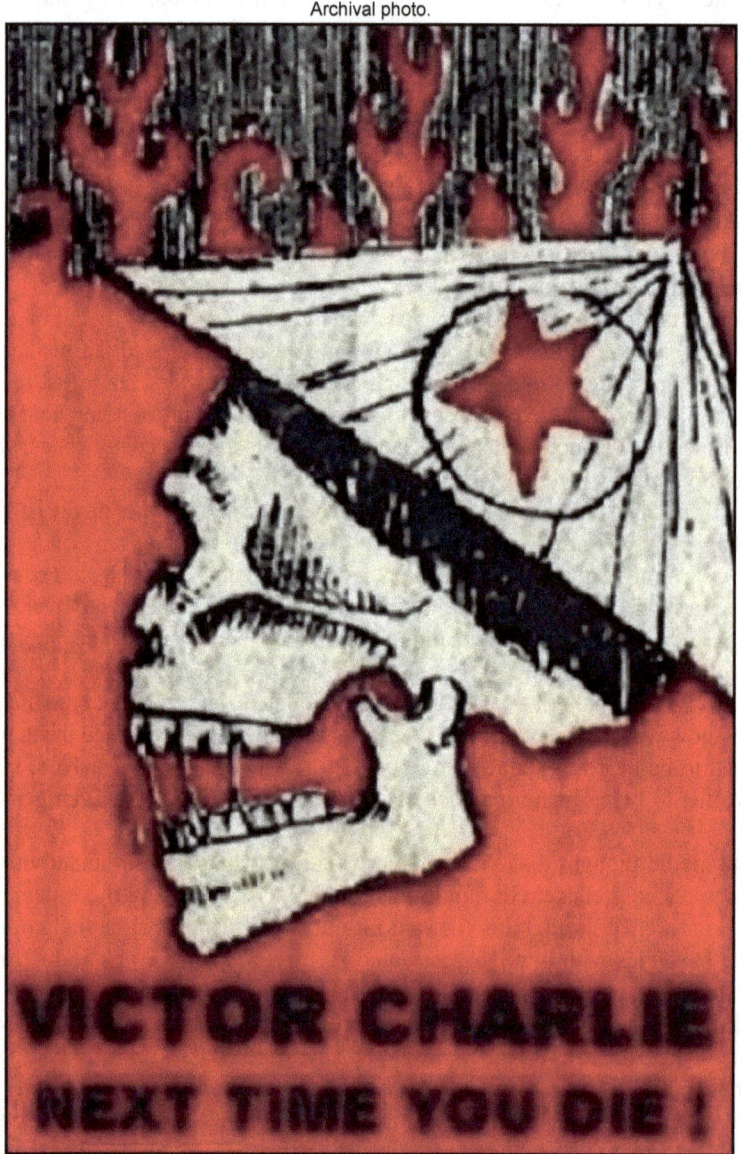

Archival photo.

No Rest for the Wary

Another day, our squad paused for a rest in the shade of a grove of coconut trees while the remainder of the company advanced to the perimeter of a village that we happened to be passing on the way to our primary objective. Standard operating procedure required that we conduct a cursory examination for enemy sympathizers.

The general definition of "sympathizer" was anyone who supplied the enemy with food, shelter, supplies, or information of military value. The specific definition varied according to viewpoint. To us, sympathizers were unarmed peasants who lent aid to the VC or NVA under threat of death or rape, in which case they were slain, and the village was destroyed by American troops under orders.

On the other hand, unarmed peasants who offered no resistance to American incursion or who otherwise minded their own business while American troops passed through their village, under threat of death or the destruction of their village, were executed by the VC or NVA for sympathizing with the invasionary forces. By these contradictory formulations, every Vietnamese peasant was characterized as a sympathizer by one of the warring factions – a lose-lose situation for the populace no matter how they looked at it.

I was having fun knocking coconuts out of a tree – one use for an entrenching tool that was not covered in the training manual. I left my rifle leaning against the trunk in order to have both hands free so I could chop a hole in the husk with my bayonet, and drink the cool refreshing succulent within. Suddenly there came the crackle of gunfire nearby. I grabbed my rifle and charged into a path where, 40 feet away, a VC guerrilla was climbing out of a spider hole, spraying bullets. He was gunned down immediately from two sides.

After that incident, I vowed never to let my rifle out of my hands again. I already related how I slept by hugging my rifle as if it were a teddy bear. I didn't let go of my rifle even when I was crouched to take a crap; instead of laying the rifle on the ground next to me, I placed it across my thighs against my abdomen. I know it sounds quirky, but the Vietnamese bush was a life or death environment that I learned not to take lightly.

This incident also changed our company's directive for the day. Now we concentrated on closely examining the village in view and the people who lived there; or rather, the people who remained there in the absence of the men who should have been there.

I spotted a storage bin the size of an outhouse; it was half filled with rice to the height of my hips. Such rice cribs were commonly found in occupied villages.

I poked through the loose rice with my bayonet, detected nothing untoward, so I stuck in my hand and felt through grains of rice. To my horror, I uncovered a booby-trap from which loose wires dangled more than a foot. For several seconds I stood stock-still – waiting for the blast to take off my hand or my face – until I determined that the device had not yet been armed. The village was definitely "hot," yet no reprisals were taken against the villagers.

The partially completed booby trap could just have well have been hidden by a VC guerrilla – such as the one who had been gunned down – without the villagers' knowledge. I never learned who made the decision that a village was hostile or not, or why one was destroyed while another was left alone.

"Ours is not to reason why . . . "

Search and Destroy Mission

Another day we entered a village that was occupied only by women, children, and leathery old men who squatted on their haunches in typical Vietnamese fashion. We found no signs of the enemy, no concealed weapons, no buried booby-traps – nothing that would indicate collusion with the VC or NVA other than the absence of virile young men. Nonetheless, this village was sanctioned for destruction.

After the 'ville was thoroughly searched and considered safe, Hueys arrived with 50-pound wooden cases of dynamite sticks, which we distributed throughout the 'ville, inside bamboo hooches and mud-walled bunkers. The bunkers proved to be too strong to destroy.

Vietnamese bunkers were equivalent to American bomb shelters; they served the same purpose. In the event of a B-52 bomber attack, villagers crammed inside the bunkers in the same way we (men of my squad) crammed into our sandbag shelters when hostile fire drove us there for protection.

Local bunkers were shaped like puptents but were made from mud instead of canvas. The single entrance was located at one end. The mud was anywhere from 8 to 10 inches thick. Once the mud dried, it maintained the hardness of concrete, which in effect it was.

My platoon was instructed to assist the explosive engineers, mostly by doing the grunt work of carrying the dynamite cases to specific sites where the engineers wanted them placed for the most destructive effect. The engineers were easy-going non-coms (non-commissioned officers; that is, sergeants), and easy to work with.

I was with them when they experimented with "demolishing" a bunker. First they started with half a dozen sticks of nitroglycerin. The explosion blew the dust off the mud walls. Then they tried half a case of dynamite. The explosion did considerable cosmetic damage to the inside of the bunker, but did no structural damage. The bunker was just as staunch as it was before the blast. Finally, they placed an entire case of explosive at the bunker's entry, every stick rigged to detonate simultaneously.

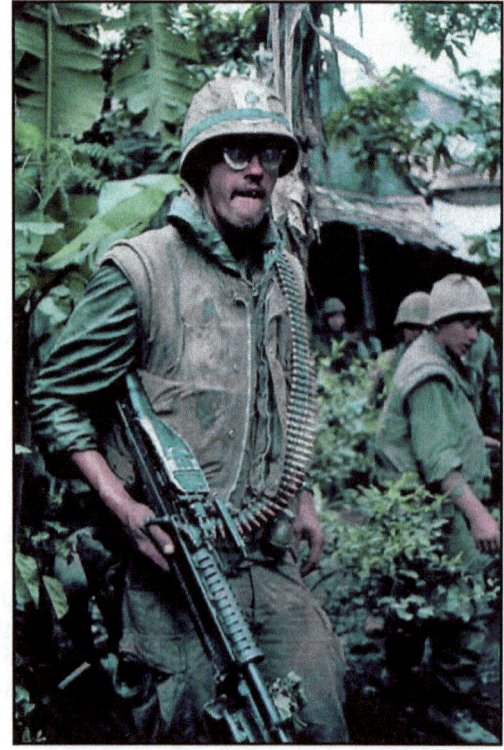

While I was toting an M-16 that weighed a mere 7 pounds, the machinegunner was hefting a weapon that weighed 23 pounds, plus at least one bandolier filled with 100 rounds of 7.62 millimeter cartridges. The reader should understand that everyone of us was trained to fire the M-60. An infantry company consisted of interchangeable soldiers, all of whom were trained to handle every hand-held weapon, and all of whom could serve in every combat role. Mortarmen were the only infantrymen who required special training and handling.

I watched this explosion. The entry was partially caved in, but the body of the bunker – some 10 feet in length – was otherwise untouched. The engineers gave up at that point because they did not have enough dynamite to destroy all the bunkers – not if they wanted to make the hooches uninhabitable. I was dismissed and told to continue transporting cases of dynamite.

By the way, the Hueys did double duty that day. As soon as we completed unloading the cargo of explosives, the villagers were place onboard and flown to the firebase, where they were interrogated and issued identification cards (about the size of a credit card). Then they were taken to another village with all their belongings – which could fit in a canvas sack the size of a pillowcase. They were not harmed in any way, just relocated.

Meanwhile, back at the 'ville, the ultimate irony was that we ran out of dwellings before we ran out of explosives. We couldn't save the six extra cases of dynamite for another job because the Hueys had already departed, except for one to carry the engineers back to base camp. We placed all three hundred pounds of explosives on the dining room table of a pristine stucco house that had been built during the French occupation, when Vietnam was known as French Indochina.

Now that I had time to rest after the hard work was done, I noticed that the coops and pens were still closed and latched. I asked the captain for permission to release the animals before the village was destroyed. In a rare moment of sanity and sensibility, permission was granted. I ran from stable to stall to henhouse, letting out pigs and goats and chickens till the hardened dirt roadways were choked with squeals and bleats and clucks as well as the curses of American soldiers who disdained farm animals running amok.

We still had one more job to do: string roll after roll of primacord throughout the village until every case of explosives was wired together on one continuous string. The troops gathered outside the village perimeter while the final splice was made. When the electrical contacts were touched, the detonator ignited the primacord.

According to the explosive engineers, primacord was a flexible detonation cord (often called detcord) which burned at 27,000 feet per second; that's 5 miles per second. It looked so much like clothesline that if left lying around a house, some people might be tempted to hang wet clothes on it to dry. It cannot explode on its own, even if you beat it with a hammer; it needed an electrical impulse for ignition to occur.

When the engineer pushed the plunger that created the charge – like a miner in an old-time cowboy movie – all the dynamite exploded in less than a second. The separate charges sounded like a single titanic blast. The entire village seemed to lift into the air intact. Then it came down in pieces of bamboo, thatch, dirt, dust, and debris. There was nothing left of the stucco house but the splintered concrete pad.

I hoped that most of the animals had gotten away in time, before they were killed by the concussion.

Cooking off Grenades

One ville resisted our reconnaissance with automatic weapons fire. The shooting was by no means hot and heavy, but it was consistent. We beat through the brush past the first row of now-vacant hooches, behind which fortified bunkers protected the central square of the ville and impeded our progress by the possibility of their occupation.

My squad was given the job of "securing" the bunkers. To do this, we had to ensure that the bunkers were empty, so that no enemy soldiers could emerge later and attack us from the rear.

As the grenadier, it was my job to "secure" each bunker. A bunker was secured by tossing a grenade into it, thus killing everyone inside. But it wasn't as simple as it sounds. Civilians might be hiding inside so as not to get caught in the crossfire between Vietnamese and American troops. On the other hand, a VC guerrilla might be waiting inside for an American soldier to walk into his sights. My job was to determine which was which: that is, to save the first "which" and to kill the second "which."

Of all the hazards that I faced in Vietnam, this was the one that scared me the most. It went like this.

The men in my squad lay side by side on the ground with their rifles (or machine-gun) pointing toward the opening of a bunker. They fired a few shots not into the opening, or doorway, but alongside it. Yawn waved for me to run forward until I was adjacent to the bunker, turn toward the bunker and proceed to its side (preferably the left side), then to work my way toward the front of the bunker. At that point all gunfire ceased so that I would not be struck accidentally.

From my position alongside the bunker, I leaned past the side and pointed my rifle toward the opening. From this position I could not shoot into the bunker, only past the opening. I yelled, "Di di! Di di!" If there was no answer, I yelled, "Di di mau."

I didn't know the words for "come out," or "hands up," so "run" and "run fast" had to suffice. If I saw hands protrude from the opening, I would hold my fire. If I saw a rifle muzzle, I would open fire.

Meanwhile, from a position of safety, Yawn peered into the darkness of the opening to look for movement inside the bunker. If he saw no movement after several seconds, he waved for me to proceed.

I shifted the rifle to my left hand. I yanked a grenade from its clip on my web gear suspender. Using my teeth, I bit down on the pull ring and yanked out the safety pin.

I was not trying to act macho. Macho was for movie actors who greatest danger was in ingrown toenail. I removed the pin with my teeth because I was holding my rifle in my left hand, and my trigger finger was on the trigger. The safety lever was on auto.

Again I yelled for people to come out of the bunker. When no one came forward, I had to presume that either the bunker was empty or it was occupied by an enemy soldier. I nodded to Yawn. He gave the order to provide covering fire. The men fired into the opening from various angles. This would cause the bullets to ricochet off the sloped walls.

At this point I could still call off the assault by inserting the pin into the arming lever. After the short fusillade I nodded to Yawn. He ordered a reduced fire.

Once the arming lever has been released, the grenade *will* detonate. There is no way to stop it. The genie cannot be put back into the bottle. At that point, replacing the pin has no effect on the arming mechanism. After the fuze has been activated on an Mk 2 fragmentation grenade, the grenade will detonate in 4 and a half seconds (give or take).

Now fir the scary part. *I had to hold the live grenade in my hand for 3 seconds.* You might be thinking, *"Are you crazy?"*

That's beside the point. The purpose of the delay was to prevent a nimble adversary

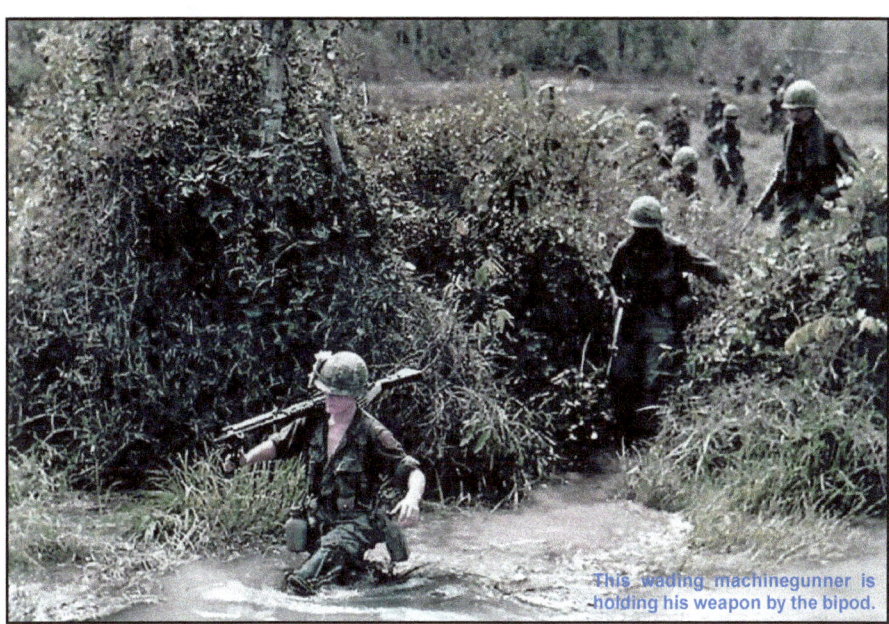
This wading machinegunner is holding his weapon by the bipod.

from catching the grenade or scooping it off the floor and tossing it back outside the bunker, with obvious deleterious results for me and my squad.

This was a precision maneuver that called for split-second timing and execution from everyone in the squad. For two seconds they maintained fire while I counted seconds in my head, starting with zero when I released the arming lever. As I reached number 2, I swung my throwing arm back. When the squad members saw my arm moving, they stopped firing so they wouldn't shoot off my hand. My arm swung forward so that when I counted the number 3, I was in a position to release the grenade at an angle that would cause it to bounce inside the bunker like a billiard ball on a 3-dimensional pool table. At the same time, I rolled around the edge of the bunker and dropped into a crouch, so I was out of the blast zone.

I did not –I repeat, *not* – yell "Fire in the hole!" the way actors do in the movies. That is as stupid as hollering, "Look out, Charlie. I'm about to throw a grenade at you."

Nor did I put my hands on my steel pot as you will sometimes see in the movies. The purpose of the steel pot was to protect a soldier's head from being struck by shrapnel (although a well angled bullet might pierce a steel pot). No real soldier puts his hands on his steel pot in order to prevent it from getting scratched during an explosion.

I digress. As soon as the grenade's explosion died down, I stood and rolled back in front of the bunker and leaped into the doorway. I could see nothing until the dust settled, but I wasted no time in feeling around the floor for victims. There was none.

However, a sheet of plywood lay flat on the dirt floor. It could have been cover for a spider hole. Immediately I lifted it with my left hand as I pointed my rifle underneath as I lifted the plywood into the air. I had to act swiftly while someone in hiding was still stunned by the concussion. There was nothing under the plywood but a horde of ants, which did not seem to have been bothered by the explosion.

I breathed a deep sigh of relief. The plywood flooring could also have concealed a booby-trap that was rigged to detonate the moment I lifted the wood.

Another thing that I should mention in regard to Mk 2 fragmentation grenades is that most of them were leftovers from World War 2. I don't know how they were stored for more than two decades, but there was an instance in which one of them detonated as soon as the arming lever was released. This resulted in the instant death of the grenadeer. Talk about a short fuze. I'm glad that I didn't learn about that until after I left Vietnam. I was scared enough as it was. Upon examination, it turned out that the entire case of grenades was short-tempered.

Overkill

All the bunkers were vacant, but Tye had the misfortune of finding a spider hole in a grassy clearing that was surrounded by shrubbery. As soon as he did, he backed away quickly and shouted his discovery. We all dropped to the ground in offensive positions along one side of the hole. Yawn quickly checked to ensure that no one in our company was in the line of fire on the other side of the spider hole.

Yawn and Tye discussed strategy. It was assumed that the spider hole was occupied by an enemy soldier. On the other hand, it could have been occupied by a male villager who was simply hiding until Vietcong and American troops finished fighting and departed. As I have already mentioned, villagers were not always treated with kindness by American soldiers who were necessarily suspicious of their allegiance.

It was also possible that the spider hole could be a gateway to a vast underground complex.

I was placed in the open about 20 feet from the hole, in a slightly lower position. The other riflemen and the machine gunner were located on either side of me but farther back.

Tye approached the spider hole and performed the recognition ritual: "Di di! Di di! Di di mau!" (Keep in mind that I cannot confirm the spelling nor the translations of Vietnamese words. I am spelling phonetically words that I only ever heard from my fellow soldiers.) This was the way in which Vietnamese people were asked to surrender.

When no answer was forthcoming, Tye stepped stealthily through the grass toward the spider hole. His rifle was aimed at the leading edge of the camouflaged lid. His finger was on the trigger. Slowly he bent over, extended his rifle, slipped the barrel under the lip – and flipped up the lid.

I heard two rifle shots followed by an explosion as a puff of smoke or dust erupted from the open spider hole. Tye stumbled backward so fast that he lost his balance and danced sideways as he twisted his body in order to regain his footing. He squatted between Yawn and me, breathing hard.

"He had a grenade in his hands. I fired two rounds, then the grenade went off."

I was shocked. Literally shocked. This VC guerrilla chose death over capture. It made me wonder what kind of vicious propaganda the Vietcong employed to make their soldiers avoid capture by committing suicide. Were they told horrendous stories about how the Americans tortured their captors, inflicted excruciating pain, drove splinters under their nails, peeled off their skin, burned the bottom of their feet to the bone, cut off body parts? What?

The platoon sergeant arrived. He eagerly jumped into the spider hole and irreverently tossed out body parts: a foot, a hand, a bloody glob of something that was unrecognizable. He ordered two of his men from our other squad to grab the body by the arms and drag it out of the hole. The sergeant searched the hole diligently for weapons, ammunition, enemy paperwork, whatever he could find.

Meanwhile, the other elements of the company had secured the village without finding anything else of interest.

I was standing next to the body when the medic wandered into view. Because the grenade had detonated in the man's lap, shredded organs lay exposed in a gory hole that stretched from crotch to rib cage. His manhood, both feet, and both hands had been severed from the body; the sergeant had found one hand and one foot, but the others must have been blown into the shrubbery.

Was he an enemy soldier or an innocent villager in hiding? Because he wore nothing but a pair of bloody shorts, there was no way of ascertaining the facts. His only weapon had been the grenade.

The medic casually crouched down on one knee. I couldn't believe what he did next. He put his hand on the lower left arm that must have been the remains of the wrist. I thought his action was insane. He squeezed the shredded stub with his fingers.

Incredibly, he whispered, "This man's still alive."

He let go of the truncated forearm. He must have felt a pulse or seen blood trickling from torn blood vessels. I didn't ask.

With excessive zeal, my platoon sergeant put the barrel of his rifle to the soldier's head, and pulled the trigger twice, splattering bone, brain, and blood everywhere. He gleefully uttered four words that will forever be burned into my brain: "He ain't alive now."

I have related this incident in precise detail so that my readers will understand how bloody was the fighting in Vietnam. And how bloodthirsty some of the soldiers acted. Combat was a grand opportunity to let the dark beastial side of a person's psyche run rampant; to literally get away with murder without having to suffer any consequences.

All I could do was shrug. Est quod est, as the Romans used to say. It is what it is.

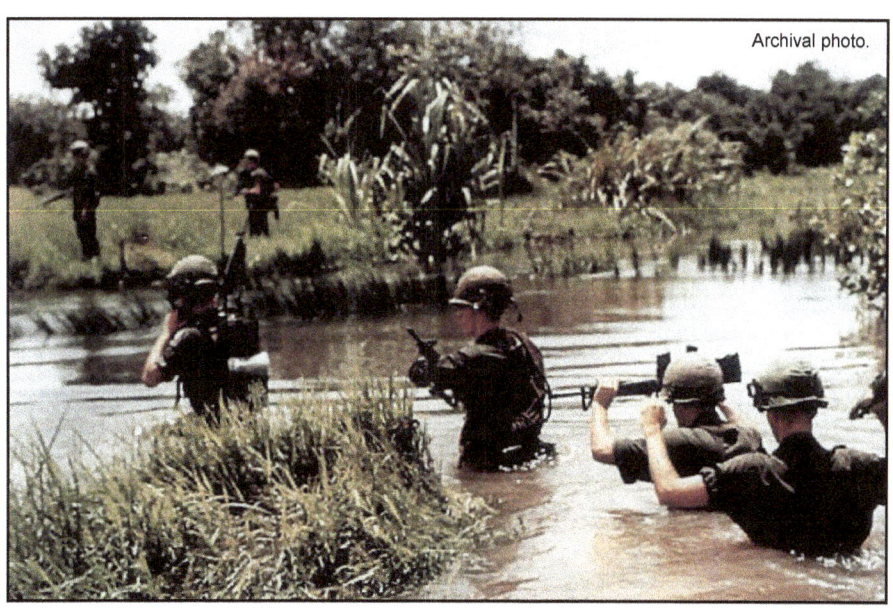

Archival photo.

Failed Leadership?

Sometimes I carried tear gas grenades and a gas mask in addition to my usual gear and ammunition. As I forced my way through dense jungle foliage, a branch pulled open the snaps of the canvas case, which I wore around my neck on a strap, and the gas mask fell out unnoticed. Not until we stopped for a break did I realize that the gas mask was missing. I told my squad leader about it, and Yawn sent me to report it to our platoon leader who, with the other lieutenants, was talking with the company commander. The captain ordered me to go back and find it, not because it was so valuable, he said, but because he did not want it to fall into enemy hands and be used against us. He detailed two men to accompany me.

After a quarter mile of retracing our steps, one of the men started balking; he didn't want to go any farther. He was scared, and in retrospect, I can't say that I blame him. The only reason that I wasn't scared was because I was still a newbie. I was not yet aware of all the queer machinations that combat in the bush could take. I wasn't taught everything about combat in Vietnam. I was learning by OJT (On the Job Training).

Without the advantage of full company backup, our situation could be perilous should we make contact with a superior force. No one knew where the enemy was located. The enemy could be following us, it could be surrounding us, it could be ambushing us, it could be *under* us. After another quarter mile the jungle opened onto a

The soldier in front (to the right) is heavily burdened. The smooth-walled hand grenades that are clipped to his waist belt are M26 fragmentation grenades. These were first used in the Korean War, then adapted for use in Vietnam, presumably after the Army expended all the Mk 2 models in stock. The cylindrical can that is located high on the web gear suspender appears to be a smoke grenade. Smoke grenades were used to inform a Huey pilot where to land. They contained different colors of smoke for the purpose of confirmation that a pilot spotted the correct landing zone. That was because Charlie could intercept radio messages, then pop smoke, attract the pilot to the wrong landing zone, and shoot down the helicopter. The identification process went like this. "Ground control: "I just popped smoke." Pilot: "I see purple." Ground control: "That is correct." Or incorrect. The process did not start with ground control announcing, "I popped purple smoke," because then Charlie would pop the same color smoke. We all carried at least one smoke grenade in our fanny pack. As for the two soldiers behind the first one (to the left), I have no idea what they are carrying. Sorry. (Archival photo.)

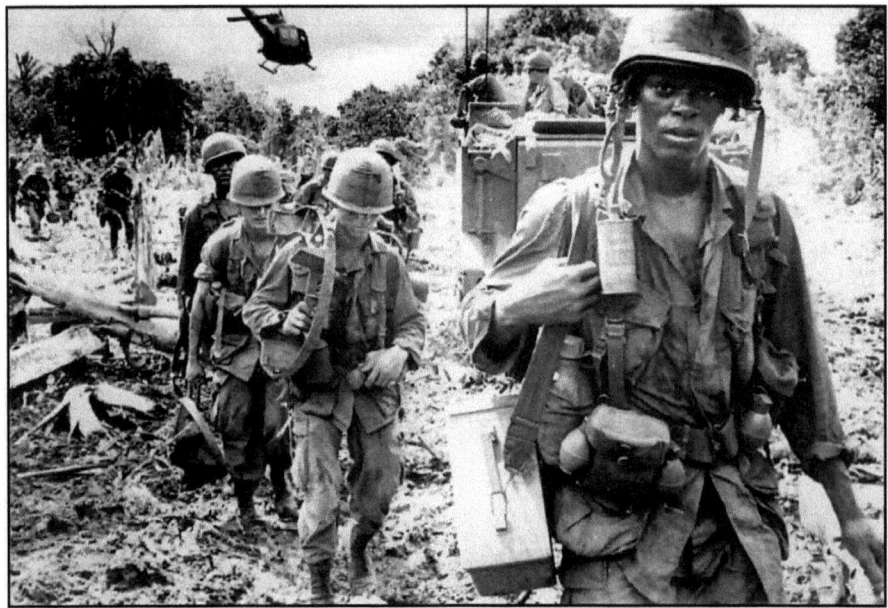

dry paddy which the second man refused to cross. It was too open, he said, and we would be too easy a target for a sniper. I argued the point, but the most I could get from the man was a promise to cover me and to wait ten minutes for my return.

"We worked this area coupla months ago and got shot up bad."

The other one agreed. "Lost a lotta men. Goddamn gooks was everywhere. I ain't goin' in the open."

"Me either."

That was gist of how they described the situation. They were adamant against crossing a hundred feet of open air without the company standing nearby to help. The narrow jungle trail was somewhat comforting because we couldn't be seen. The tangled foliated limbs closed overhead and created a tunnel effect. If I wanted to continue, I had to do it alone.

I wasn't as scared as they were because I hadn't been involved in the massacre that had decimated their company a couple of months earlier. It was impossible for them to convey to me what they were feeling, just as it was impossible for me to convey those feelings to my readers. The written word can express only so much. So don't think that I proceeded because I was braver than they were. The truth was that I was only more ignorant. Plus, I didn't want to fail in my mission to recover the gas mask. I didn't want to go back to the captain empty handed. At that moment I was more concerned about humiliation than I was about meeting an enemy soldier, or two, or more.

I crouched down low and ran across the open paddy to the opposite tree line, where the company had only recently pushed its way through. Within five minutes I found the gas mask lying in the underbrush on the side of our original trail. I tucked it into the case and fastened the snaps. I held onto the closure with my left hand; my right hand held the rifle with my finger on the trigger.

Back at the edge of the field, I waved. I was relieved to find that my reluctant companions were still waiting for me. One of them signaled for me to cross. When I reached the "safety" of their company, I was stunned to see how jittery they were. They were happy to see me alive, but they were happier that we could now rejoin our outfit. No longer looking on the ground or in the brush for the gas mask, we now jogged until we reached the rear guard of the company.

I reported the success of my mission to the captain. He said, "Let that be a lesson to you." Break time was over. He called for the troops to get on the move.

Was he truly concerned about Charlie obtaining a gas mask, or did he want to teach me a lesson to be more careful with army equipment? In retrospect, I think he made a poor tactical decision to risk the lives of three men simply to prove a point.

Crack Shot

According to an intelligence report, the NVA was massing in our area for a major assault, and there existed the possibility of being overrun. That night, while standing observation post, I witnessed the predicted action begin but against our neighboring company. Across several miles of open paddy came the cacophony of gunfire, mortars, and artillery as the attack proceeded, along with flashes of light from tracer rounds. I detected the presence of a Huey gunship by the light of its tracers as it spewed solid streams of lead beyond the perimeter of the outfit that it was protecting.

It must have been firing a minigun: a six-barrel minigun or Gatling gun that was

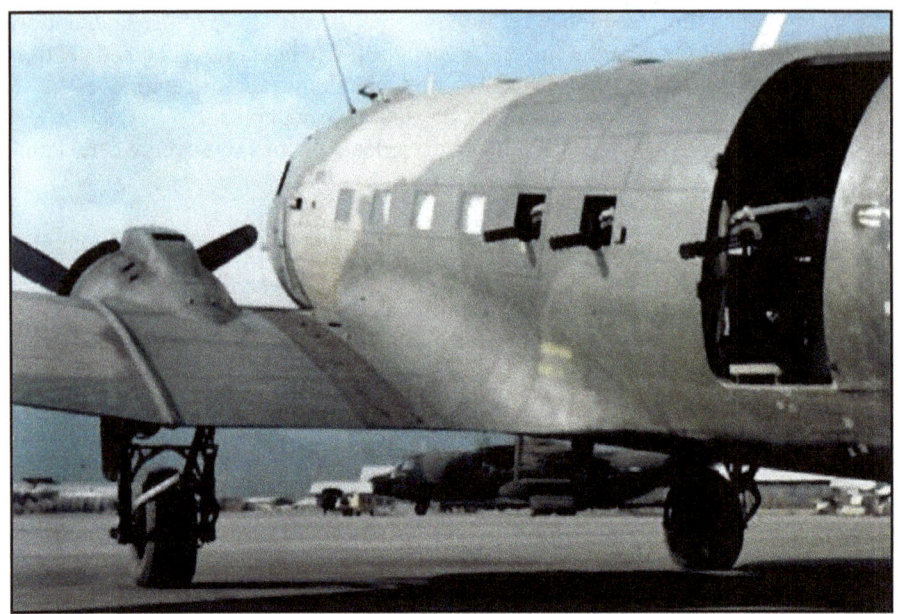

If you thought a Huey-mounted gatling gun was bad-ass, this Douglas AC-47 close air support gunship carried three of them. Different configurations could carry two that were rear mounted. In combat support, this fixed-wing aircraft generally banked and made a pylon turn over its target with all three guns blazing. As one sergeant described it to me, when this gunship fired at a football field, not even a rabbit could escape death. This modified DC-3 was often called Spooky, or Puff the Magic Dragon. I don't know why.

operated by an electric motor. It could spew nearly 6,000 rounds per minute.

I felt some relief in presuming that Charlie's forces were spread too thin to attack two positions at once, and that while our fellow soldiers were fighting nearby, we should survive the night unscathed. It might be our turn some other night.

While standing observation post and watching the distant show, I thought about the deserted hooch I had spotted before dusk. Our defensive circle was like wagon train in old-time western movies. Along one quadrant the jungle began only a few feet from the perimeter. The other three quadrants faced dry paddies that were miles in extent. Patches of jungle broke up the monotony and blocked the view of a curved horizon. The deserted hooch sat secluded on the edge of a small patch of jungle, and one side had a clear field of fire facing our temporary encampment.

Our nighttime routine was to launch a grenade about every half hour, in order to let the enemy know that we were on the alert. The whumping of grenades did further service by keeping awake the men who were on guard. It was easy to fall asleep after a long day "humping the boonies"

Whenever someone decided that enough time had passed to launch the next grenade reminder, the others on guard did the same. It might seem that this constant but sporadic explosive uproar – from grenades, gunfire, mortars, and claymores – and the agitation that was consequently aroused, would make nighttime slumber impossible. On the contrary, I found it difficult to remain vigilant even with a starlite scope glued to my eye. I was constantly drowsing despite the potential proximity of death.

With my nerves on edge from the attack in progress against our fellow troops, and the possibility of imminent attack against our own company, the more I thought about that secluded hooch, and the more uneasy I became. After a lengthy period of silence, I shifted the grenade launcher in my lap. It was not the over-and-under model, secured beneath the barrel of an M-16 but sharing a common stock. The rifle and the grenade launcher had separate triggers, not unlike a two-barreled shotgun. The Hispanic soldier carried that multi-use weapon. I held a dedicated M-79 grenade launcher.

In the pitch blackness of night, I couldn't see the hooch. I knew where it was located with respect to the jungle silhouette behind it: tall trees to its left and slightly shorter trees to its right.

I extrapolated its range and bearing from memory. I estimated the distance as four hundred yards: nearly a quarter mile, and close to the maximum range when the barrel was elevated to nearly 45 degrees. I adjusted the barrel for windage. The can-shaped grenade left the tube with a whoosh, lobbed like a badminton shuttlecock, and – after a lengthy flight along its ballistic path – detonated with a dull thud. That was normal.

But the dull thud was followed a few seconds later by flashes of light and long tongues of flame, then by a massive explosion which sent blazing thatch and bamboo splinters high into the nighttime air.

Incinerated debris showered down for many minutes, like a movie in slow motion, and burning ash floated a hundred feet or more into the air. The remains of the hooch burned for hours with occasional bursts of brilliance. A person used to viewing Hollywood pyrotechnics might think that such a discharge was normal, but in reality, fragmentation grenades were anti-personnel devices that blasted shrapnel through flesh like its hand-thrown brethren and ground-hidden claymores. In this case, a secondary explosion triggered by the sparking of metal on metal must have accounted for the titanic blast that followed.

I had made a perfect shot into the hooch, which must have been an enemy ammunition dump, perhaps in anticipation of an attack against our compound, coordinated , ,with the attack against our fellow company. The next morning, we retreated in the opposite direction without investigating the remains of the hooch.

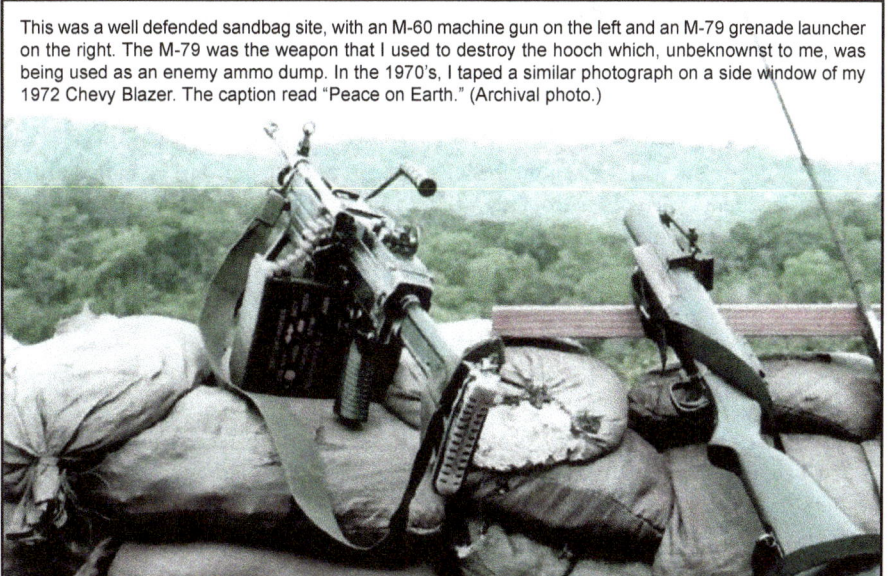
This was a well defended sandbag site, with an M-60 machine gun on the left and an M-79 grenade launcher on the right. The M-79 was the weapon that I used to destroy the hooch which, unbeknownst to me, was being used as an enemy ammo dump. In the 1970's, I taped a similar photograph on a side window of my 1972 Chevy Blazer. The caption read "Peace on Earth." (Archival photo.)

Sleep Deprivation

The next night our company was the target of an artillery attack.

I admit to being aroused by the first incoming round, but because it exploded some 300 yards away from where I lay on the ground, I merely opened my eyes without otherwise stirring. The jungle erupted with a brilliant flash of orange. Leaves were shredded from trees and torn limbs fell in flames.

We had no tents or blankets, no mosquito mesh. We slept under the stars. With ostensible detachment, I watched men dash madly for the safety of the sandbag shelters. I was determined not to quit my earthen berth until the rounds landed close enough to be a sure danger to life and limb. I luxuriated in complacency born of the youthful sense of invulnerability and the practical necessity that was demanded by fatigue.

When the next round landed 50 yards closer, I heard shrapnel whistling through the air, followed by thumps and sizzles as jagged, fist-sized chunks of metal struck the damp sandy soil or landed in our wash-up puddle less than thirty feet from my head. I calmly detached my helmet liner from my steel pot – which I had been using as a pillow – lay my head down on the helmet liner, then balanced the steel pot on the side of my face. I pulled my rifle tighter against my chest, made sure that the safety lever was not on – and fell into much needed sleep.

I opened one eye when I heard the whistle of another artillery shell on its way. This one landed another 50 yards closer than the previous one. It seemed to me that the enemy must have had a pre-determined aiming solution, then relied on someone who was stationed nearby to relay additional aiming instructions. In this manner, the shells were "walked" toward our camp.

I decided that I would not head for the sandbag shelter until the artillery shells closed to 200 feet.

After the concussion of the third round, I closed my eyes, then knew no more till dawn, when my squad leader kicked my leg with his boot. I had slept through several more minutes of artillery fire, none of which came close enough to arouse me. My team members saw me lying on the ground but thought that I was dead. I shocked the heck out of them when I yawned and nonchalantly asked about breakfast.

One who has never been subjected to the exhaustion due to constant combat might find it difficult to accredit such a story. In the tranquility of an ordered and sane society, people are often roused by the slightest sound – the dripping of a faucet or the creak of a board or the tick of a clock. But in the bush, we were so spent from the long daily patrols, the frequent awakenings from nighttime gunfire, and the hours spent on nighttime guard duty, that I seemed to exist in a constant state of exhaustion.

I was the only one who arose refreshed that morning.

Body Count

The fighting in Vietnam was different from that of conventional modern warfare in that there were no strict lines of confrontation. Nor was there any way to distinguish territory dominated by friendly forces from territory dominated by the enemy. The country belonged to whomever occupied the land at a particular moment in time. Dominion changed hands according to a semi-circadian cycle: American troops and the Republic of Vietnam held tentative command by day, while Charlie controlled the night. All was enemy territory.

Against this backdrop of exchanging supremacy there was no way to gauge the progress of the war. So the United States established a scoring system of attrition called the "body count." According to this scheme, every dead enemy soldier brought the friendly forces one step closer to victory. But the system got out of control when the definition of "soldier" was expanded from arms-bearing warrior to include unarmed civilians called "sympathizers" and, all too often, women and children caught in the line of fire. This ultimately led to a pathology for which, to American shame, the Vietnam conflict will forever be remembered.

Shoot to Kill

I experienced this morbid abnormality firsthand on a patrol during which my squad was temporarily detached from the company and sent to investigate three women wearing white ao dais (ankle-length dresses) white, wide-brimmed hats, who, upon the appearance of American troops, withdrew from a group of peasants harvesting rice in a far-off paddy that was barely visible through a break in the jungle. Taking a perpendicular route, six of us plodded along a tree-lined trail while the rest of the company continued toward the day's primary objective.

After a few minutes travel we broke out of the jungle into a vast open area of wet and dry paddies that were separated by dikes a foot or so high: a patchwork quilt of green and brown. I could see the three women in the far distance, running full speed away from us. They were already half a mile away, and the network of paddies stretched on for so many miles that I couldn't see the end of it.

Burdened as we were, with a day's worth of ammunition and a wealth of other equipment, they were easily outdistancing us. Yawn called for us to run. He set the pace. We couldn't run at full speed. We loped along as best we could with our equipment bouncing and clanging. We managed to keep the women in view but we were not gaining on them.

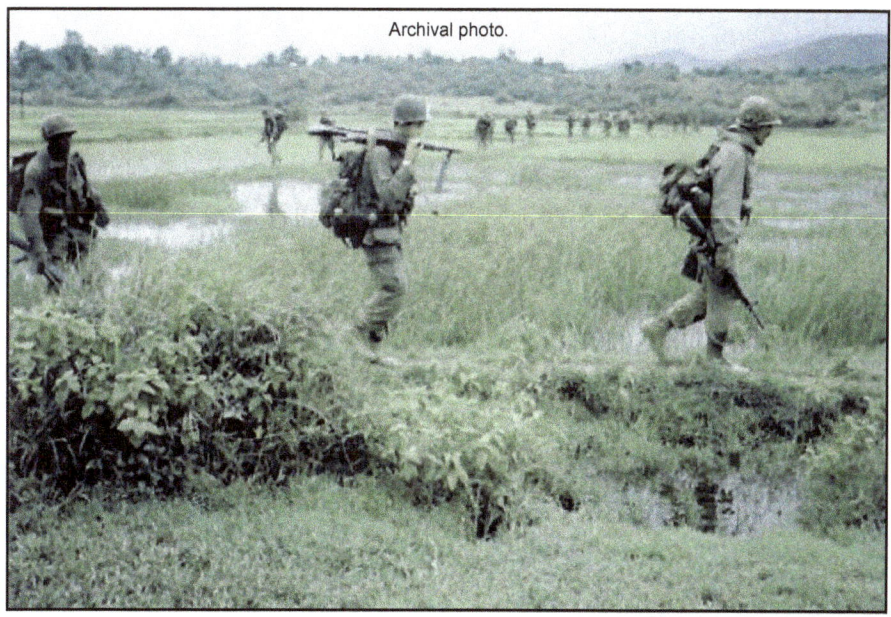
Archival photo.

Peasants looked up from their work at picking rice. They watched us in awe as we passed. Each partially flooded paddy had its own crew: mostly barefoot women wearing shorts and tops.

I don't know how long or how far we ran. The women in white were always in view, at the same distance, as if they were teasing us to catch them. Finally, they turned left onto a perpendicular dike. By the time we reached that dike, they were about to reach a tree line half a mile away.

Yawn ordered us to halt. A dozen female peasants bent over at the waist, stood ankle-deep in water nearby while a middle-aged man in an adjacent dry paddy tended a water buffalo. The three slender white figures shaded by straw conical hats scurried toward the trees in front of them.

"Shoot them!" shouted Yawn, indicating the women in white by aiming his rifle and pulling the trigger.

It was a long shot, but certainly within range of an M-16 in the hands of an expert marksman. Obediently I raised my rifle, jammed the plastic stock against my shoulder, and melded my eye to the rear sight. Taking careful aim, I squeezed off half a clip – ten bullets – and watched the tiny puffs of dirt where my bullets hit the ground. When I finally lowered my gun to look over the scene of battle, the field was clear of white fleeing figures.

The rice-harvesting peasants were crying and shouting and scampering out of the way. The man in charge of the water buffalo lay groveling on the ground, and the domestic bovine was pirouetting crazily with fear and pain. Yawn had shifted his aim to the water buffalo – about a hundred yards away – and peppered its broad brown hide with slugs. At that distance he could hardly miss such a car-sized target. The water buffalo was being stung by the projectiles, and its circular dance instantly turned into fierce frenzied leaps much like those of a bucking bronco. When the beast's owner stood up and ran after his charge, Yawn hastily shot at the man.

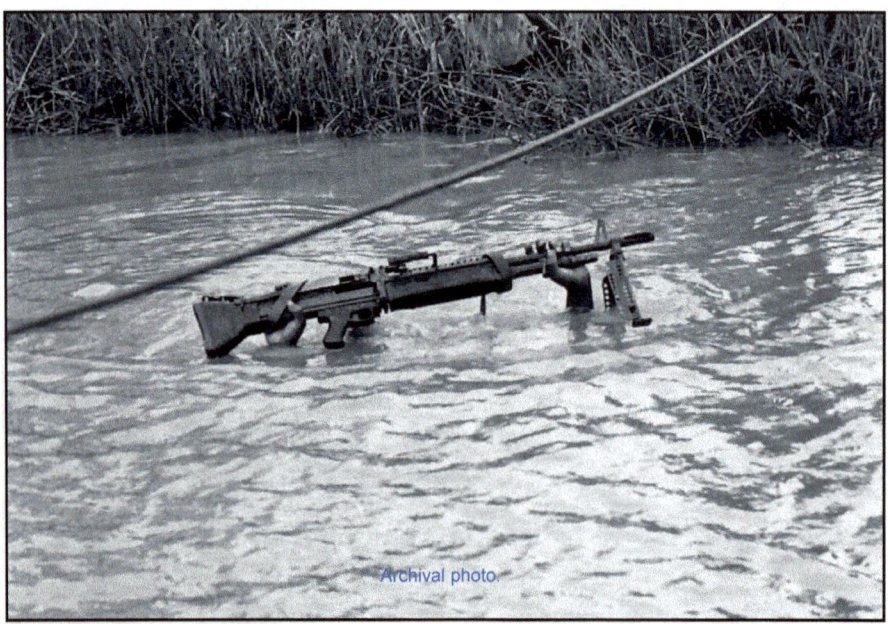

Archival photo.

Why? Because he was running. Not running away, but running after the water buffalo that Yawn had wounded.

I trotted past the mob of screaming, scrambling women along a dike that separated two wet paddies. With each running step my web harness rose clear off my shoulders and slammed back down with a jolt. Half a dozen hand grenades crashed together on my chest with a sound like clanging church bells. The weight in front shifted the harness balance forward. The bottom two grenades kept slamming into my groin; I was forced to secure them with one hand as I ran with my rifle in the other.

I didn't splash diagonally toward the man and the water buffalo because running through muddy water would have impeded progress tremendously. I knew from experience how the suction of the mud could completely stop a man at a full run. When I reached the intersection of a perpendicular dike, I turned right and ran for all I was worth. I saw Yawn's bullets kicking up dust around the water buffalo and its owner, but so far the man, who was running around the crazed, wounded animal and was snatching for the reins, had not been hit.

When I reached Yawn's line of fire I shouted and waved my rifle over my head. I stood between him and the peasant. Yawn flung down his arms in disgust; my action had robbed him of a kill. Yawned finished off his magazine at the water buffalo, then ceased firing. After the cacophony of barking rifles, the sudden silence was deafening.

I tried to keep myself between Yawn and his target, but this was difficult to do because the man kept springing after the water buffalo's reins. My shouts finally got his attention. He jabbered in Vietnamese and gesticulated wildly at the rampaging water buffalo, and continued to sidle after it despite my vociferous threats. He didn't appear to be intimidated by me or my swinging rifle, or by the squad of armed American soldiers. His water buffalo was all important to him.

I shouted and pointed toward Yawn. "Don't run because that man wants an excuse to kill you!"

We stood as close to face-to-face as we could get considering the difference in our heights – the top of his head barely reached the middle of my chest. I yelled at him and he yelled at me; I cursed in English, he cursed (I presume) in Vietnamese. We continued this senseless babble for nearly a minute, neither understanding the words that the other was shouting, but both comprehending the meaning. When he started to amble after his water buffalo again despite my gesticulations and loud protestations, I added might to my threat.

I aimed my rifle at the ground between the peasant's feet, and pulled the trigger. When the gun fired, he leaped like a cat at least two feet into the air, and when he came down, he had a different opinion about who was in charge of the situation. His volubility ceased, and he meekly permitted me to march him back to where the squad had gathered around the group of crying, cowering women.

Yawn was furious. Somehow a young girl had gotten shot in the back. She lay on the ground bleeding while the older women wailed. Frenetic grilling revealed that none of the other squad members had discharged their weapons despite Yawn's order to shoot. Only he and I had fired, so any blood spilled lay on our hands alone.

Referring to the fleeing women in white, I admitted, "And I didn't shoot *at* them. I shot over their heads."

I soon realized that my plan could never have worked. I reasoned that Yawn's order to shoot down the three women in white was predicated upon the fact that they were running away, and that to save them I had only to bring them to a halt. I laid down a precise pattern of fire directly in their path, my bullets kicking up dust and clods of dirt whose message was intended to demonstrate the futility of escape. I could just as easily have killed them in a trice. They fled all the faster and vanished into the foliage. Fruitless as it was, in the split second in which I had to make an important decision, I just couldn't think of any other way to try to save their lives.

Yawn's rounds never got close.

When I explained this to Yawn, he became apoplectic. "When I say shoot, I mean shoot to kill!" he screamed.

"But the only reason they ran was because we were chasing them and shooting at them. They weren't armed."

He was not impressed by my logic. Furthermore, it now became obvious that he and I were the only two who had fired a weapon. None of the others had obeyed Yawn's order to shoot. This was a silent communication that the rest of the squad thought as I did: not to shoot unarmed women.

Worse for Yawn, it meant that he had to have been the one who sprayed bullets at the innocent rice pickers, and was therefore responsible for shooting the girl in the back.

Now that the shooting was over, the women who were crouching on the ground gathered around the wounded girl, waiting silently, almost expectantly, for a similar fate.

Our squad was in a difficult situation. We were miles away from our company. We did not have a radio. We did not have a medic. We were on our own and in the open. Our rifle reports had given away our position. Already, enemy guerrillas could be closing in on us from every quarter.

"Let's get out of here," Yawn grumbled. "And bring those two men along."

In addition to the man I had dragged away from his water buffalo was another one who had been harvesting rice with the women. Both possessed identification cards and should have been left alone, but Yawn wanted to turn them in for questioning about the fleeing women in white. This made no sense to me because the running women had merely run past this group of farmers. They had not interacted with them.

Yawn marched off along our return path without a backward glance.

I motioned to the wounded girl on the ground. "Hey! What about her?"

The girl was sobbing softly, and the women around her were cooing. My bringing her condition to his attention only infuriated him more.

"Leave her there," he scowled. "She'll die."

I crouched by the girl's side and examined the wounds. The bullet had entered her back beneath the left shoulder blade, had angled upward and outward, and had exited from the front of the upper part of her arm, which hung limp. Other than the mild sobbing, she did not act as if she were in too much pain. I had no dressings, not even a spare cloth or rag, and neither did anyone else.

I ripped off her shirt and tore it into lengths, which I tied around the entry wound and the exit wound to stop the bleeding. I fashioned a sling which I tied around her neck and arm in such a way that it held her arm against her naked chest.

After my meager first aid, Yawn and I had another confrontation. I argued that we needed to have a medevac fly her to an aid station. He argued – quite reasonably – that we were deep in enemy territory, were separated from our main force, had no medic, no radio, and no way to get help.

"Then we'll take her with us," I said.

He still wanted to leave her there. He argued that we had no stretcher.

"I'll carry her." I laid my rifle on the ground and scooped up the girl in my arms. She didn't weigh more than eighty to ninety pounds: a slender twig of a thing with tiny bare breasts that looked like a pair of fried eggs sunny side up. She couldn't have been more than eighteen years old.

By defiance I had committed military sacrilege.

The girl never flinched as I hefted her in my arms. I cradled her head on my left side so her wounded arm did not press against my chest but instead lay inert across her belly. Yawn shouted angrily that I couldn't leave my rifle behind. But I couldn't hold onto it because of the girl, and I couldn't sling it over my shoulder because we had not been issued slings, an artifice which ensured that our rifles were always in hand and ready for instant use. Up to this point not one of the other men had uttered a word, offered to help, or come to my defense. They were cowed by Yawn's overbearing domination.

"Someone else can carry it."

The Hispanic instantly said, "I'll carry it." He stooped down and picked up my rifle.

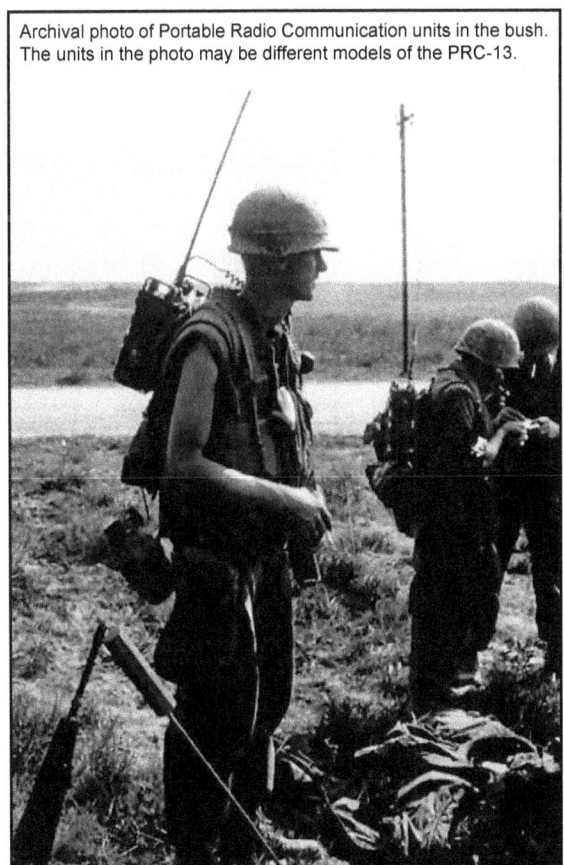

Archival photo of Portable Radio Communication units in the bush. The units in the photo may be different models of the PRC-13.

In the bush, the most inportant person in the company was not the captain, not even the medic, but the radio operator. Without him, there was no way to contact base camp for help or back-up, or to commiunicate with aircraft. He was not unique. Everyone of us were trained to operate the PRC-13 (pronounced Prick-13). The only difference was that he had to carry the radio and stay close to the captain. I don't know the exact weight of the unit, but I think it was between 25 and 30 pounds. A radio operator generally carried an M-16, as did the medic. In combat, each doubled as riflemen unless his specialty was needed.

I have a pet peeve about radio lingo. I often hear movie and television actors signing off with the phrase "over and out." In radio lingo, the word "over" means "I have finished speaking and am awaiting your reply." This informs the corrospondent that it is now his turn to speak. "Out" means "I am finished speaking and am signing off." This informs the correspondent that the conversation is over and no reply is necessary, nor wanted; the conversation is ended. I is equivalent to saying, "Good-bye." You can understand how ludicrous it is to say "over and out," which would mean "I have finished speaking and am awaiting your reply, and I am signing off and saying good bye."

Yawn and I glared at each other in a wordless contest of wills: my contempt against his authority. None of the other men spoke , and even the Vietnamese seemed to sense the explosive danger of the clash. After a long, uncomfortable moment in the hot sun, Yawn yielded. He turned and started walking.

We left the women in the paddy behind us. Yawn led the way to our point of departure from the company, which by that time was a couple of miles away on a search and destroy mission. I struggled with my burden weighing lighter in my heart but heavier on my arms. Sweat poured down my forehead and into my eyes; my throat was parched; my biceps were weakening. I didn't know how many miles I could take the strain, and Yawn did not look back to see if I was maintaining the pace.

After an indeterminate time, which I estimated was a mile or two, we came upon an oasis: a two-story house in the middle of a vast open paddy. For a moment I thought I had drifted through The Twilight Zone and gone back in time to the country home of my grandfather's birth. The house sat inside a large, all-around grassy yard enclosed by a wooden fence; a stone-walled well pump occupied a cool place under the shade of a large deciduous tree. Simply dressed women eyed us warily as a host of children gamboled over the grounds. It might have been a school.

Yawn led the troops through the gate and announced that we would take a break in the shade. Gently I placed the girl on the ground near the well pump, and let her drink from my canteen. The well pump was functional. One member of the squad pumped the handle up and down until water spouted out of the nozzle. We all drank our fill and topped off our canteens under the watchful eyes of the locals, who neither interfered with us nor exhibited curiosity. They simply watched. We did not exchange greetings nor ask permission for anything.

I unbuttoned my shirt and let the sweat evaporate from my chest. It was deliciously cool in the shade of the tree.

I noticed an abandoned door propped against the tree. I was ecstatic, for here was my stretcher. I appropriated it at once. When Yawn gave the order to go, I placed the door on the ground next to the girl, slid her onto it, then motioned for each of the two captured men to take up a corner of the foot of the door as I picked up the head with my arms behind my back: like moving men hauling a heavy piece of furniture. The procession filed out of the yard with scarcely any reaction from the inhabitants.

With renewed vigor and with much of the weight off my arms, I thought I could carry my precious load until we caught up with the company, but after half a mile of walking in the hot sun my muscles ached horribly, and I began to stumble. I went down on one knee, managed to pick myself up, and kept going for another quarter mile. I went down on both knees, jolting the girl horribly, and when I tried to stand, I found that I didn't have the strength to do so. By breathing deeply for a moment to recuperate my energy, I finally managed to stand.

Yawn ordered two men to relieve me. Each one took a corner at the head of the door while I carried their rifles in addition to mine. I walked alongside in order to keep the girl in the shade that my body created. We walked a couple more miles before catching up with the company's rear guard. A dispatch was sent forward to the commanding officer for the radio operator to call for helicopter evacuation for "two prisoners and a wounded civilian." This brought the company advance to a halt.

I knelt by the girl's side in order to keep her face protected from the sun. I propped her head in my lap, put the mouth of my canteen to her lips, and let her drink. None of

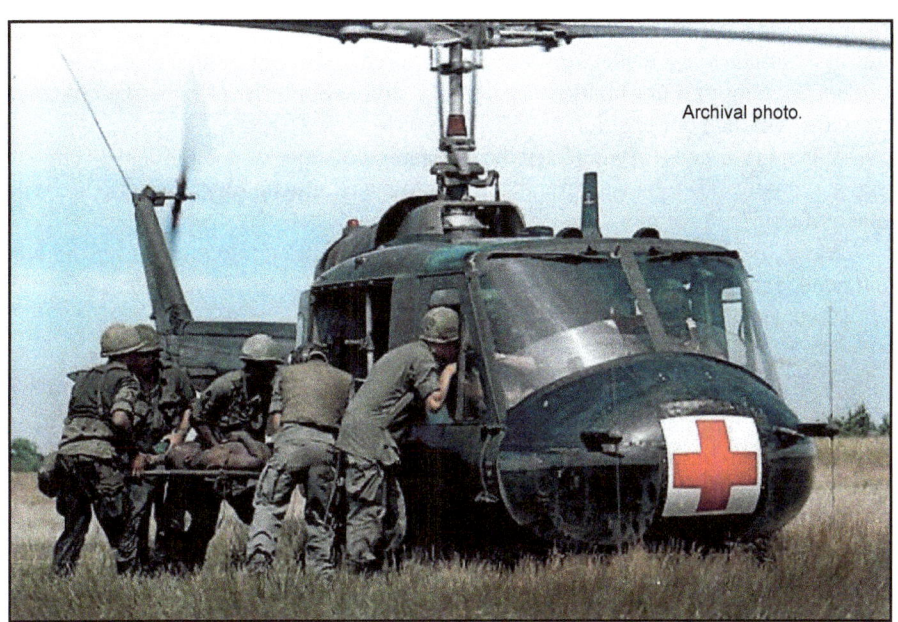
Archival photo.

the other squad members wanted to let the captured peasants drink from their canteens, so I let them have my other one. All our water was soon gone. The four of us carried on light conversation, the language barrier being partially overcome by gestures and hand signals. The girl spoke in a soft lilting voice that carried no hint of the pain she must have felt.

Little time passed before I heard the whup-whup-whup of an approaching Huey. It touched down amid a storm of propeller-driven dust. I lifted the girl in my arms. A medevac team jumped down from the cargo deck hauling a stretcher. I walked toward them slowly.

The girl yanked my sleeve with her uninjured hand. I looked down and realized that she was trying to tell me something. Most of her sing-song tones were drowned out by the noise of the Huey's engine and whirling blades, and I couldn't understand her language anyway, but I fully appreciated her meaning by her action. My shirt was still unbuttoned, so she leaned up and kissed me on the chest.

Then the stretcher bearers arrived. I placed her on the stretcher as gently as possible, folded her injured arm across her middle, and looked for the last time into her dark, fathomless eyes. As the stretcher bearers ran back to the Huey, Yawn shoved the two prisoners past me toward the cargo deck. They clambered aboard, the Huey took off, and I watched till it disappeared over the trees and toward the horizon. I never saw the girl again or heard what happened to her.

Remembrance of that emphatic kiss has often surfaced in my mind.

For Your Actions . . .

For the rest of the day the men in my squad avoided me as much as possible. The object of Yawn's wrath was a stigma that no one wanted to share. After we returned to our sandbag compound, Corporal Yawn assigned me to dig a deep pit that was intended to be used as a latrine, even though the other one was nowhere near full. I thought that this assignment was a make-work job whose purpose was pure vengeance. I dug with my entrenching tool until dark, after which I stopped in order to plant the claymore mine that guarded our position.

When I returned and connected the detonator, the other men in the squad commiserated with me. They all suggested that I try to make up with Yawn because he could make life difficult for me.

Yawn lived up to their predictions. Later that night he told me that he had recommended me for court-martial.

Vietnam was a crazy, fucked-up war.

Capture, not Kill

The next day started like any other day. We ate breakfast at first light. We took care of personal business. We stood around waiting for the orders of the day.

Yawn told me to exchange four of my fragmentation grenades for teargas grenades, and to carry the gas mask without losing it. Our primary objective today was to gather intelligence by interrogating villagers of local hamlets. For that reason, we were taking with us an ARVN interpreter. (ARVN stands for Army of the Republic of Vietnam.)

We hiked for an hour in a totally new direction by entering the jungle next to our camp, and quickly turning left. This was a direction that we had not taken since I joined the company. But my fellow squad members assured me that they had gone that way before, and that it was a particularly hot zone where casualties had been high.

On the outskirts of a hamlet that they had searched the month before, lay a large area of dry paddies that could be flooded from a stream through a tunnel in a tall dike. The dike stood ten feet high, with a broad flat top that doubled as a cart trail. The narrow tunnel that pierced the bottom of the dike stretched a full thirty feet through compacted dirt.

Arichival photo.

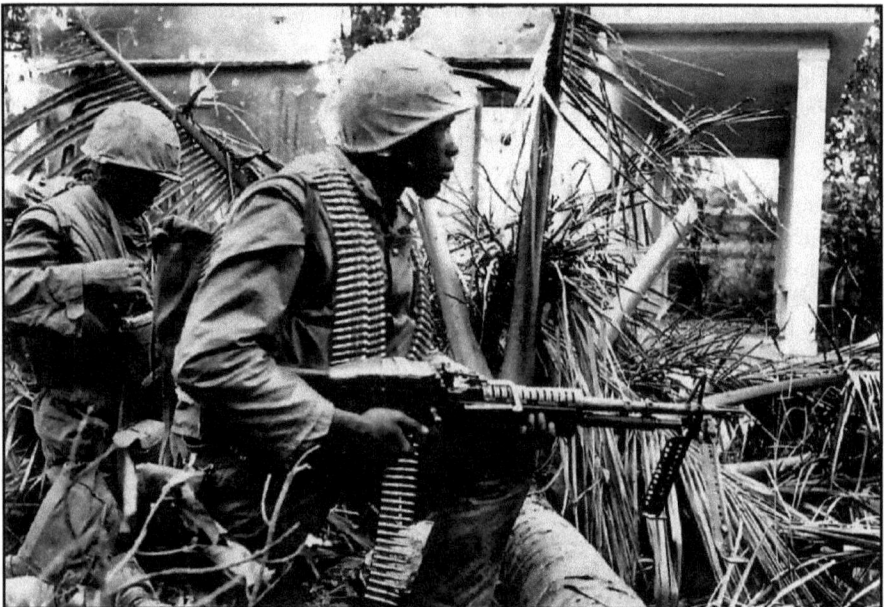

As a matter of routine, two men crawled into the tunnel, one from each end. Suddenly there came shouts of fear and warning. Both men crawled out backward faster than I thought possible. Once clear, each fired shots into the entranceway that faces him. In the middle of the tunnel, they had found an alcove dug into one side, and in that alcove a man sat calmly in the dark. They hadn't taken the time to notice how he was armed.

The usual procedure in such a case was to toss grenades into the hole and fragment the enemy to death, or kill him with the concussion, then crawl in and pull out the body parts. But this day I was called in to effect the capture.

Yawn explained the procedure to me as my squad members positioned themselves around the two openings to provide cover. I donned the gas mask, slithered along the side of the dike to the streamside entrance, tossed a tear gas grenade inside, then ran behind a nearby tree. As tear gas filled the tunnel, a few rounds were pumped into the opposite end, in order to prevent the man from escaping in that direction and to herd him toward me.

"Di di," I yelled through the sweat-filled mask. "Di di mau." (Literally, "Run. Run quickly," in Vietnamese, but also used by American soldiers to mean "come out now.")

I was poised with my rifle jammed hard against my shoulder and with my finger tight on the trigger. I expected the man to come out shooting or, possibly, tossing grenades. If he did, I was prepared to fire. Dense clouds of gas billowed out of the tunnel opening, turning the advantage toward the enemy. No longer would I first spot the man crawling out on all fours. Instead, I might see grenades bouncing along the ground or hear bullets tearing through the air. I was nervous as I ran scenarios through my head.

To my relief and complete astonishment, the man announced his forthcoming by first calling out in Vietnamese and then walking slowly out of the tear-gas fog with his eyes open and his hands held high over his head, reiterating something in his language and shaking his head from side to side. He wore no uniform and carried no weapons on his person. He was dressed in shorts, T-shirt, and sandals.

I grabbed him and pulled him aside in case someone else emerged from behind. An improper seal caused my mask to leak. I was nearly blinded by tears, yet the man demonstrated no signs of discomfort, but kept up his singsong litany. He looked like a civilian in hiding: an innocent villager who didn't want to die.

The ARVN interpreter took the man away. As the smoke cleared enough to see, I crawled into the tunnel to look for weapons and booby traps. I found nothing but an empty alcove. When I reported my negative findings to the captain, I saw that the ARVN had tied the prisoner's hands behind his back and had tightened a rope around his neck. He screamed obscenities at him as he yanked on the rope and slapped him across the face. I couldn't bear to watch.

The company was called to a halt for lunch while the interrogation proceeded. I ate quickly, then ambled into the hamlet to rid my pack of some of its weight. The troops in the bush were well supplied with sundries provided by the Red Cross – more than we could ever hope to consume. It was my habit to collect all the surplus sundries, stuff them in my shirt pockets and knapsack, and distribute them to the village youngsters during patrol. Whenever I appeared with proffered gifts, I found myself surrounded by little, outthrust hands. The children never smiled, but they gratefully accepted candy, toothpaste, toilet articles, and cans of rations. The women usually looked on passively.

62

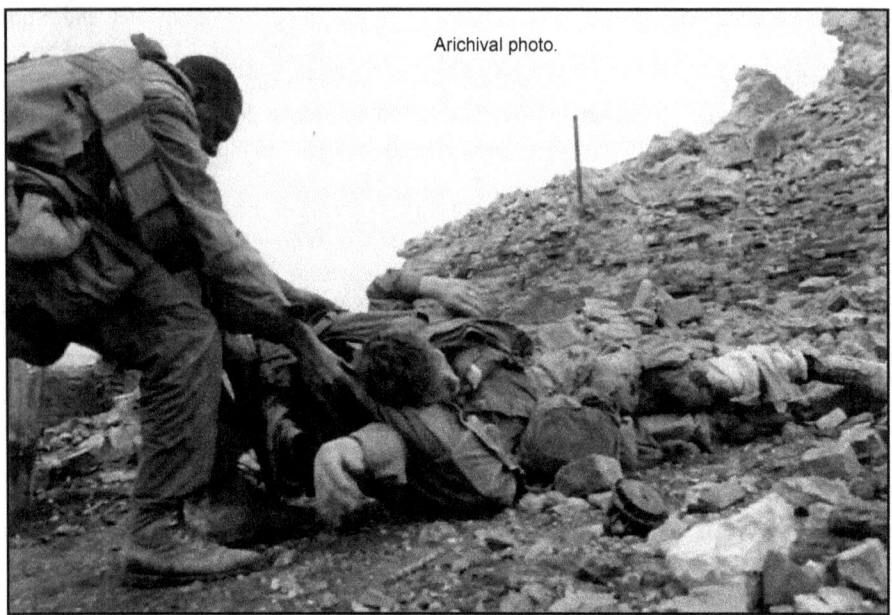
Arichival photo.

This day I came upon two bawling children, a boy and a girl, clinging to their mother's dress. I stared as I handed out presents under the mother's watchful eyes. She began talking in Vietnamese. I shook my head to communicate that I did not understand her language. She pointed to the distance where the prisoner was being led along the edge of the jungle by violent jerks on the rope, like a stubborn farm animal, then pointed to herself and to the children by her side. I replied with hand signals, and quickly interpreted her gesticulations to mean that the man was the woman's husband and that these were their children. He was another peasant caught in the war of political domination; he had hidden from the American troops the same as he would have hidden from Vietcong insurgents.

The lump in my throat was so large that I could barely swallow. I gave away the rest of my food. The woman accepted my tributes, then turned and walked back into the hamlet, crying, while I ran to tell the captain what I had learned. Firing broke out before I arrived, and my first thought was that the prisoner had been executed. But then I saw action on the other side of the river that bisected the paddies. Two men flipped the lid off a spider hole and pulled out a dead guerrilla.

"Take cover!" Yawn yelled.

I saw the prisoner on the opposite bank indicate a grassy patch of dirt. More shooting broke out as M-16's on semi-automatic chopped thatch away from the lid of another spider hole. The prisoner knew where the VC were hiding, and he was pointing them out! Almost immediately came the rat-tat-tat of an AK-47, followed by the crescendo of responding M-16's. Grenades whumped in the ground as machine-gun bullets scythed through the trees. Shots and shouts filled the air.

"Watch out! They're everywhere!"

On the other side of the stream I saw armed men rising out of the ground like soldier's sown from the Hydra's teeth. Instinctively I lunged for cover with the other men in my squad, behind a foot-high dike overlooking the water through a natural bamboo barricade. The village was not simply sprinkled with isolated spider holes, but stood atop a major underground complex of intersecting tunnels. Our forces were mixed like two football teams after scrimmage. We couldn't fire into the mingling mass across the river for fear of shooting our own men.

"They're comin' outa the riverbank!"

Armed soldiers poured out of the muddy slopes at the water's edge, bursting out of the ground like earthworms in a rainstorm. The fusillade that erupted was deafening. Now I had a clear shot at the enemy. Bullets chopping through the bamboo forced me down.

"They're on your side! They're on your side!"

Either the tunnel complex extended under the river or a separate system existed on the side where my squad happened to be located.

"Look out! They're behind you!"

Popping sounds came from our rear. The entire squad leaped up from behind the dike and charged for the bamboo thicket half a dozen paces in front, temporarily forming a line. I was spinning to glance behind when I spotted a pair of NVA regulars climbing up the bank toward our left flank, no more than forty feet away.

At the same time, another VC regular unseen by me enfiladed our rank from the right, boxing my squad in a four-way crossfire.

As I ran toward the bamboo thicket, I made eye contact with the enemy soldier in the rear. He raised his gun to shoot me, but I was faster. I put three bullets into his chest.

I was shifting my aim to the man in front, in the middle of a step with my left leg in the air, when an enemy bullet from my right struck the inside of my upper leg, tore through the femur, and splattered blood, muscle, and bone chips out the other side. The force of the bullet spun me halfway around. I crashed to the ground on my right side, landing on top of my rifle. The pain was instant and excruciating.

"I'm hit! I'm hit!"

With extreme effort I pushed myself up onto my right elbow. I tried to crawl toward cover, but my injured left leg lay across my right leg, and I felt numb and paralyzed from the waist down. I couldn't move.

My upper body pressed hard against my right arm, and my elbow was pinioned, but I still retained my grip on the trigger. Then I perceived that the front man of the two-man team was running in a crouch along the perpendicular dike. His partner – the one I shot – lay still on the ground. The enemy soldier turned his head as he ran and looked straight in my eyes. No prescience was required to read that look.

In sheer terror I screamed at my teammates who were digging furiously into the bamboo thicket. "Get him! Get him! He's gonna shoot me!"

I twisted back just as Charlie drew to a halt. With controlled and deliberate intent, the man faced me, dropped confidently to one knee, rested his elbow on his other knee, and sighted down the barrel of his gun directly at my heart. He was so close – barely thirty feet away – that I could clearly see the wooden stock and protruding banana clip of the AK-47.

My terror turned to panic which I instantly restrained. I couldn't move the rifle to my cheek in order to aim it at the enemy, so I leaned back and raised my forearm barely enough to elevate the barrel off the ground. I started pulling the trigger. What is hundreds of words in the telling was only seconds in the occurring. All the while I stared at the black round hole of the enemy muzzle, I looked to see where my bullets were hitting the ground in relation to my target. I didn't see any tell-tale spurts of dust, so I reasoned that I must be shooting too high.

Near-Death Experience

I pressed my arm down flat against the ground, pulling the trigger all the while. I managed to fire eight rounds before he fired one. My last round must have been awfully close to his head, because I saw the man flinch and the muzzle jerk upward a fraction of a second before I saw the muzzle flash.

I felt something solid and incredibly cold penetrate my chest like a sharpened icicle, formed a mental image of the bullet drilling completely through my body, was slammed back against the ground so hard that I bounced upward and forward onto my face, found my viewpoint suddenly shifted to a point inside my skull, looked down upon the convolutions of my brain, observed a thin white mist separating from the gray matter and coalescing into a cotton-like ball which shot out of the top of my head and into the sky, from which I looked down upon my body lying on the ground, then my viewpoint proceeded upward through the stratosphere until I could see the entire blue and white planet hanging beneath me against the black backdrop of space. I moved faster than the speed of light: past the Moon and planets and out of the solar system into the distant interstellar reaches. As I zoomed by thousands of stars every second, I found myself approaching a gigantic orb of brilliant white light: a living galactic core in which souls found final solace.

I felt strangely at ease. Somehow, I knew that when I reached that central sphere I would be absorbed by the light, and in the process of absorption I would find freedom from pain, would find surcease from sorrow, would find everlasting tranquility, would find ultimate peace, would find – death!

Although the fear and anticipation of death can be torturous, death itself is not a terrible experience for the one who dies. It is the living and the loved ones who suffer.

But I was not ready to die. I refused to yield. By means of some mysterious mental force, I willed myself to screech to a stop on the fringe of that specious sphere of light. Slowly I accelerated away from the deceptive illusion of serenity, back through space, back through the solar system, down through the atmosphere, and back into my skull, where the ball of mist that composed my essence drifted apart, and the thin etheric wisps remaining perfused into the folds of my brain.

I awoke to a world of mortal suffering.

My right eye lay pressed against the dirt. With my left eye I could see no farther than a few inches beyond the rim of my steel pot. The rattle of rifle fire and the bursting of grenades told of the battle that still raged. Because of the nerves that were torn away by the slug, my left arm jerked spasmodically over my head, as if some mad marionettist were yanking frenetically on invisible strings. I yelled "Medic!" in a voice that barely croaked. My call was an instinctive response that sounded ludicrous under the circumstances, even to me as I said it. It was blatantly stereotypic.

I seethed with anger that my companions had dived for cover and left me to face the enemy alone. "He shot me again," I lamented.

"Gentile, lay still and maybe he'll think you're dead!" The machine gunner's stern advice comes across humorously in print, but it was not intended to be funny and in fact it was good advice in light of my predicament: exposed atop a dike with my arm

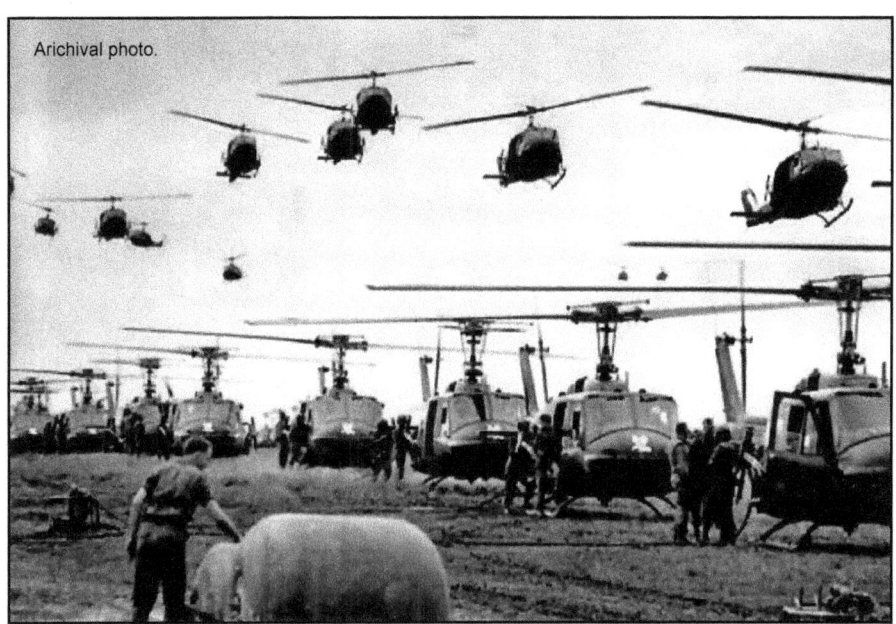
Arichival photo.

twitching crazily, and attracting attention.

The fighting gradually died down. The sharp chatter of automatic weapons fire yielded to the howls and moans of the wounded. I lost all capacity to cry out, but I remained conscious. Boots thumped the ground nearby, shadows cast across my face. PFC Tye grasped my left shoulder and rolled me over onto my back. I screamed at the excruciating pain induced by the movement.

Tye unbuttoned my shirt to look at the tiny hole in my chest. He also examined my leg, which was bleeding profusely. During his ministrations I continuously asked for the medic and morphine. The best he could do was give me a sip of water, which I craved.

Corporal Yawn's face swam into view. When he said he was going to remove my web gear, I cried for him not to touch me. He said that he would not touch me, but just unclip the suspenders and pistol belt. Gently he separated my suspenders from my pistol belt and unclipped the pistol belt so I could be lifted out of my gear when the medevac arrived.

Reinforcements were landing en masse. Helicopter gunships flew so thick overhead that they darkened the sky like a horde of locusts in migration. The battle was very much in progress, but the position occupied by my squad was no longer in the arena. A colored smoke grenade marked our location so the medevac could home in on it. Twenty feet away, a fellow platoon member bawled like a banshee. He had been shot in the same enfilade that took me down.

A Huey touched the ground in a cloud of dust. A stretcher was thrown by my side. Four men grabbed me by the arms and legs – I screamed again in pain – and lifted me onto the stretcher. The two stretcher bearers raced for the hovering Huey. The bearer at my feet threw the end of the stretcher into the cargo bay, but he didn't lift it quite high enough. My left heel caught the edge of the platform. The bearer at my head was already shoving me in. This forced my broken leg to bend up at a sharp angle, knee

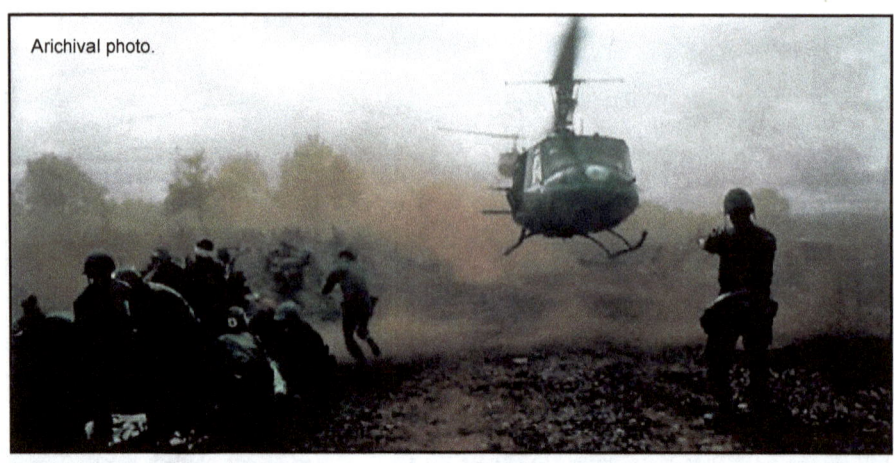

Arichival photo.

pointing skyward. I shrieked in agony despite the sucking chest wound.

The helicopter took off as soon as my companion was tossed in. The Huey banked at an altitude of five hundred feet, and as my head lolled to the side I stared straight down at the battlefield, where olive-drab troops scurried over the ground like ants whose nest had been invaded. Then, mercifully, I lost consciousness.

Last Rites

I regained consciousness in a forward aid station attached to the firebase that gave artillery support to my company. There were no doctors there. Two medics were holding my left leg away from my right leg. One of them held my foot as the other wrapped an inflatable splint around my leg and secured it with Velcro. The other one yanked a cord that was attached to a CO_2 bottle. The plastic bladder inflated almost instantly. The pressure of the bladder against my leg performed a twofold operation: it put pressure on the wounds – entry and exit – while it put pressure on the bullet holes to stop the bleeding.

I didn't feel any pain.

Fade out.

I regained consciousness just in time to see a medic straighten and turn to someone beyond my field of vision. He barely missed seeing me open my eyes. "You better go get a chaplain. This guy's not gonna make it."

Everything beyond the medic was a gray nothingness.

Fade out.

My eyes closed and opened.

A chaplain stood by my side, looking down at me in evident distress. I saw him make the sign of the cross over his face and chest. His mouth moved, but I could not hear any words. The gray nothingness surrounded him.

My senses were shutting down. My eyes were dimming out so that I could see nothing but the chaplain's face. My ears could not detect any sound. I didn't feel any pain. I was on the brink of mortality.

I knew what was happening to me, but I didn't have the energy to care. I closed my eyes for what I thought would be the final time.

Fade out.

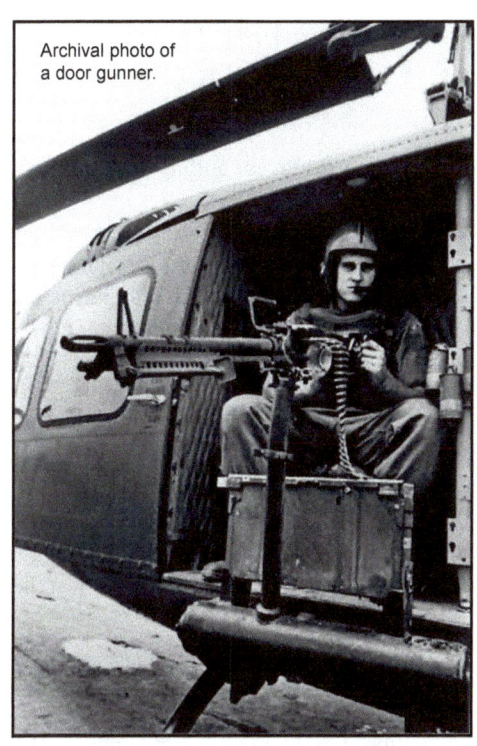

Archival photo of a door gunner.

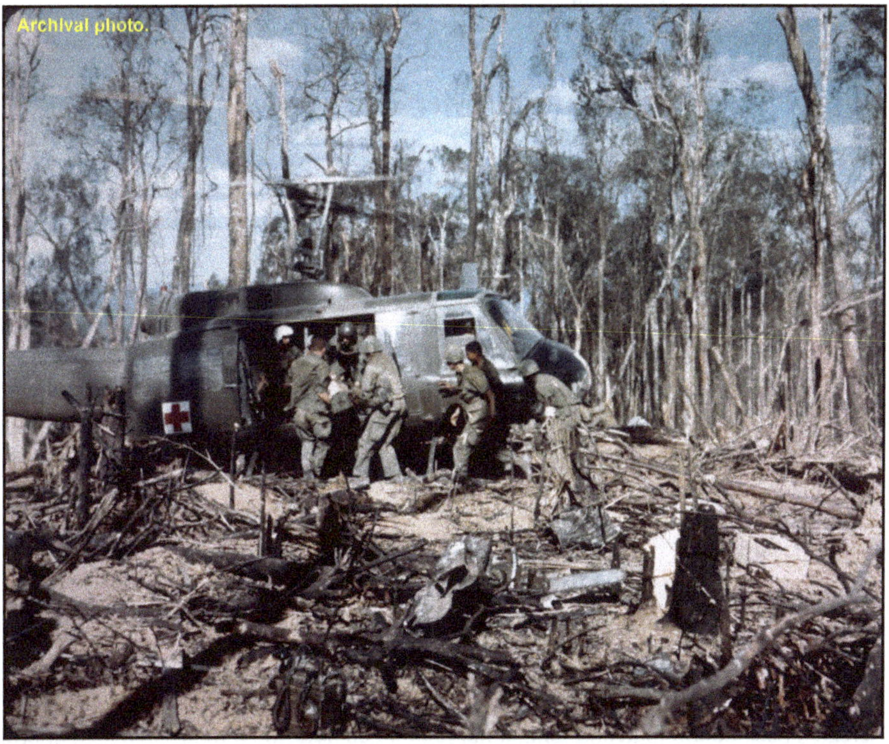

Archival photo.

Part 2
Hospital

The bright sun burned into my eyes, adding discomfort to the pain that I felt throughout my body.

My vision had improved enough that I could see that I was being carried on a stretcher under a deep blue sky. I could also hear indecipherable noise.

In addition to four stretcher bearers, on each side of me a soldier scurried along holding aloft a bottle from which a tube ran down into my arm.

"Where are we going?" I muttered hoarsely.

The soldier on my left bent down, although he continued to hold the bottle high. "To the hospital in Qui Nhon. It's about a forty-five-minute flight."

"Can I get a shot?" Meaning morphine.

"When you get there."

It didn't matter. I lost consciousness immediately without ever seeing the plane. Not that it made any difference to me, but I learned later that it was a C-130 cargo plane called the Hercules. It was the workhorse of the Vietnam war. It is still flying military missions today.

I awoke in an emergency room just as a nurse put her hand on the St. Christopher's medal that I wore around my neck in place of dog tags. The Catholic symbolism meant nothing to me, but the sentimental value was great because Bill Reese had given it to me on the day of my induction. I grabbed her wrist harshly. "Do you have to take it?"

"Yes," she said firmly but soothingly. "But I'll see that you get it back."

Fade out.

The pain was unbearable when two orderlies hoisted me onto a cold metal table beneath an X-ray machine. I screamed in agony when they lifted my broken leg.

Fade out.

Doctors and nurses stood shoulder to shoulder around me. Their masked faces were bathed in stark white light. Giant shears cut through the legs of my fatigues and through the tongues of the jungle boots. Needles went into my arms.

My body was wracked with pain. "Can I have a shot now?"

A tall man wearing a white surgical gown secured a vial of clear liquid to a hanger. "That's what this is." He connected the vial to a tube coming up from my arm, then turned a spit cock handle. "Bye."

The anesthesia hit me fast. My head lolled on the operating table just as a doctor lifted my left shoulder to examine the exit wound. I heard a sucking sound and saw a thick clot of bloody pulp gush from a hole in my back: a mixture of lung tissue and coagulated blood the size of a golf ball. It splashed off the table into the doctor's face. He let go of my shoulder and jerked away . . .

Fade out.

Back from the Dead

My world became one of sleep, pain, darkness, pain, spectral faces, pain, shadowy shapes, pain, pain, and more pain. I suffered wakefulness from shot to shot. When my screams became too loud and long, a nurse plunged a needle into my upper right arm and injected me with Demerol. This semi-conscious state went on for days – perhaps weeks. I remember snatches of events and to some extent the sequence, but have retained little awareness of the lapse of time.

At first my vision extended only inches from my eyes, so that it was necessary for doctors and nurses to lean into my face in order to get my attention. Days must have passed before I recognized that the indistinct form in the fog at the limit of my vision was my leg. It was suspended from a metal trellis. Eventually I ascertained that a stainless-steel pin had been drilled through my shin bone and was wired to a heavy weight at the foot of the traction bar. Because the bullet had demolished a large chunk of the femur and left a gap in the bone, the weight had been installed in order to stretch the leg muscles apart; otherwise the muscles, acting like powerful rubber bands, would pull the shattered ends of the bone together and my leg would heal several inches shorter than its original length. By keeping the leg stretched, the bone could not knit until each end grew out far enough to reach the other end.

The bullet had narrowly missed the femoral artery; had that artery received the slightest nick, it would have resulted in almost instant death as the blood would have been pumped out of my body.

That was the good news. The bad news was the fact that the bullet had damaged the sciatic nerve. This accounted for extraordinary pain that I was suffering.

During one of my conscious moments, a doctor informed me further about my condition. The operation took four and a half hours. Part of that time was spent removing bone chips from my outer thigh. He told me that if I hadn't been in such excellent

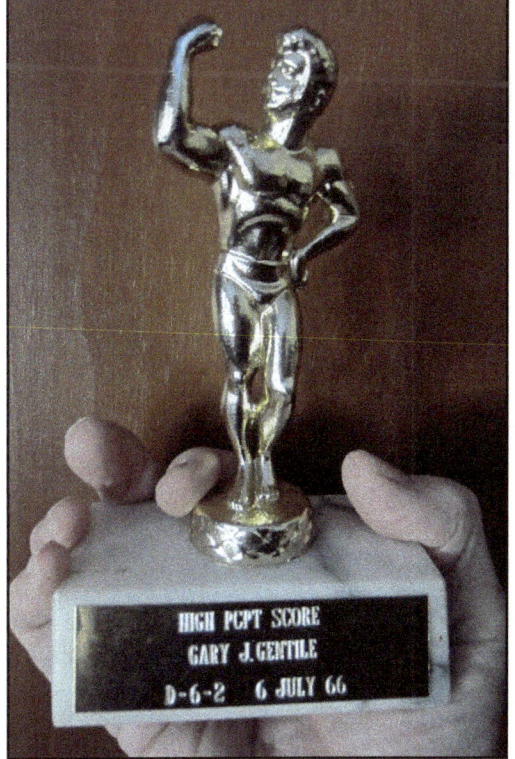

This was the award that I received in basic training for achieving the highest score in my company for the Physical Combat Physical Training test: 492 out of 500. Of five aims, worth 100 points each, I flubbed a perfect score only on the hand grenade accuracy aim. The other aims were running a 6-minute mile (while wearing combat boots and fatigue pants); overhead bars (where I completed the required number of 72 bars in 37 seconds, and totaled 116 bars in the allowable time of 1 minute); low crawl (I think); and I don't remember the fifth one.

I had never fired a rifle until basic training. The shooting range test consisted of 84 pop-up targets at distances that were scattered from 25 meters to 450 meters. I hit 69 targets with the M-14. But a kid from Winston-Salem, North Carolina hit 70, so he received the marksmanship award.

physical condition, I would have died either on the ground or during surgery.

The bullet that had been intended for my heart had missed that essential organ by barely two inches. It had entered my chest between the second and third ribs without breaking either one, passed barely an inch under the aortic arch – a pierced aorta would have proven instantly fatal – ripped through the lung, broke several ribs in my back, and tore through the middle of the scapula (the shoulder blade), breaking the bone and drilling an exit wound the size of a silver dollar.

Nerve damage was extensive. My left arm was paralyzed and totally without feeling. For weeks the doctors stuck pins into my fingers, palm, and back of the hand – without obtaining any response. If I was distracted by one doctor while another tried the procedure, I wasn't aware that I was being tested. The consensus of medical opinions was that I would never be able to move that arm again. It was permanently dead.

Nerve damage in my leg created a contrary condition. As noted, intense, burning pain enveloped my foot as if it were buried in a bed of hot coals, or fettered in a furnace. Phantom flames shot up my lower leg, sometimes raging out of control, at other times smoldering slowly. Ironically, the wound itself was relatively painless. I retained partial movement of my toes. Most of my leg was numb to pin pricks, yet the burning pain was continuous, a result of damage to the sciatic nerve.

Every breath was torture. My lungs expanded with each inhalation, which in effect was equivalent to stretching all my chest wounds, internal and external, created by the bullet's passage through my torso. Consequently, I breathed short and shallow.

Nurses made me breathe through a tube in which a floating ball rose higher as I breathed deeper. They urged me to ignore the pain while blowing harder and harder. The purpose of this excruciating exercise was to prevent pneumonia: a condition in which fluids filled the air sacs in the lung and caused infection. In my current condition, I could not afford to have less capacity to transport oxygen throughout my body.'

After the enemy bullet passed through my lung, the lung deflated like a punctured balloon. Thus I was breathing on only one lung. This condition was called a "sucking chest wound." Even had the field medic been near enough to treat me in the bush, he would not have given me morphine to alleviate my pain. This was because morphine – and other opioids as well – reduced the rate of respiration. As I was receiving oxygen from only one functioning lung, a further reduction of respiration would have been fatal.

Yet for all the damage done to my body, I was lucky to be alive. For that I have to thank the unnamed medic who, in a last-ditch attempt to save my life, performed an operation that he was not qualified to perform. He took such a chance most likely because he – and I – had nothing to lose. I was going to die. So he performed the cutdown that saved my life. Unable to locate a vein in my arm due to the massive loss of blood, he sliced open the flesh in the inner crook of my right elbow, reached in with a finger and pulled out the vein – which he managed not to nick – and stabbed it with a needle to which he connected a bottle of plasma.

This timely transfusion had brought me back from the edge of death.

I was told that field medics received only an eight-week course in emergency first aid. A medic's prime function in Vietnam was to dispense salt tablets and anti-malaria pills, and, in the extreme, slap a compress on an open wound. They were not trained to perform surgical procedures, especially such a delicate operation as a cut-down. I guess he figured that I was going to die anyway, so what did he have to lose by trying?

How close had I truly been to the oblivion beyond? No one can say. Had my heart stopped beating, stunned into paralysis by the trauma of the enemy bullet's close passage? I don't know. Did I see God? Definitely not. My trip through space to the white galactic core was a hallucination induced by the lack of oxygen and blood sugar in the brain, and by the release of organic chemicals such as adrenaline and endorphins – all of which affected the brain and, by extension, the mind, which was a construct of the brain.

Studies have shown that given a similar stimulus, almost any human being would see a white light. Studies of near-death experience (NDE) and consequential out-of-body experience (OOB) have established that fact. The reason that some people see their creator or dead family members was due to their religious convictions and preconceived notions – they saw in that final moment what they hoped to see, or what their cultural heritage led them to expect to see.

My near-death experience did not convert me to spirituality. My acceptance of reality remained unchanged. I suppose that because I had a scientific bent, and had read a number of books about the planets and the stars, I had an astronomical hallucination.

A World of Pain

As my sphere of awareness expanded, I noticed a profusion of plastic tubing that surrounded me like a spider web. Two tubes snaked down from hanging bottles and fed blood and liquid into my arms intravenously. One drainage tube was sewn into the outer gash on my leg, another into the huge hole in my shoulder blade. They siphoned pus from the wounds. To drain fluid from my punctured and deflated lung, a thin plastic tube had been inserted through the side wall of my chest and pleural cavity. A catheter drained my bladder. This mass of tubing compelled doctors and nurses to approach my bed from my right, where they had to contend with only one aerial tube during examinations.

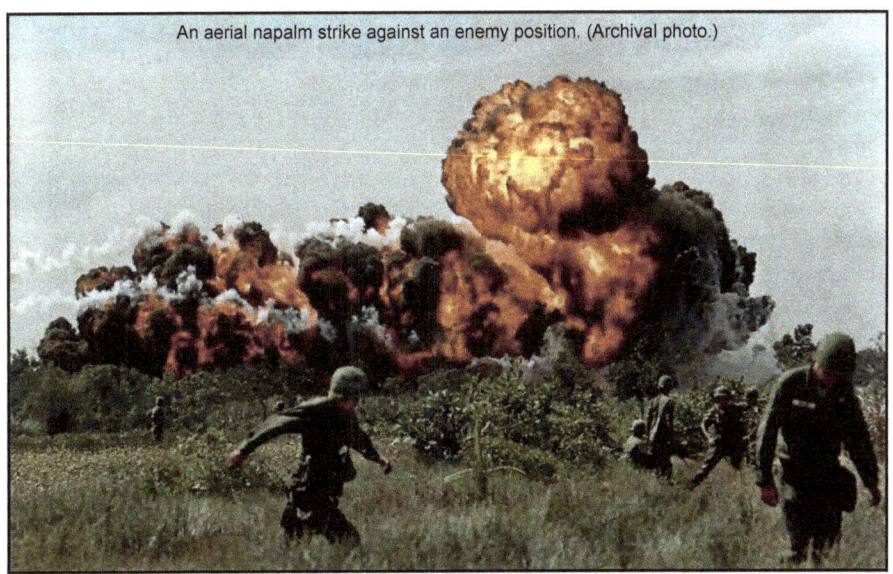
An aerial napalm strike against an enemy position. (Archival photo.)

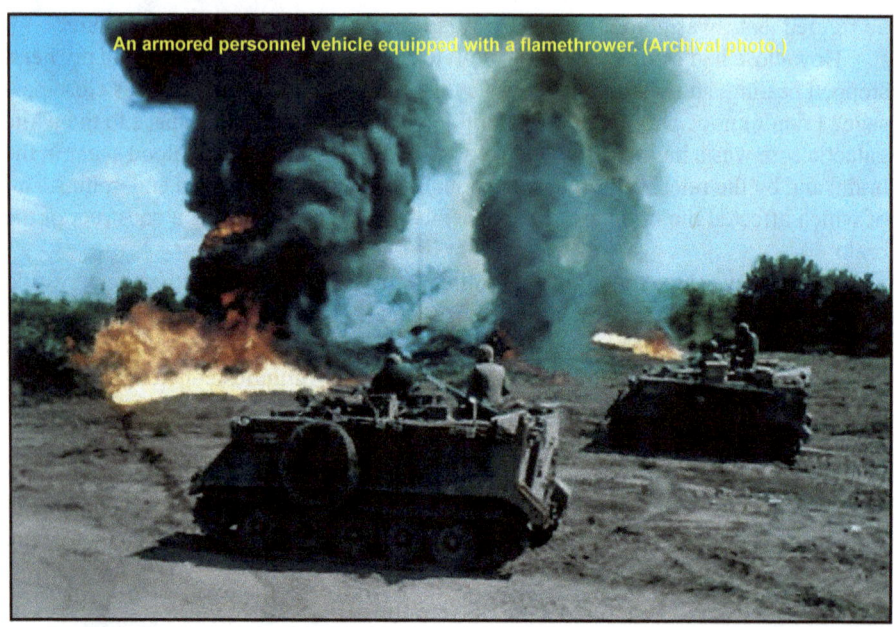
An armored personnel vehicle equipped with a flamethrower. (Archival photo.)

Changing sheets was a complicated job as IV bottles and drainage bags were shuffled, and the coils of tubing were temporarily rerouted. Two nurses lifted me from one side while another nurse, on the other side, pulled out the soiled sheets from underneath my body, then pushed clean sheets back. They did not start this procedure until after I have been given a pain shot.

The dim, distant shadows slowly resolved into recognizable objects. For a long time, doctors and nurses appeared abruptly in my field of view like off-camera effects. After a while I was able to distinguish the nursing station from the background gloom. As the most critical patient in the ward, my bed was positioned right next to it. Later, I could see all the way across the aisle. The patient in the bed opposite mine had suffered severe shrapnel wounds. The flesh had been stripped from one whole side of his torso, revealing an ugly mass of raw tissue, the white bones of the rib cage, and nearly exposed organs. He screamed louder than I only because both of his lungs were functional.

A war zone hospital is a place of unspeakable horrors.

Eventually I learned that the hospital consisted of a series of interconnected Quonset huts, whose corrugated metal walls held the tropical heat at bay as long as the air conditioners ran continuously.

One day a Vietcong guerrilla was rolled into the ward. He had been napalmed, and every square inch of skin had been burned off his body. He was wrapped in white bandages from head to toe, including his face, except for slits for his mouth and nostrils. He reminded me of Boris Karloff in *The Mummy*. He screamed constantly at the top of his lungs for hours and hours on end. During that time, I forgot my own pain because I couldn't imagine what exquisite torment could make a person cry so pitifully. I was deeply disturbed by his agony, and just as deeply relieved when he died. I saw his body being wheeled out late that night. In the sudden shocking silence, I felt relief that such ineffable suffering had ceased. Death was a desired pardon.

Two officers appeared at my bedside wearing dress uniforms, the first I had seen since arriving in-country. They explained that they had visited twice but that both times I had been asleep. With little pomp, one read official orders and the other presented me with two Purple Hearts. They stayed less than five minutes. Judging by the stack of medals they were carrying in a cardboard box, a busy day awaited them.

The army had just paid me off for my wounds with a cloth ribbon and a lead medallion which was painted to look like gold. I was barely conscious enough to appreciate the gesture.

Then came more surgery. I don't know what they did to me other than to remove the catheter and one of drainage tubes; I don't know which one. (I still had the IV tubes in my arms.) At the very least the doctors had to restitch the wounds. How they dealt with the large exit wound in my scapula, I never learned, and was too fuzzy-minded to think to ask.

I was also prepared for transportation by being encased in plaster from just below the armpits: a full body cast that immobilized both legs and left only my toes exposed. The crotch area was open front and back, and covered with a white sheet. I have a faint recollection of awakening while being encased in the cast in a room with bright lights. The caster, or cast maker, assured me that everything went well during the operation.

I have no recollection of eating or drinking since the firefight. I presume that I was given saline solution through one of the IV's. I don't know the purpose of the other IV. Nor do I have any recollection of urinating or having a bowel movement while I was in the body cast – which, by the way, was called a spica. The purpose of a spica cast was to immobilize the hips and upper legs.

The traction pin through my shin bone was held in place by the plaster wraps. A metal spanner between my thighs maintained the angle of spread of my legs, and doubled as a carrying yoke. Two men could lift me like a packing case, each with one hand on the yoke between my legs, and the other hand gripping the top edge of the cast over my chest.

The Red Cross gave me some toilet articles and a ditty bag in which to carry them. The bag was also big enough to hold my wallet and St. Christopher's medal – the only personal items that I possessed – and the Purple Hearts.

Another purple heart

I was moved to a new location inside the Quonset hut; or perhaps to a different Quonset hut. I was unconscious during the move, due either to the anesthetic that I was given before the operation, or to a subsequent dose of Demerol.

I was sleeping peacefully when I felt someone shaking me hard by the shoulder; my good shoulder. The shaking didn't hurt, but it brought me into consciousness in a world of wracking pain. My bad leg felt as if it were on fire.

Two uniformed officers were standing in front of me. The closest one told me that they were there to give me another Purple Heart. I was in so much pain that I screamed at him for waking me. I remember yelling something like, "I've already got two Purple Hearts. I don't need another one. Get out of here and leave me alone."

After a moment, they about faced and left, taking the Purple Heart with them. That is why I have only two Purple Hearts in the attic.

Transport

I was wheeled out of the Quonset hut into the hot, bright sun. My only covering beside the plaster cast was a sheet. A truck drove me to the airport where I was loaded onto a C-130 cargo plane that had been specially converted to carry wounded soldiers. Non-ambulatory patients on stretchers were stacked in tiers like bunks on a troopship. The restricted head room didn't bother me because I could neither rise up nor roll over.

Early in the flight my pain medication wore off. In the ward I was given injections of Demerol every four hours, day and night. I needed the shots desperately and on time because the pain-relieving effect always wore off before the next dose was due. I suffered horribly as the end of the fourth hour approached. A nurse was in attendance on the plane, but no doctor. She explained that she was not authorized to give prescription medicine. The most she could offer was aspirin. This was absurd in light of the seriousness of my condition. I had undergone extensive surgery only the day before.

The rest of the flight was a nightmare. And the nightmare grew worse when we landed in the Philippines, a stopover on the way to Tokyo. During my conscious moments I was wracked with pain. An ambulance took me to a holding ward for the night. I kept asking for a doctor to prescribe pain medication, but it took hours for the only one on duty to wade through scores of new arrivals and to read all their files. When a doctor finally reached me, he explained that my medical file contained no orders for pain medication, and that I would have to wait until I reached my final destination before having my file reviewed. I groaned at this information.

His only concern was that the jostling of travel may have dislodged the set of the femur. He sent me to another building for X-rays. I waited for hours for the technicians to get to me, by which time it was long after dark. Then I was rolled back to the holding ward, which was the size of a gymnasium but with a slightly lower ceiling. Here the non-ambulatory cases were left for the night on gurneys.

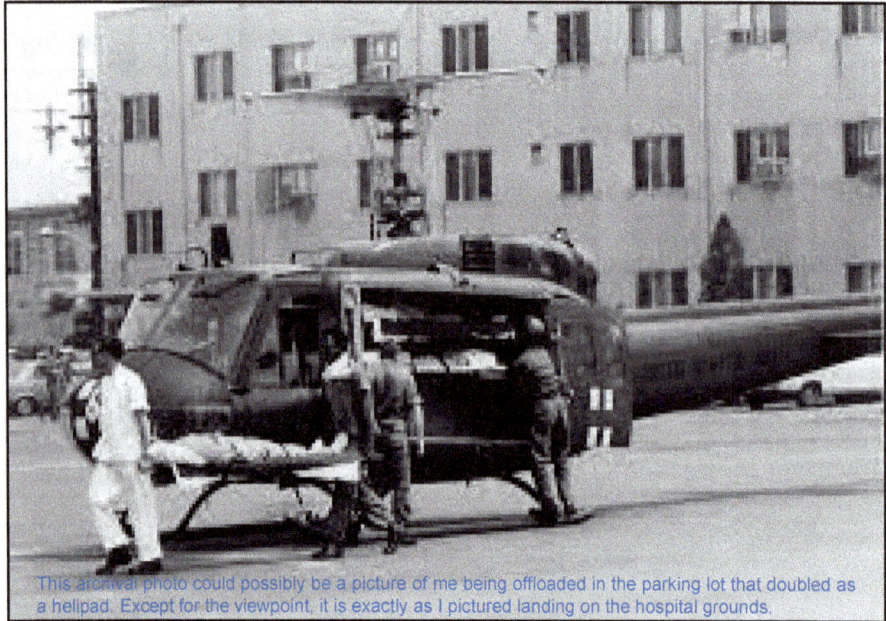

This archival photo could possibly be a picture of me being offloaded in the parking lot that doubled as a helipad. Except for the viewpoint, it is exactly as I pictured landing on the hospital grounds.

I had been given some food that morning, but I was too sick with pain to eat. The room stank with the odor of unchanged drainage bags, and was filled with the moans and the cries of patients who, like me, were given no medication to alleviate their pain. To add to the overall agony, the bright ceiling lights were kept on all night.

I did not sleep at all but spent the entire night writhing in pain. A towel draped over my face kept the lights out of my eyes. The next day I was put on a plane for Tokyo. I remember nothing about the flight except chronic pain. After landing, a Huey medevac, which was equipped with doors and frames on which stretchers could be stacked, flew me and several other patients across Tokyo, providing a grand aerial view of Japan's capital metropolis. Mount Fuji, whose summit was white with snow, towered like a painted backdrop behind a cramped, crowded city that was stereotypically Japanese in design and construction. The narrow streets and conical houses were identical to those that were trampled by the prehistoric Godzilla.

106th General Hospital, Kishine Barracks

The U.S. army hospital in Tokyo was a collection of modern, multi-story steel-and-concrete buildings that offered medical treatment and surgical procedures that were not available in Vietnam. If a soldier could be cured or healed in less than two months, he was returned to duty. If, in the opinion of a board of doctors, a patient required more than two months for complete recovery, he was rotated home permanently.

I was placed in an overcrowded ward whose medical and management staff were totally dedicated to the comfort of their patients. During my stay, I received the best care that it was possible for them to provide. When I arrived in late afternoon, it was obvious to the staff how much I was suffering. No doctor had yet been assigned to my case so injections were not allowed, but staff orderlies obtained special approval for the administration of codeine in tablet form.

Codeine relieved my pain, but it also induced hallucinations. Late that night I came out of my stupor in the middle of a jungle scene. A firefight was in progress. As our position was about to be overrun, the officer in charge gave the order to move out. I was unable to walk. I bellowed, "Don't leave me! Don't leave me!" When no one paid any attention to my plea, I struggled after them, screaming.

An orderly rushed into the ward and found me standing beside my bed. I had managed to shove myself over the side of the bed where by great good luck I had pivoted over the edge and landed on the linoleum floor with both feet of the cast. Instead of toppling to one side, I remained upright like an ancient stone statue, leaning back against the tall frame of the bed. Single handedly, the orderly levered me back onto the bed, then raised the side rails, which had been left down in the belief that a person in a full body cast and with one arm paralyzed could not get out of bed on his own. I managed to overrule that belief.

The tubes that were sewn into my body had been held in place by the plaster, but the IV and drainage bags had torn loose, creating a mess that the orderly had to put back together. Although he assured me that I was safe in the hospital ward, my eyes perceived things differently. Gradually, over what seemed like an hour or so, the battle scene gradually transformed from jungle to hospital. The sandbag bunkers morphed into beds, the palm trees resolved into concrete columns, the men in the squad became sleeping patients, none of whom had been roused by the tumult. I was the only patient awake in an otherwise quiet hospital ward.

The next day I was wheeled into the preparation room to have the cast removed and additional surgery performed. Prior cases took up too much time and they didn't get to me. I was alarmed because until I was thoroughly examined by a doctor, I couldn't get shots for pain. The nurses and orderlies pressed my case until a doctor took it upon himself to authorize the injection of morphine. I passed a tolerable night – without hallucinations – and had my surgery the following afternoon.

When I regained consciousness after the operation, I found myself castless but restrained in a new traction assembly that kept my broken leg angled nearly forty-five degrees to the left. The torsion was intended to help the bone heal straight. A new traction pin had been inserted through the shin bone. This one was drilled through the middle of the bone, for greater strength. Heavier weights beneath the pulley assembly stretched the leg muscles farther apart. The weights tipped the scale at 25 pounds. Yet I could not feel any pain or discomfort that I could attribute to traction assembly, not even from the traction pin in my shin bone. All the pain that I felt originated from the damaged sciatic nerve.

The drainage tubes had been removed and the holes had been stitched. A single IV dribbled saline solution into a vein in my left arm. My right arm was free to move in case I wanted a drink of water. A water pitcher and a glass stood on a table whose tray rested on a swivel whose height was adjustable. A box of tissues stood on the tray.

At mealtime, I could raise the back of the bed and swivel the tray over my lap; although, I didn't eat much. I pretty much picked away at the food and sent most of it back to the kitchen.

During the days and weeks that followed, I was preoccupied by pain. My only alleviation came from injections of Demerol. Occasionally I was switched to morphine so that my body would not become dependent upon the drugs. I avoided addiction, but my body produced a tolerance to the drugs such that relief no longer lasted for four hours from one shot to the next.

Once injected, a delicious numbness engulfed my foot and surged up my leg and body until a cloudlike, insensate wave swept over my head, at which point I drifted peacefully to sleep. This feeling was not a "high" in the junkie's sense of the term, but a sense of well-being that resulted from the release from intolerable pain. The effect perhaps is similar. The difference lies in the reason for taking the drug.

Increasing waves of pain racked along my leg as the analgesic wore off. Suffering miserably, I watched the clock as the seconds ticked by with agonizing reluctance toward the time appointed for the next hypodermic injection, which brought diminishing relief. The period and potency of sedation dropped with each succeeding shot, until finally I was fully conscious and in torment for more than half the time. Instead of increasing the dosage or decreasing the time between shots, the doctors decided to wean me from the drugs by permitting injections only at night. During the day I was reduced to mild medication in pill form.

Along with this increased sensitivity to pain I found certain positions uncomfortable, as if a bed spring were digging into my backside. This forced me to lie more over to my right, where I was soon covered with bed sores. When I complained about this newfound agony, a doctor enlightened me about the wound in my buttock. This came as a surprise to me. He assumed that it was a shrapnel wound, but I knew that no grenades had gone off in my vicinity during the firefight.

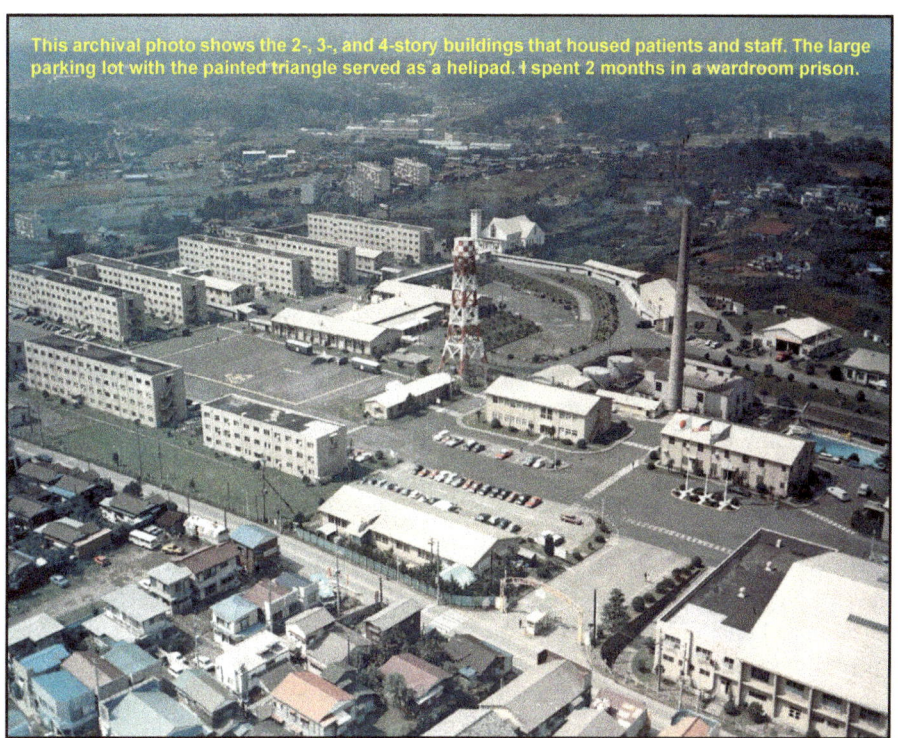

This archival photo shows the 2-, 3-, and 4-story buildings that housed patients and staff. The large parking lot with the painted triangle served as a helipad. I spent 2 months in a wardroom prison.

I pondered over this wound for several days until I came to this conclusion: I think that as I lay on the ground with my arm jerking madly over my head, the enemy gunman realized that I was still alive, so he hastily plunked another round into me, perhaps while he was crouched and on the run, and that the bullet passed through the meat of the gluteus.

That also explained why those two officers awakened me that day in Qui Nhon to give me another Purple Heart. Somehow, they had learned from the doctors that I had a third wound.

At the height of my medicinal intake, I swallowed as many as 29 pills a day, of various prescriptions.

I had received so many injections – some analgesics but mostly antibiotics – that my right arm became so callused that the needles could no longer penetrate my skin. I watched as a highly skilled nurse – whose injection technique was to toss the needle like a dart at a dartboard – bounced a needle off my arm three times without making penetration. The needle acted like a rubber ball. She had to switch to my left arm.

Eventually, my left arm grew so callused that it would no longer take a needle. The nurses then gave me needles in the upper right thigh. Needles didn't bother me. They were nothing more than pinpricks amid a world of ineffable agony.

Then came the day when I learned that instead of medical sutures made of thread, my wounds had been stitched with wire. The wire must have been thin but to me it looked like coat hanger wire.

I learned about the wire stitches on the day of preventable agony, when it came time for a medical sergeant to remove the stitches. When he told me that the stitches were made of wire, I expected that I would be given a general anesthesia to knock me out for the procedure. Wrong. The sergeant showed up at my bed with what I recognized from working with my father in the electrical trade, during summer vacations, as diagonal pliers (called dikes in the trade, or nippers). The pliers had two cutting edges like scissors, but they were angled and made of hardened steel for cutting copper wire.

Without preamble, the sergeant bent over my wounded leg, snipped a suture below the twisted knot, grabbed the knot with the pliers, and *yanked*. The suture came out along with pieces of skin and drops of blood. It goes without saying that the scars were the most tender parts of my body, and hurt just by being touched lightly. Yanking out sutures in that manner hurt more than I can describe. My scream must have been heard in Washington, DC, but there was no one there who cared about me.

I endured this torture about 30 more times. (I was not in any frame of mind to keep count.) By the time the sergeant was done, my wounds were a bloody mess. A nurse bathed them with a damp cloth that soaked up the blood but did not make me feel any better. I don't know why the sergeant didn't coordinate this procedure with my Demerol disbursement. That would have reduced the pain somewhat. It must have interfered with his schedule.

One day my temperature got so high that my body was packed in ice to reduce the fever. I think they said that my temperature reached 105 degrees. Nurses stood by to ensure that I didn't move or remove the painful ice packs against my skin. Throughout the day, nurses exchanged the ice packs with fresh ones, straight from the freezer.

After what seemed like eternity to me, but which was more in the order of several weeks, the chronic pain felt worse because the Demerol was not working as well as it had been. Usually, within seconds after the injection, I started to feel relief. The relief started at my left foot, then gradually moved along my leg, past my lower body, past my upper body, then up my head, at which point I fell asleep.

I would awaken a couple of hours later and find that I was pain free. Initially, this condition lasted almost until it was time for another injection, four hours later. By that time I was starting the feel pain again.

After a couple of weeks, the medication lasted only three and a half hours. For the final half hour until my next shot, I was in excruciating pain. After a while, the pain free condition lasted only three hours. Then it dropped to two and a half hours. Finally, the medication relieved my pain for only an hour and a half. Then I spent two and a half hours in misery. No amount of pleading convinced the nurses to give me another shot before the four-hour deadline. Nor would they increase the dosage.

The doctors increased the alternation between Demerol and morphine, figuring that the medicines became less effective because my body had adjusted to Demerol. This helped a little but not as much as I would have liked.

Those were horrible days but worse was yet to come. Came the day when I was cut off completely from the injected painkillers that I so desperately needed. The following days were a constant torment until the healing process of my own body reduced the level of pain. I was given pills as a replacement for the shots, but they didn't help.

I would have suffered far less pain if the bullet in my thigh had not damaged the sciatic nerve. I was having pain that was equivalent to sciatica. As the doctors had already told me, damaged nerves did not heal; or, in the rare circumstances when they did heal, the nerves took a long time. By "a long time" I mean years.

The pain finally became endurable without strong painkillers, but barely so.

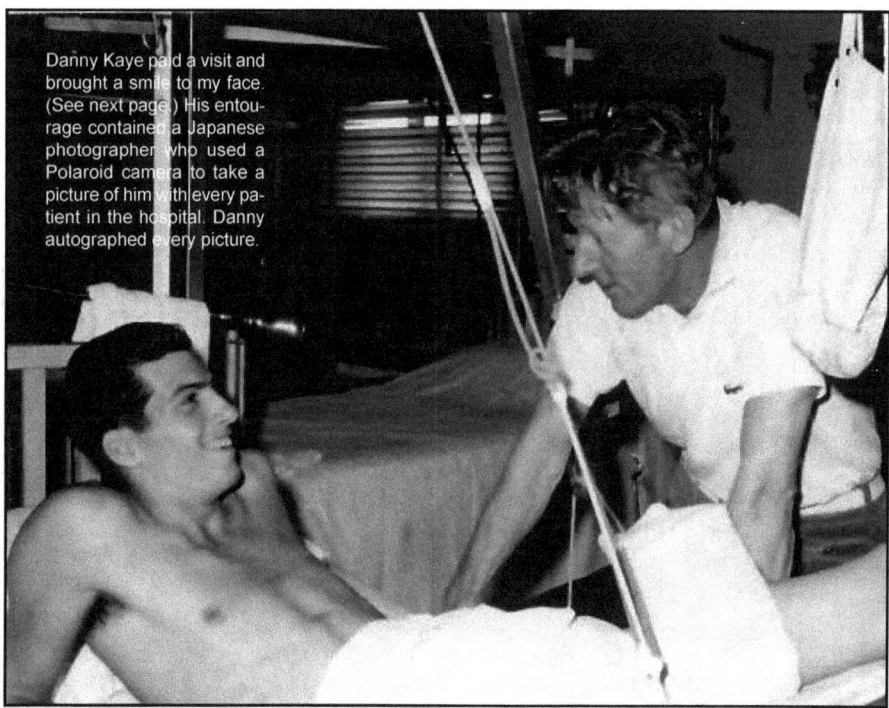

Danny Kaye paid a visit and brought a smile to my face. (See next page.) His entourage contained a Japanese photographer who used a Polaroid camera to take a picture of him with every patient in the hospital. Danny autographed every picture.

The only treatment that didn't hurt was the cleansing of the hole left by the first traction pin. Every day a nurse – whose surname was Yates – squirted antiseptic solution into one end of the hole, then dabbed it as it flowed through the bone and spilled out the other end. This was done until the skin healed over the opening.

My leg slid back and forth along the traction pin in use without any pain whatsoever. I guess there are no pain receptors inside the bone.

Then came the day when I felt something sharp on my left buttock, where the third bullet had left a 4-inch scar. I mentioned it to the orderly. He felt it too. It was like a thorn sticking through the skin. He knew what it was, so he told the ward sergeant, who examined me at once.

"Looks like we missed one."

"One what?"

"One stitch."

"It must have broken in two when I pulled it out. The skin grew over top of it."

He got his trusty pliers, bit down on the wire that protruded through the skin about a sixteenth of an inch, and *yanked*. You guessed it: no pain pills, no local anesthetic, no Novocain, just blood and guts. My blood, his guts.

Worse yet, he examined the other wounds and found two more stitches that were buried. As long as he had the pliers, he yanked out those hidden stitches as well.

Day to Day Humdrum

My level of external awareness increased to the point at which I could hold a conversation, listen to music on the radio, watch Japanese television, and read a book. I recognized my surroundings and knew what was going on in the ward, which was my

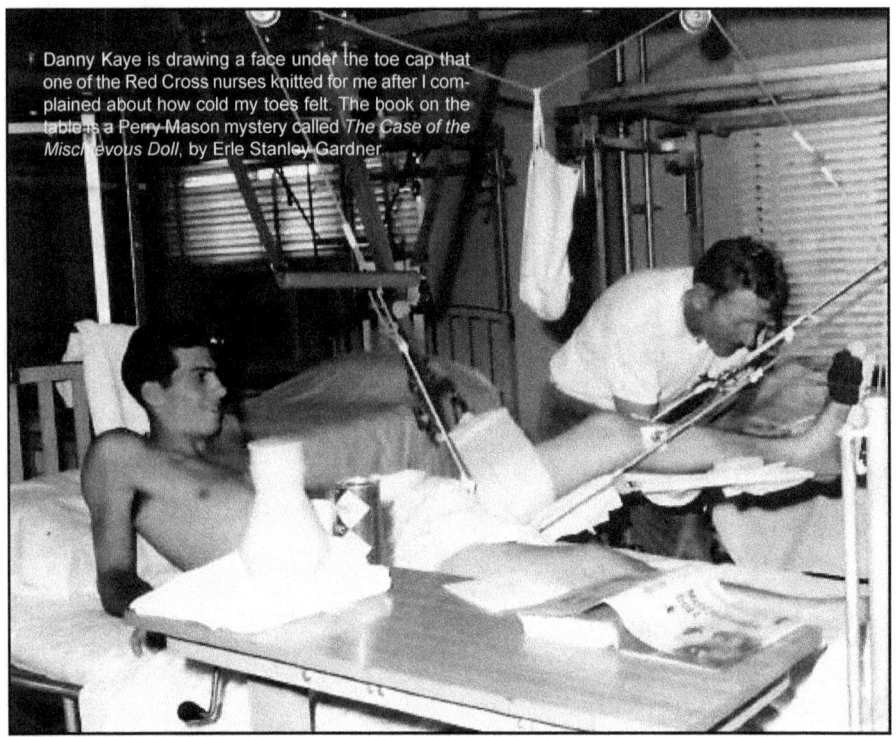

Danny Kaye is drawing a face under the toe cap that one of the Red Cross nurses knitted for me after I complained about how cold my toes felt. The book on the table is a Perry Mason mystery called *The Case of the Mischievous Doll*, by Erle Stanley Gardner.

only frame of reference.

Most of my solace I found in the pages of books that were circulated by a Red Cross nurse, whose "bookmobile" made rounds twice a week. It was difficult for me to hold the book in one hand, but it was even more challenging to turn the pages. Then I had to lay the open book face up, use my fingers to turn a page, then pick up the book again and use my thumb to hold the pages flat.

Japanese television was broadcast in the Japanese language. Programs consisted largely of sumo wrestling, in which two incredibly fat men wrestled as they tried to push each other out of a circle whose radius measured 10 to 15 feet. There were entertainment shows that specialized in singing and dancing. And there were popular American shows in which the dialogue had been translated into Japanese.

The highlight of the week was *Rawhide*. Everyone in the ward either cheered or sang along with the theme song, because it was broadcasted in English. However, the rest of the episode was spoken in Japanese, so we never understand what anyone was saying. The funniest part was listening to Eric Fleming and Clint Eastwood speak in high-pitched squeaky voices.

Unexpected Visitor

One afternoon there was a buzz of activity that occurred when a group of people entered the room wearing neither uniforms nor hospital garb. Since the head of my bed faced the hallway door, I had to twist around in the traction harness to see what was causing the ruckus. If I had been given a choice of celebrities I would most like to see in person, without hesitation I would have picked the very person who entered the ward unannounced. He was my teenage favorite television entertainer, Danny Kaye.

With an entourage of Japanese dignitaries, reporters, and photographers, the famous nightclub comedian, movie star, and prime time television idol, stopped and chatted with every patient. The photographer took a Polaroid picture of each patient with the comedian, which Danny Kaye autographed on the spot.

When he reached my bed, he smiled and shook the hand that still functioned. When he asked me how I was doing, I lied - I told him I was okay. He offered words of encouragement. Then he saw my toe cap and his creative talent emerged.

I lay naked except for a sheet and, when I was cold, a couple of blankets. Because the traction assembly prevented my leg and foot from being covered, and due to restricted arterial circulation because of the elevated posture, my toes were always cold. A Red Cross nurse had knitted a red woolen cap with a tiny tassel on top, which she planted on my toes for warmth. It was my only piece of apparel.

Now Danny Kaye took a felt-tipped pen and drew a happy face on the top of my foot beneath the cap. My skin was hypersensitive from damaged nerves so that each stroke of the pen felt like the scratch of a knife, yet I never winced or complained. I was happy to have him draw on my foot not only because of who he was but because of what he represented.

Someone back home cared about us. And, as I later discovered, there weren't too many of them who did.

Another Unexpected Visitor

I received another visit from an unexpected quarter, this one from Corporal Yawn. While in Tokyo on R & R (rest and recuperation), he came to the hospital to see me and the other man who had been wounded in the same crossfire. He was perfectly affable and exhibited no signs of animosity over our past differences. He filled me in on the details of the firefight, and assured me that they enemy soldier who had shot me in the chest did not survive the onslaught; he was finally mowed down by sheer American firepower. Yawn also wished me luck in recovering from my wounds. He didn't say anything about turning me in for court-martial. I presumed that it had been dismissed.

I have never understood why he bothered to visit. I didn't think he was capable of feeling guilt or compassion.

Nor did I understand why I was so happy to see him. After all, we parted on less than friendly circumstances. Such is human nature.

After my wounded companion recovered enough to become ambulatory, he rolled his wheelchair into the ward to visit me. (I have forgotten his name; he belonged to my platoon's other squad.) We compared notes of that awful day on the battlefield. The bullet that took him down in the first fusillade went through his calf between the two bones without breaking either one. Then the VC marksman who shot me through the chest tried to do the same to him. His bullet hit my companion directly in line with the heart, but he – you're not going to believe this – was saved from death by an extraordinary combination of circumstances: the bullet struck at an oblique angle and ricocheted off his dog tags. The force of the bullet broke his sternum and fractured some of the surrounding rib cage, but he lived to tell the tale.

I could almost imagine that incredible guerrilla picking off toy ducks in a shooting gallery. I have often wondered why he chose to remain in the open and fight when he could have run for cover from an overpowering force. Was he deranged or patriotic? Or do both words mean the same?

Slow Recovery

Things did not always go smoothly in the ward. One day, I was scheduled for a fasting blood test. This meant that I could not eat breakfast until after my blood was taken. Breakfast came and went, but no one showed up to take my blood. By 9 o'clock I was getting mighty hungry.

A man in black stopped at my bed; he was holding a tray full of crackers. "Would you like to take communion?"

Although I wore a St. Christopher's medal in combat, I was not Catholic. As I noted above, the medal was given to me by my close friend Bill Reese. He was Catholic. So were some of my other friends. So was my father. I went to Baptist Sunday school only because my mother and my maternal grandparents were Baptist. I was raised Baptist, but declined to be baptized because at the age of 14. I repudiated religion and became a realist.

I would have eaten anything because my tummy was growling, so I said, "Sure."

He used tongs to pick up a cracker and place it over a tiny silver platter which had a long handle. I opened my mouth, he inserted the tongs into my mouth, and he let the cracker fall onto my tongue. When I tried to chew the cracker, it immediately stuck to the roof of my mouth. But at least I got some sustenance.

Half an hour later, the ward sergeant wandered into the ward. When he looked at me, I said, "Any word about my blood test. I'm pretty hungry."

"Haven't you had breakfast?"

"No. They said I couldn't eat until after the blood test."

He erupted like a volcano. "GET THIS MAN HIS BREAKFAST." He turned to me. "Blood test is canceled." He turned and tore along the corridor to the staff area, where he picked up a phone and called for delivery of a meal IMMEDIATELY.

We all hated doctors' visit day. The docs seemed to enjoy hurting patients by poking, prodding, and squeezing their wounds. They didn't really enjoy it; it just seemed that way. They had to check everyone's wounds to ensure that they were healing well and were not getting infected. To check the wounds, they had to press them hard.

The fellow whose bed was perpendicular to mine had most of the skin torn off his left side and stomach, courtesy of flying shrapnel. He was in constant pain without being touched. He howled whenever a doctor pulled off the wrappings to inspect this wound, which was mostly red and raw.

I got off light because my wounds were exposed and not bandaged.

One day, a fellow patient who was ambulatory bought a Polaroid camera at the PX (Post Exchange). He walked around my bed and took a bunch of photographs of me, some holding one of my Purple Hearts. He wouldn't take any money for the film.

There wasn't much excitement in the ward. But one day the glass on my nightstand chattered. Soon the water in it was splashing and the glass vibrated across the tabletop. Then the windows rattled, dishes and glassware fell and broke, my bed danced across the smooth linoleum floor, IV racks toppled, pandemonium reigned. Someone yelled "Incoming!" Several ambulatory patients – one in a wheelchair and another missing a leg – dived for the floor and crawled underneath the nearest bed, cowering and crying

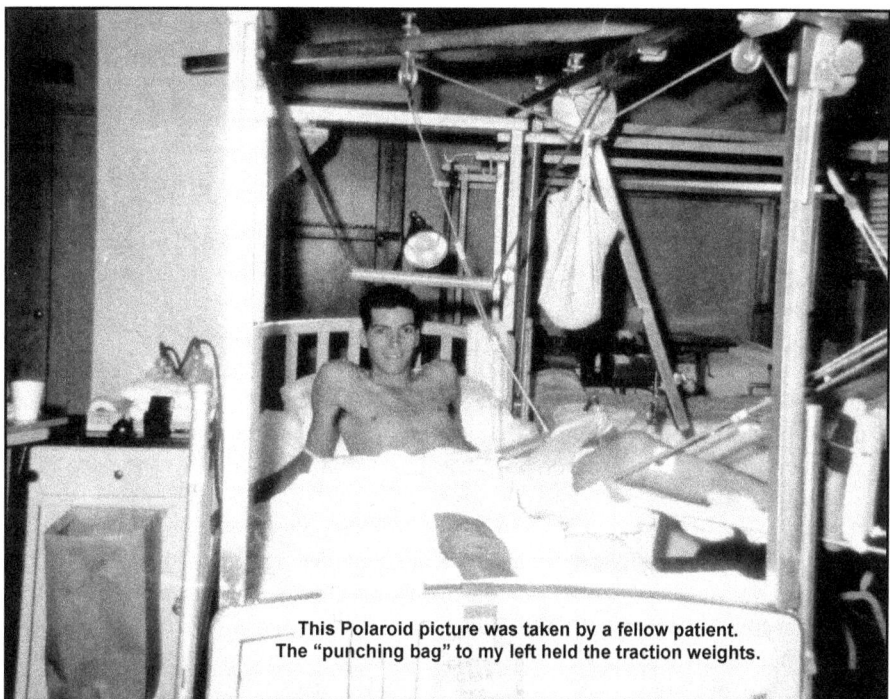

This Polaroid picture was taken by a fellow patient. The "punching bag" to my left held the traction weights.

in fright.

The rumbling lasted for nearly half a minute before subsiding. Orderlies rushed into the ward to quiet the patients in alarm before they hurt themselves in their fear-crazed belief that they were back in Vietnam and under attack. The situation was under control by the time the aftershocks struck. The earthquake had moved the beds several feet from their allotted positions. There was no structural damage to the building.

The only other excitement in the ward was an upcoming marriage between nurse Yates, who tended the unused traction hole in my shin bone (as well as handling urinals and bedpans, and assorted wiping jobs) and the head nurse (who once refused to give me pain shots when I needed them). What made this military marriage particularly unusual was that Yates was a corporal while the head nurse was a lieutenant.

We all joked about the disparity by noting that now he was going to have to salute his wife as well as take orders from her. He didn't seem to mind.

A Miracle

The most exciting thing that happened to me (other than meeting Danny Kaye) was that one day I felt a twitch in my finger. I looked down and saw another twitch. The last joint on the index finger of my paralyzed hand moved a sixteenth of an inch.

I yelled for an orderly to look at what I could do. The problem was that I couldn't do it again. No amount of mental power could force the finger to move again.

"It's just a nerve reaction. It doesn't mean anything. Don't get your hopes up."

I didn't.

The next day I felt another twitch. I picked up my hand and placed it where I could watch it. The finger twitched irregularly several more times. When I tried to make it twitch, I couldn't. The fingertip twitched on its own several times throughout the day.

The next day, the entire finger twitched. That is, the finger stayed rigid and slightly bent, and twitched at the knuckle of the hand. I still could not make it twitch. It just twitched erratically on its own. My entire arm, hand, and fingers still had no feeling.

On the day of the doctors' rounds, I told them about the twitching. They said the same thing that the orderly had said. It was merely reflex action from the nerve damage.

Despite the dire predictions, day by day I felt more movement until after a week, I could move my whole hand by wishing it to do so. The doctors were astonished. They had never seen nerve damage heal itself with such celerity.

I still could not move my arm, but as I gained strength in my fingers, I could use my left hand to turn the pages of a book. Other than reading, there wasn't much else I could do in the hospital. I couldn't even get out of bed and go for a walk. I couldn't see outside. The ward had a balcony, but because of the angle of the traction assembly, my bed couldn't fit through the doorway. I was trapped in the room; I was trapped in the bed.

I had never been able to sleep on my back. I had always slept on my right side, with my left leg bent, with my cat named Kitty snuggled against my belly: my cat instead of an M-16. Now I was stuck on my back in a constant state of pain and with no way to get comfortable. I couldn't roll over or change my position in any way.

The pain in my bad leg was slowly decreasing. This implied that the damaged sciatic nerve was healing.

Despite the constant pain and discomfort, I was getting better. I was also becoming more conscious of my surroundings; more mentally aware. Because I could do nothing

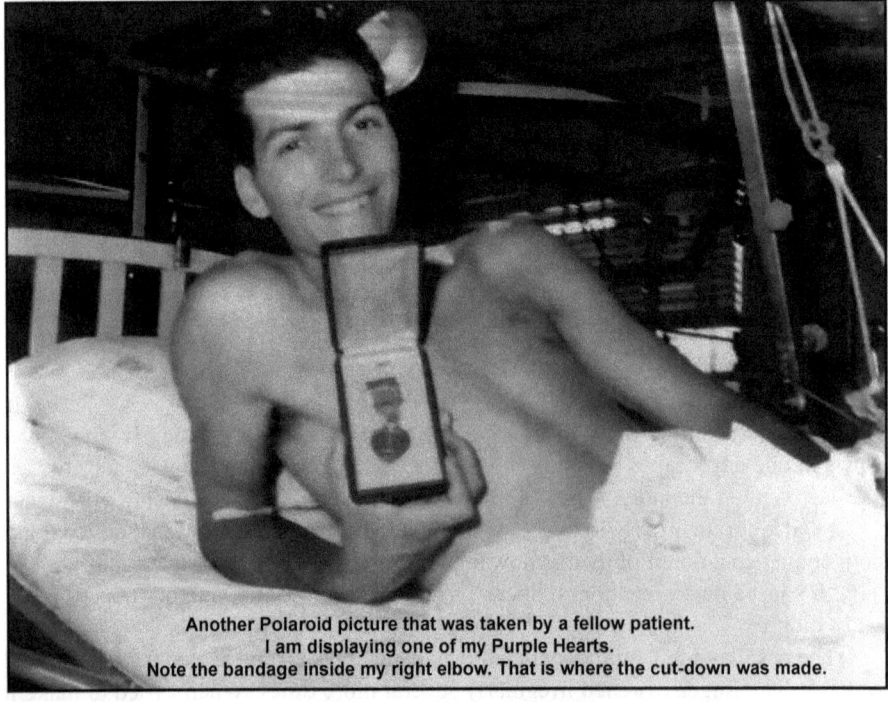

**Another Polaroid picture that was taken by a fellow patient.
I am displaying one of my Purple Hearts.
Note the bandage inside my right elbow. That is where the cut-down was made.**

to rush the healing process, I read voraciously. The Red Cross nurse let me borrow three to four books at a time: more over weekends. I eagerly looked forward to her twice-weekly visits. She had a plentiful supply of mysteries but a pitiful supply of science fiction (my favorite topic since 7th grade). I read a slew of Perry Mason books by Erle Stanley Gardner, and loved every one of them.

Meanwhile, I had full sensation in my fingers, which enabled me to grip a book but not to bend my wrist.

Way Station

The 106th General Hospital maintained a constant turnaround of patients. Soldiers came and soldiers went. According to protocol, a patient did not stay in the hospital for more than two months. If a patient could be healed withing 60 days, he was sent back to his unit in Vietnam. If he could not be healed within 60 days, he was sent to an Army hospital in the States, preferably one that was nearest to his home.

Due to this rotation procedure, I never made any close friends. I knew the given names of only a handful of patients. One patient who became mobile during his stay used to park his wheelchair next to my bed so we could chat. He had fallen off his APC (Armored Personnel Carrier – kind of like a passenger tank that could disperse a squad on a battlefield while providing cover from a 50-caliber machine gun). His foot got caught in the track while the APC was in motion and was ripped off above the ankle.

Speaking of feet, a strange thing happened to my good foot: the skin started to peel off the sole. When I first noticed the condition, I didn't think much about it. But I became alarmed as the condition worsened. The peeling was much like sunburned skin in that I could tear off thin sheets that measured several inches in length. My foot did not hurt, nor did I feel any pain as I peeled off sheets of skin.

First orderly Yates and then the ward sergeant examined my feet after I alerted them to the condition. The left foot – which I could not reach due to the traction gear – was not affected. (That is, I have no recollection of it being affected.) Both medical men agreed that I had a mild case of jungle rot (called trench foot in World War 2) from traipsing through rice paddies and wading across rivers.

I concluded that Vietnamese rice pickers had healthy feet because they worked barefoot, and therefore their feet aired out on dry land; whereas American soldiers wore constantly soaked socks and jungle boots. Combat boots were fitted with grommets that served as drain holes, but socks stayed wet throughout the day.

In any event, after the outer layer of skin peeled off, the underlayer was soft and unaffected. I had no recurrence once the condition healed.

By bed was originally located close to the center of the ward. Of the beds on the floor, I could see about half of them if I twisted my neck right and left. After a month or so, my bed was relocated to a corner. Instead of being positioned so I could see across the room, the bed faced the corner. From this position I could see only a few of the patients to my left; the outer wall of the building was to my right. I never learned why my bed did not face outward, so I could have a view of the entire ward. I was distracted by too much pain to think of asking for the reason.

There was never a doubt in my mind that I would not be sent back to my unit. I had a long way to go in the healing process. My pain level was no longer severe; I would call it moderate. I was able to move my lower arm but I was not able to lift it.

Came the day that the ward sergeant told me that I was scheduled for transport. The first part of the process was to get me packaged in plaster.

Most of the staff members were employed in disassembling the traction rig. They had to be extremely careful with my leg because the femur might not be completely knitted. Only an X-ray could make that determination. I don't remember exactly how they did it, but here is a close approximation about how it had to be done.

First, my leg had to be extracted from the traction rig. To do this, the 25-pounds of weight had to be removed so that there was no pressure on the pin that passed through the hole in my shin bone. Then the side bars that straddled my leg had to be disconnected from the pin without letting my leg drop or straighten. This meant that one or more people had to hold the padded extension that supported my leg while someone else disconnected the hanging support below my hip. After my leg from freed from the contraption, my leg could be swung inboard and lowered onto the bed. Finally, the pulleys and cables that held the weight bag (now empty of weights) could be disassembled and removed.

For the first time in two months my bed was narrow enough to fit through doorways. One of the orderlies pushed my bed through the staff area to the elevator bank. From there we went down to the basement where the cast master was waiting to build another spica cast around my body. The orderly and the caster shifted me from the bed to a narrow table with indentations for reaching under my torso.

When the previous cast was made, I was still unconscious from the anesthesia that had been administered for the surgical procedure. This time I was conscious so I could see how the cast was made.

Mostly it was a matter of wrapping gauze around my legs, over my hips, and up to my armpits. After the dry layers were applied, the following wrappings of gauze were coated with wet plaster of Paris. The gauze was unrolled like toilet paper. A spacer was placed on my chest and stomach, so I had space to expand my lungs as I inhaled. As before, a post was placed between my legs in order to enable handlers to lift me. The shin pin was kept in place by poking the pin through the gauze and then covering it with plaster. The whole process took an hour to an hour and a half.

(I did not have a watch, so I never knew the time. Neither did I have a calendar, so I never knew the date. I knew that I was wounded on July 14, 1967. I also knew that the present month was September. Closer than that I could not hazard to guess.)

After I was returned to the ward, an ambulatory patient wheeled my bed out the side door of the ward onto the balcony, where I could breathe some fresh air. That night, after dinner, someone wheeled my bed down the elevator and outside the building to a "drive-in" theater where a movie was being shown. In English!

I don't remember what movie was playing, and I didn't care after living in a cave for two months. It felt great just to be outside.

Flying Home, Almost

The next morning I said goodbye to the staff who had helped me through so much pain. Two orderlies picked me up by grabbing the post between my legs and the top of the cast on my chest. They transferred me from the bed to a gurney, then rolled me into the elevator. From the ground floor they took me to a waiting bus. The back of the bus had been fitted with stretcher mounts three tiers high. I was placed on the top tier.

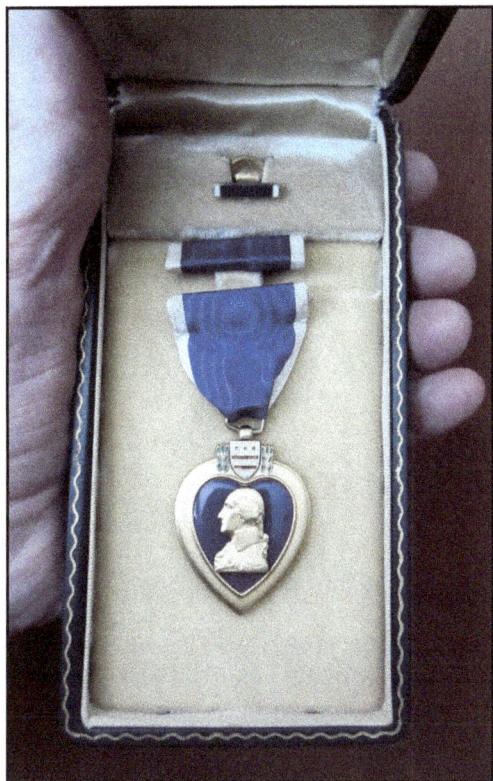
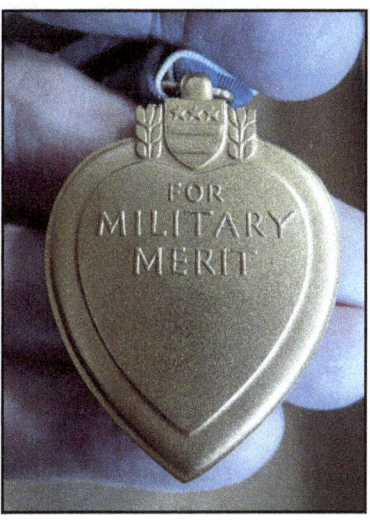

Purple Heart in its presentation case. The top device is a lapel pin. The middle device is worn on the upper left chest of a dress uniform. The obverse of the bronze-alloy medal shows a profile of George Washington. The shield above his head is his coat of arms. Below is the reverse of the medal.

My sole possessions were a sheet, and my ditty bag that held my wallet, St. Christopher's medal, Purple Hearts, and toiletries.

I didn't have the grand view of the city and Mount Fuji as I had from the Huey on the way to the hospital. Traffic was heavy on the way to the Tokyo airport: not just bumper to bumper but also fender to fender. The bus driver drove with remarkable patience and care so that the patients were not tossed about like jungle boots in an electric dryer.

Delays meant nothing to me. I could heal just as fast on a stretcher in the bus as I could in the hospital that I just left, or on the plane that I was supposed to board. I had a feeling, though, that the plane wouldn't depart without a whole busload of patients.

Speaking (or writing) of healing, I could now lift my lower left arm from the elbow. I no longer had to roll my body to the right, then push my left arm under my shoulder, as I did when the Polaroid pictures were taken. I still had to roll over, but now I could move my left arm by itself. The damaged nerves were healing at an accelerating rate.

Eventually the bus reached the airport. The ambulatory patients departed the bus in quick order, while those of us in stretchers were each carried by two soldiers to the plane. I was manhandled into the bottom bunk of a tier of beds, likely because I was too heavy and too difficult to lift to a higher bunk.

I slept all the way to Anchorage, Alaska. Anchorage was the same city where I stopped when I flew to Vietnam from Fort Dix, New Jersey. (Technically, I flew from McGuire Air Force base, which shared a border with Fort Dix, but I was stationed at Fort Dix.)

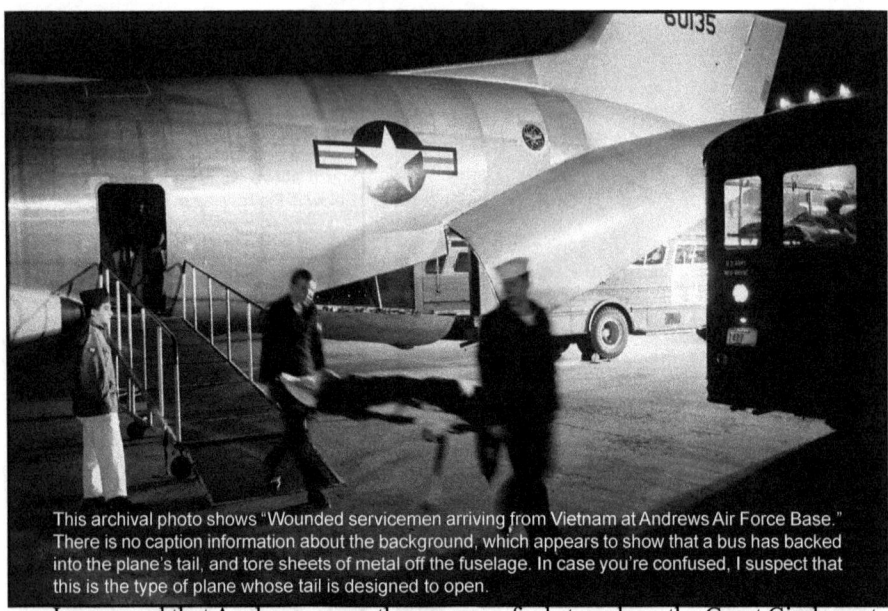

This archival photo shows "Wounded servicemen arriving from Vietnam at Andrews Air Force Base." There is no caption information about the background, which appears to show that a bus has backed into the plane's tail, and tore sheets of metal off the fuselage. In case you're confused, I suspect that this is the type of plane whose tail is designed to open.

I presumed that Anchorage was the common fuel stop along the Great Circle route between East Coast airports and Japan and the Philippines. What I remembered the most about my previous stop at Anchorage was entering the airport and walking straight ahead until I saw a pair of white kneecaps in front of me. As I bent over backward and gazed toward the ceiling, I saw that the legs belonged to a polar bear that must have stood 16 feet high. The polar bear was stuffed.

On this flight, when the plane touched down on U.S. soil, Red Cross nurses swarmed aboard to cheer the non-ambulatory patients with their presence and welcome-home smiles. Praise the Red Cross! That organization was always on hand to make up for the humanitarianism that the military lacked.

I awoke in my bunk as a nurse asked me if she could help in any way. I requested a blanket and medication for pain. She hurried away and returned almost immediately. She tucked a thick off-white blanket around my body from feet to shoulders. She lifted my head, placed two pills on my tongue, then held a paper cup of water to my lips. It's not easy to swallow water and pills in a supine position.

I don't know what kind of medicine she gave me. I slept the rest of the way to Andrews Air Force Base, in Maryland, outside of Washington, DC. I don't remember eating anything during the flight. I don't remember being hungry either. I suspected that instead of pain medicine, I was given something that would help me to sleep. It worked.

I am certain that many of my readers must have seen television broadcasts of soldiers returning from the Gulf War, Afghanistan, and Iraq. They arrived on American soil to be feted by reporters and crowds of well-wishers who welcomed them home and who honored them for their service overseas. Wives, children, parents, and friends ran to their related soldiers and gave them hugs and kisses.

By contrast, Vietnam veterans were generally greeted by raging and booing civilians who expressed nothing but contempt for returning soldiers. These unappreciated soldiers were exhausted from fighting an aimless conflict that most American citizens didn't want. After a number of mob scenes, a new protocol prohibited citizens and news teams from meeting homecoming veterans.

There were no parades, no bands, no flags, no smiling faces, no overjoyed wives to welcome their husbands home.

To avoid bad press, we were sneaked unannounced through a back door of the base where no one could see us struggling on crutches, being pushed on wheelchairs, being carried on stretchers, being wheeled in caskets. There was no hurrah as Johnny came marching home. There was nothing but grave silence.

We were loaded onto olive drab buses in a parking area where non-military personnel were not allowed to go. The buses transported us to the rear entrance of nearby Fort George G. Meade.

I was first placed in a small room with two beds. This semi-privacy had advantages, such as a television and a telephone. I asked the orderly if I could use the phone to call home. The phone was connected to a long wire. He placed the phone on a table next to the head of my bed.

My mother answered the phone. We chatted for a while, then she told me that my father was in the hospital with hepatitis, and might be there for several more weeks. She gave me his phone number. After talking with her, I called my father. We commiserated with each other's medical issues. During our conversation I happened to mention that at least I came home in one piece and had no missing parts.

After we disconnected, the orderly, who was on the left side of the bed, asked, "But, what about your leg?"

The spica cast enveloped my entire left leg and most of my foot except for the toes. Plaster covered the right leg only to the knee. During the phone calls I was dangling my lower leg off the edge of the bed, where it was out of sight from his perspective. I swung it up and onto the mattress.

He took a deep breath. "I thought you were an amputee."

A couple of hours later, an officer entered the room to confirm my identity. He glanced through a roster sheet twice without finding my name. He left unceremoniously.

The officer returned a half hour later. He told me that I had been sent to the wrong hospital. I was supposed to have been flown to McGuire Air Force Base (in New Jersey, where I had started my journey to Vietnam), and transported from there by the regular Army bus service in adjacent Fort Dix to Valley Forge General Hospital, in Phoenixville, Pennsylvania.

The room I was in was not for transients but was reserved for patients who were assigned to the base. He left the room before I could ask any questions. Soon, a pair of orderlies arrived. They picked me up as gently as if I were a portable toilet – perhaps because I smelled like one – and placed me on a gurney. They rolled me out of the room and along a hallway to an open ward that was not much different from the one in Japan, except that it was larger.

So much for privileges for a wounded Vietnam veteran.

I felt less cramped in the open space. The ward was a mixture of bed-ridden and ambulatory patients; many were missing an arm or a leg, or a combination of both. Or worse. The ward resembled a horror show of wounded patients who – as far as I could see from my location in the ward and my supine position and my cumbersome plaster apparel – were a ragtag mob of amputees. Even though I wasn't ambulatory, I was possibly in the best – or most complete – physical condition of all of them.

I spent the night in my new accommodation, wishing that I were back in the semi-private room, which was quieter. The next day, a different officer confirmed that I had been sent to Andrews Air Force Base by mistake. Because there was no regular Army bus service between Fort George G. Meade and Valley Forge General Hospital, I would have to wait until special transportation could be arranged.

Valley Forge General Hospital specialized in orthopedic medicine. It serviced veterans who lived in the northeastern United States, including New England and most of the Great Lakes region. The other patients in my ward were waiting to be flown south and to the west.

For now I was on hold.

I remained on hold for ten days.

Time Passes

I would have been more comfortable in traction, but the cast could not be removed until I reached my final destination, where I would serve the rest of my recuperation time. Meanwhile, I had three square meals per day, and a rubdown in the evening from a cadre of nurse trainees.

I didn't get as much of a rubdown as the rest of the guys. Less than six inches of my back was uncovered, and the hole in my left shoulder blade was still bandaged. That left only a few square inches of skin that was exposed, although the nurses tried to get their fingers inside the cast as far as they could reach. Plus, I suffered the indignity of having to hold the sheet in place over my exposed private parts while the nurses rolled my plaster-encased body onto my stomach, with my legs spread so wide that I was in fear of being rolled off the bed in the process. Having one lower leg free allowed me to save myself from falling overboard. I don't think that the small bit of rubdown I received was worth the effort. But the various nurses got A's for their effort.

What mattered more was that I received a surprise visit from some of my teenage friends from Philly (Philadelphia, Pennsylvania). Bill Reese drove his '57 Chevy for three hours in order to bring my wife (an impromptu marriage before I left for Vietnam) to see me. Also with him were Jay Enright and his younger brother Kenny Enright.

They were fellow members of what we called the Gang. Before we were separated by the war – er, excuse me, the conflict – we hung out at Greg Carr's mother's garage. We furnished the two-car space with multiple layers of carpets which we scrounged from the neighborhood on the night before trash collection day. We also foraged for used furniture. This method of decorating our "club house" was called "trash picking."

By the time of my return to the United States, the Gang was in the process of being split apart. The Enrights managed to avoid the draft, as did Hugh Kelly, Bill Purtle, and Charles Yearicks. Chuck Callabreese and Bill Reese enrolled in college. Greg Carr did a four-year stint in the Air Force, of which one year was spent at an Air Force base in Vietnam. Eddie Hackett and Tommy Nash joined the Marines; each did a tour in Vietnam. If this sounds like the cast of *American Graffiti*, I suspect that George Lucas had planned it that way.

Bill was shocked when I showed him the St. Christopher's medal that he had given me. I showed him how the back of it was now smeared with blood. My blood.

By the time I left Fort Meade, my arm had regained much of its motion if not all of its strength.

Valley Forge General Hospital

During the time that I waited for the army to arrange for my transfer, I itched abominably in the sweaty cast and received no medical treatment, not even inspection of my wounds. I resided in medical limbo. Nurses bathed my arms and lower right leg but could do nothing for the rest of my body – except for the private parts that I washed myself with a sponge.

After seemingly endless waiting, the army finally coordinated my transfer with the transfer of two ambulatory patients and their crutches. I was loaded into the back of an Army station wagon whose rear seat had been removed. The other two patients crawled in beside me, and had to sit or squat on the floor, but did not seem to mind the discomfort. The driver and the co-driver, who had shotgun, were affable fellows who took turns behind the wheel. Air conditioning kept us all cool.

The four-hour drive was uneventful.

Valley Forge General Hospital was a huge complex of two-story wood-frame barracks that was constructed during World War Two. In its heyday, the hospital's more than 100 buildings held over 3,000 patients. Large groups of buildings were connected by covered corridors so that doctors, staff members, and ambulatory patients could

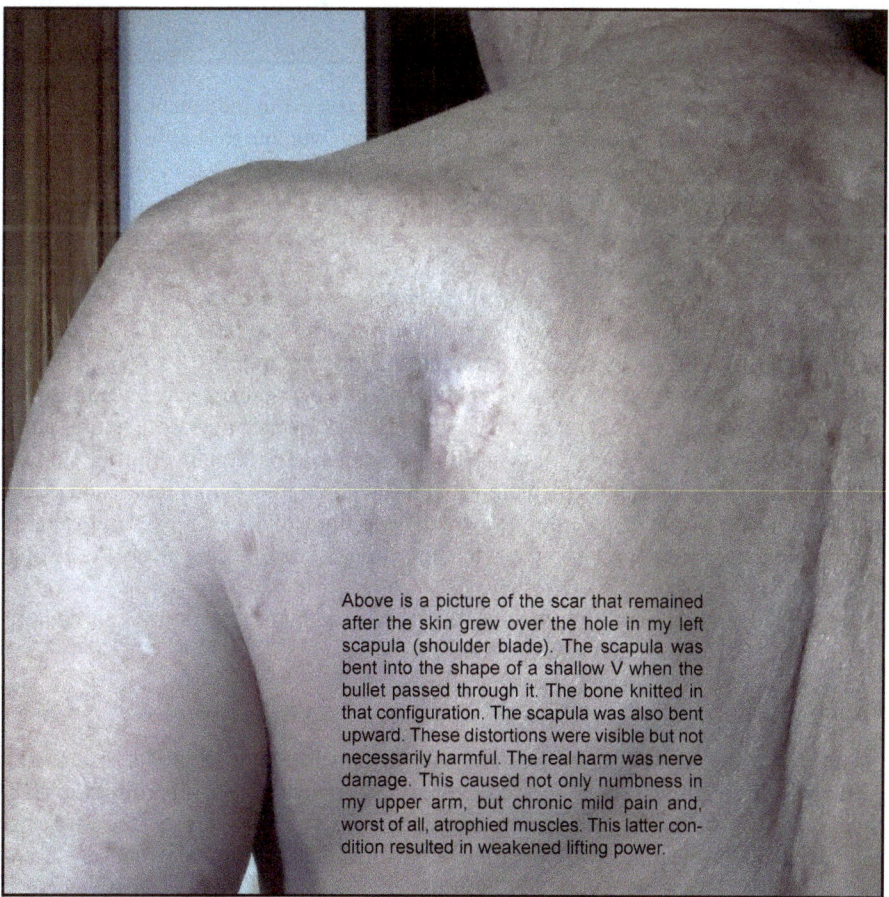

Above is a picture of the scar that remained after the skin grew over the hole in my left scapula (shoulder blade). The scapula was bent into the shape of a shallow V when the bullet passed through it. The bone knitted in that configuration. The scapula was also bent upward. These distortions were visible but not necessarily harmful. The real harm was nerve damage. This caused not only numbness in my upper arm, but chronic mild pain and, worst of all, atrophied muscles. This latter condition resulted in weakened lifting power.

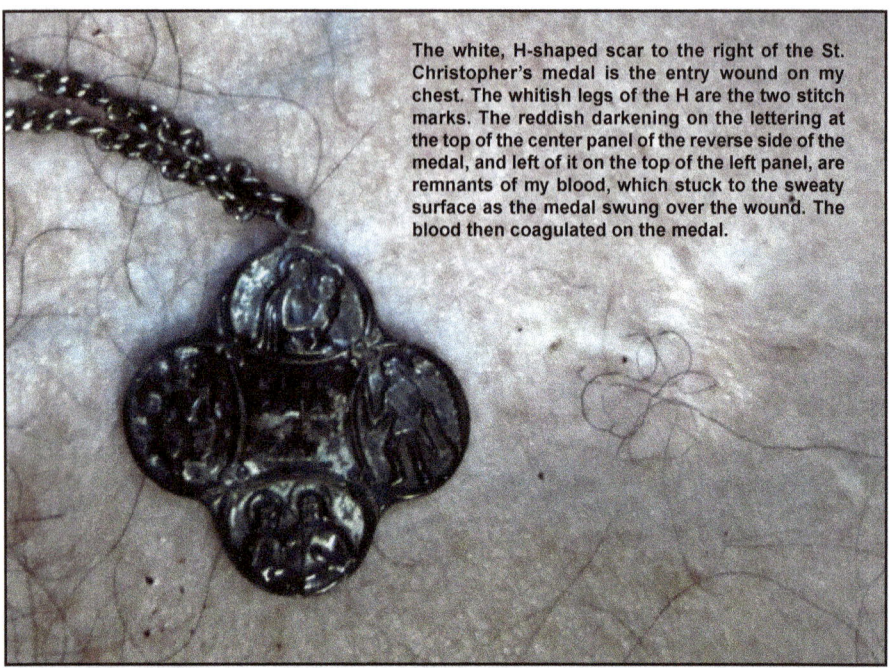

The white, H-shaped scar to the right of the St. Christopher's medal is the entry wound on my chest. The whitish legs of the H are the two stitch marks. The reddish darkening on the lettering at the top of the center panel of the reverse side of the medal, and left of it on the top of the left panel, are remnants of my blood, which stuck to the sweaty surface as the medal swung over the wound. The blood then coagulated on the medal.

pass from one building to another without being exposed to inclement weather. This was important not just to keep passersby from getting wet, but to enable them to avoid winter snowstorms which could be severe. Keep in mind that Valley Forge was the place where General George Washington and his troops camped during the fierce Revolutionary War winter of 1777/1778.

To be clear, the hospital and associated wards were not separate rooms in a single building but rather a sprawling network of previously isolated two-story wings connected by long narrow corridors that were built and adjoined later. The floor plan resembled the random lay of tiles in a completed game of dominoes.

The day after my arrival, a technician using an electric buzz saw sliced through the sides of the cast. He and an orderly lifted off the carapace to expose white, pulpy flesh that couldn't have looked much different from that of a scalped turtle. Under a doctor's direction they gently lifted me out of the plastron (the bottom mold) and placed me in bed under a traction assembly, to which I was immediately rigged. After examining my wounds, the doctor pronounced that my wounds were healing nicely. As always, I was dressed in a sheet.

My recuperation from this point was a long and boring process and not particularly noteworthy. Basically, I had to heal. Time passed slowly.

I Become Ambulatory, Almost

My uncles and aunts and friends of the family came to visit. Red Cross nurses, Veterans of Foreign Wars members, church groups, envoys from local fellowship clubs such as the Moose and Elk, and community leagues, all paraded through the wards unannounced in the evenings without predictable schedules, often passing out snacks and gifts and always spreading good fellowship.

Soon I recovered fairly good use of my arm. A physical therapist stopped by daily to help me exercise and build up my strength. X-ray examinations turned out well, so it wasn't too long before the doctors decided that I could be released from the iron maiden. Once free from the traction assembly I was able to sit up in bed. The first time I did so, I got so dizzy that I nearly passed out. In order to acclimatize to the altitude, I asked to have the bed cranked up in stages. A doctor slid out the traction pin without a hint of pain. The remnant hole had to be treated with antiseptic like the previous one.

After three months of confinement on my back, the freedom to lie on my side was sheer luxury. The doctors warned me not to place undue stress against my left leg because the surrounding musculature was extremely weak and might not provide adequate support for the still-knitting bone. They told me how another patient had rolled over and rebroken his femur, then had to spend another two months in traction. I was careful.

An orderly handed a pair of light blue pajamas to me. He helped me wriggle into the pants first, then into the long-sleeved shirt.

All this was done in the open but none of the patients seemed to care or bother to watch. The ward was nearly a hundred feet in length, with beds facing inward along both outer walls.

Another orderly pushed a wheelchair close to my bed. I needed help to get vertical because my left arm was so weak that I couldn't use it to push up my weight.

Getting into the wheelchair was an ordeal. An orderly helped to pull me upright and swing my legs over the edge of the bed. At that point I was so woozy that I turned white and went limp, and had to be laid back down. My heart wasn't used to pumping blood up to my head. I fared better on the second trial, although I would have fallen flat on my face if the orderly hadn't been holding onto me. As I slid off the bed and stood momentarily to make the transfer to the wheelchair, I found that my good leg wasn't strong enough to support my weight. It buckled like a strand of wet spaghetti. I collapsed as they eased me into the seat. All I could do at first was slouch, recoup my energy, and gasp as I caught my breath.

I felt dizzy again. The orderlies waited until I told them that the spell had passed. With one orderly on each side, they maintained a strong grip as they eased me into what should have been a comfortable position: flat on my buttocks. But the bullet wound on my left buttock instantly reminded me of its presence. I had to wiggle in such a way that most of my weight – little as it was – lay on my right buttock while the left buttock barely touched the seat.

I didn't know then that this was going to be my sitting position for the rest of my life: a slouch with a twist that elevated my left buttock off the seat, then constant maneuvering to other sitting spots when the first sitting spot got too painful to endure.

One of the orderlies wheeled me out of the ward into the central hallway, executed a slow turn, then pushed me along the interconnecting corridor past other wards until we reached the X-ray room at the end. He and the X-ray technician carefully lifted me onto the table. The technician took a number of X-rays from different angles: of my thigh bone and the scapula.

They moved a scale next to the X-ray table. They held onto me as I hunched in a nearly vertical position. My legs wobbled and I almost collapsed, but the orderly caught me and slipped me onto the wheelchair.

When I landed in Vietnam I weighed 170 pounds. Now I weighed 125 pounds. I had the body of a prisoner in a Nazi war camp.

Afterward, the orderly pushed me through the corridors on a familiarization tour. There were no maps. I was glad when he returned me to the ward and helped me onto the bed. All that activity exhausted me. It was time for a nap so I took one. The chronic commotion and the buzz of voices did not prevent me from falling fast asleep.

Step One: a Wheelchair

I became ambulatory sometime in October. I don't have the exact dates of anything that happened to me after I was wounded, on July 14, 1967. Nor do I recall the order in which primary events occurred. I organized the events in 106th General Hospital to the best of my recollection. I will do the same from here to the end of the book. I did not keep a diary because I never thought that I would want to write such a book as this. I remember the events that occurred, but not necessarily in their proper order.

The red-letter day was the one on which I was issued my very own wheelchair. This happened several days after the trial day, when I got pushed around the hospital by an orderly. I had to practice getting out of bed because the bed was so high and I was so weak. An orderly stood by while I practiced landings and takeoffs, until he was satisfied that I was able to solo without hurting myself.

By this time my left arm was almost fully functional. I went to physical therapy every other day, not only to exercise my recuperating arm, but to exercise both legs for eventual walking. No longer did I have sharp sciatic pain in my leg. I felt aching but not agony.

My shoulder pain was worse. This was ironic in that when my arm was paralyzed, I had no feeling at all in the arm or shoulder. Now that feeling was returning, I began to suffer pain; not in the arm but in the shoulder blade around the exit wound and along the muscles that compressed the lung. Those muscles had atrophied so much that I got out of breath at the slightest exertion.

What I learned over time was that the atrophy was permanent: the result of damage to the nerves that controlled the shoulder and lung compression muscles.

Getting into the wheelchair by myself without a safety was a challenge. An orderly stood by and offered suggestions. The first thing he told me was to lock the wheels before I tried to get on the seat in, order to prevent the wheelchair from rolling away from me. I had to move slowly because I still got woozy from being vertical. Three months spent lying flat on my back put me at a distinct disadvantage.

I found that by moving slowly I could slide off the bed and drop into the seat with a thump. However, I did not have the strength or the balance to climb back into bed. Even though I was the patient, the orderlies were more patient that I was. I got around the ward by pulling on the floor with my feet and by pushing the wheel grip with my hands. It felt awkward at first, but within a few days I made remarkable progress. Soon I became self-sufficient.

For days I practiced wheeling myself gently around the ward. It felt great to be mobile again, and to flex my developing muscles. At the end of a week, I was strong enough to climb out of bed on my own, with the help of an overhead bar. Soon I was able to climb back in again. I was growing less dependent on the medical staff and becoming less of a burden. No longer did I have to ask for a urinal or bedpan – I could wheel myself to the latrine and onto the toilet. Life was full of simple pleasures.

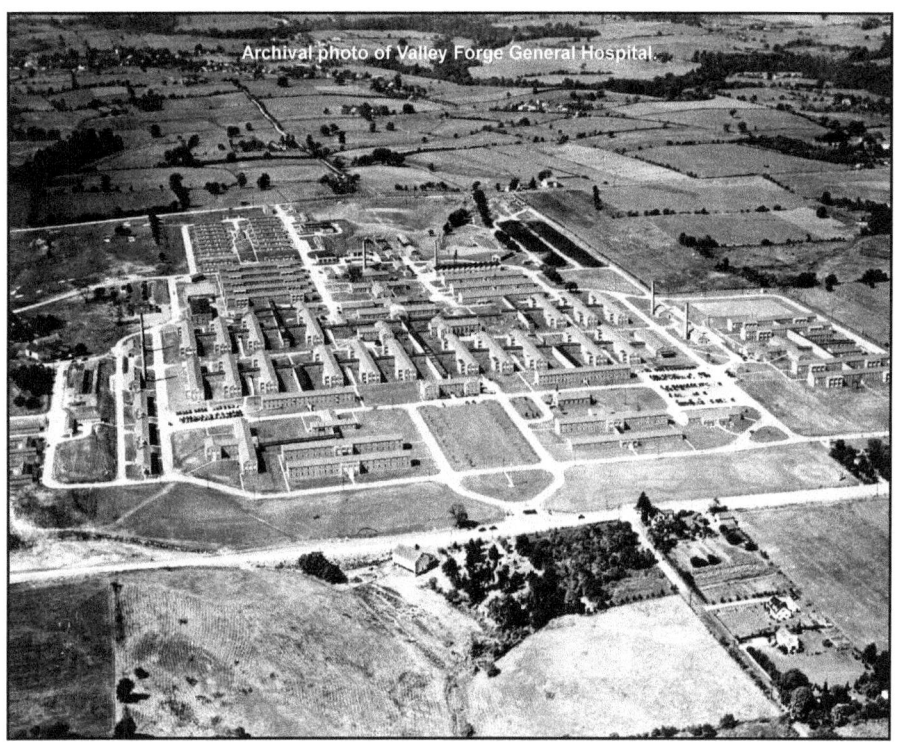
Archival photo of Valley Forge General Hospital.

Being ambulatory after a fashion meant that I could visit the hospital library. This was not a lending library; it was a paperback dispensary. The shelves overflowed with books that had been donated by individuals, local businesses, and charitable organizations. It was a free-for-all for anyone who wanted to borrow books for keeps. I have always read prodigiously, but never so much as I did during that year I spent in the hospital. Reading is still my fondest pastime.

I routinely went to the library after I had physical therapy. Additional books were always available, and there were so many donations that books were piled several feet high along the walls where there were no shelves or bookcases. I stuffed books on both sides of my legs, then jammed more under my thighs and in my lap. No one bothered about my smuggling routine because as quickly as I absconded with a wheelchair load of paperbacks, there were always more than enough to fill in the shelves that I had emptied.

I read an average of two books per day.

A hospital is a depressing place. Most of the patients at Valley Forge were not going home intact. Unlike in the movies, wounds resulting from actual warfare were seldom clean and bloodless. The quick merciful death – with time for that last smoke and a soul-wrenching message for the wife and kids – is a contrivance of theatrical fiction. The teeth-gritting flesh wound is a plot device with dramatic appeal. The short, painless rehabilitation is a make-believe story meant to soothe the souls of gullible viewers.

In reality, bullets and shrapnel caused horrible internal damage and bequeathed mutilations the nature of which often exceeded the capacity of the most vivid imagination. Wartime military hospitals were charnel houses of the living dead.

The hallways thrived with maimed and mangled bodies and with mindless brains. Here were not the heroes pictured in posters promoting the fight for democracy, but the permanently disfigured martyrs who were hidden from the eyes of the public to be the cat's-paws for the country's secret political ambitions. Here the norm was the disabled soldier: men missing fingers, hands, arms, legs, eyes, groins, organs, patches of flesh, chunks of bone, pieces of head, parts of face, and some or all of the above. To truly appreciate the horrors of war, one has only to visit the military wards and see what came to pass when Johnny got his gun but did not come marching home again.

The two patients I remembered the most were the captain who had lost his right arm at the shoulder and his left leg at the hip. He was a career soldier who in the instantaneous flash of an explosion had lost his livelihood, for Uncle Sam had no use for battered bodies and brittle bones. As soon as this patient was healed, he was kicked out of the service and left to his own devices.

The other one I remember was the man who had lost his forehead. Instead of having a convex angle above his eyebrows, he had a concave angle. The frontal part of his brain was missing. He didn't talk. His face had no expression. He was walked around the ward by an orderly as a way to keep him functional. After he was put back into bed, he stared at the ceiling and did not move at all except for blinking.

Fate had a more fortunate end in store for me. While I was going to physical therapy, others were being fitted with artificial limbs or learning how to write left-handed. While I was doing wheelies along the corridor in my wheelchair, others were adjusting to severe handicaps that would leave them crippled for a lifetime. Of all the patients in Valley Forge, I considered myself the luckiest, for I knew that one day, however far in the future, and no matter how much enfeebled, I would walk out of the hospital on my own two feet and with the anatomy I was born with.

I had no trouble remembering the words of the pastor who told the class in Sunday school, "I wept because I had no shoes, till I met a man who had no feet."

Jerry Blavat

Into this cheerless world came those who managed to shed some joy. Undoubtedly the one most remembered person of all was Philadelphia disc jockey Jerry Blavat, known at the time as "the geator with the heator" (whatever that meant). He arranged free entertainment for the troops and brought to the hospital a number of well-known singing groups whose names, unfortunately, I cannot remember, even though I used to listen to them on the radio during my high school years.

But I never forgot Jerry Blavat. The auditorium was always packed on these occasions with folding seats, wheelchairs, and movable beds – standing room only was an unacceptable circumstance considering the nature of the audience. Yet patients managed to choke the room independent of rank. In fact, there was no rank in the hospital; there were no badges on shirts and hats, and no stripes on arms. Saluting was a lost art. Equality was in vogue. Among the patients there was only one status: patient.

At a time when most American soldiers were treated like dirt, Jerry Blavat cared. That mindset meant more to me and to everyone else in the hospital than watching the groups that he brought for our entertainment.

Other groups who made rounds through the wards were the Red Cross and the Vet-

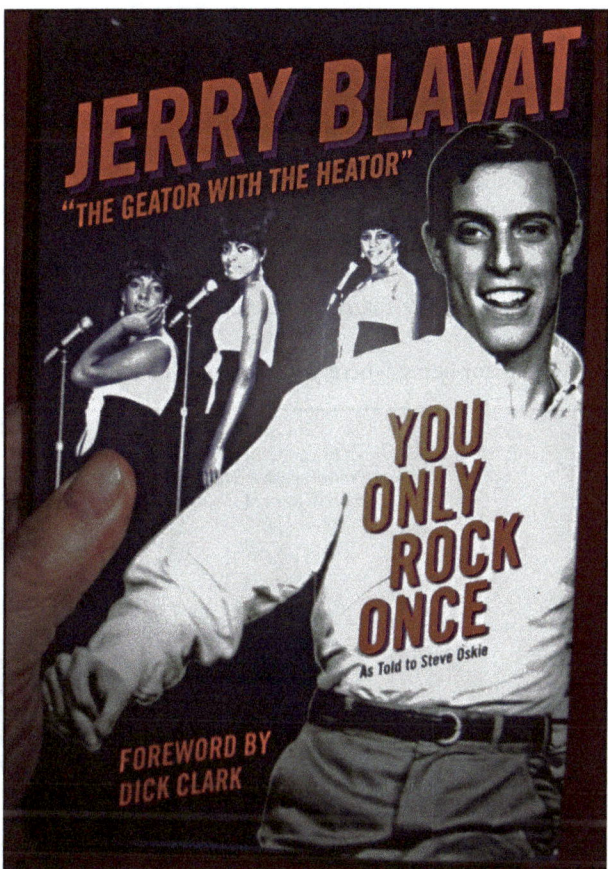

Jerry Blavat was a Philadelphia icon throughout his career. He was known mostly for his various radio programs on which he played popular records, at first when they were newly released, then later in life by which time they had become even more popular "oldies." He was often seen on television, especially Dick Clark's *American Bandstand*. He owned record labels. He also owned and operated a New Jersey nightclub called Memories. He organized dances known as "hops." He wrote a column for the *Atlantic City Weekly* and articles for other magazines. He produced concerts. He made personal appearances at record stores. In other words, he was involved in popular music for his entire life. He passed away in 2023, but he will live forever in the hearts and minds of people young and old, especially those Vietnam Veterans who were patients at Valley Forge General Hospital. One vet went so far as to leave at the Vietnam Wall in Washington, DC, a long-playing record titled "Jerry Blavat Presents / For Young Lovers Only." Who could ask for a better memorial? In his autobiography, he did not mention entertaining the troops at the VA hospital.

erans of Foreign Wars. They appeared after dinner when most patients were lying on their beds, watching television, or reading books and magazines, or – on rare occasions – talking with visiting relatives and friends.

Because Valley Forge General Hospital served patients who lived as far away as New England and the Great Lakes, distance often precluded regular visitations. My family members lived in Philadelphia; they visited me only once.

Red Cross nurses brought smiles and good cheer, along with comestibles such as cookies and candy bars and other sweets that the Army didn't provide.

The VFW had numerous posts in the area. Their members and their wives made numerous visits. They stopped at every bed where they spoke with every soldier. Many of the members had served in World War 2, so they were conversant with the effects of warfare and its aftermath. They knew from experience that soldiers suffered mentally as well as physically from their combat experiences.

Mental afflictions were called "shell shock" in World War 1. They were called "battle fatigue" in World War 2. Now they were called "post-traumatic stress disorder." Psychiatrists like to use long-winded phrases such as "postconcussionsal syndrome" and "combat stress reaction," and probably a few that I haven't heard.

As William Shakespeare might have written under different circumstances, "An explosion by any other name would stink as bad."

No matter what it's called, the presence and actions of family members and friends and even complete strangers who care are the best medicine there is for meaningful convalescence. Having a name attached to a condition doesn't make it feel or heal any better. Most of the time, the condition wasn't recognized, by neither the patient nor the doctors. That's because – in my non-professional opinion – the condition was buried deep in the subconscious mind, waiting to erupt when the hidden mental trigger was pulled. This eruption may not surface until many years later; or it may not erupt but instead it may seep to the surface in stages; or it may never make itself known.

Or it may be subdued or suppressed by people like Jerry Blavat, who contributed to the mental health of Vietnam veterans more than he or anyone else could possibly have known or predicted.

Thank you, Jerry Blavat. Thanks for being where you were needed the most.

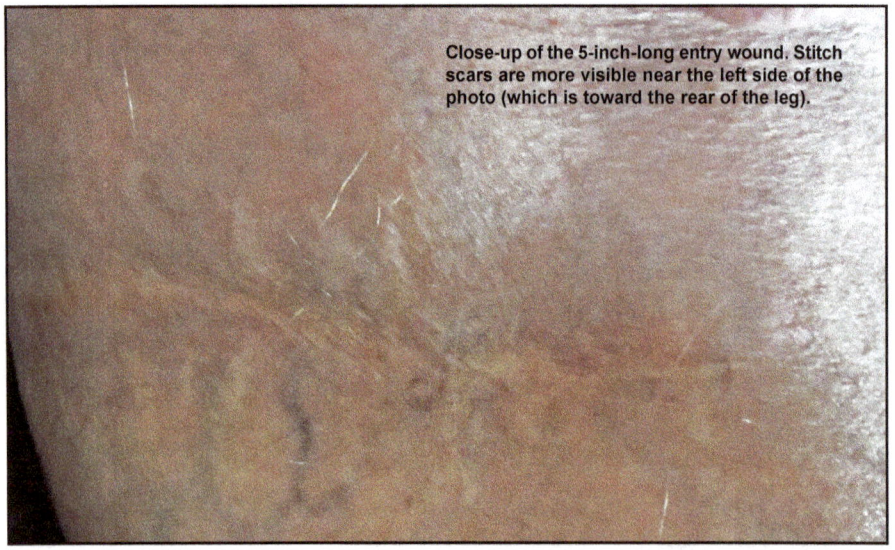

Close-up of the 5-inch-long entry wound. Stitch scars are more visible near the left side of the photo (which is toward the rear of the leg).

Getting Around

Ambulatory patients were expected to pay for their keep, so along with the wheelchair came a job. For an hour or two each morning and afternoon I sorted letters in the mailroom with the paid personnel. Although sitting upright for such a long period of time often caused me great discomfort, it felt good to be productive again. Having a fair amount of freedom in my schedule, I worked my job along with my physical therapy sessions and doctor's rounds.

I was busy. My reading routine suffered.

By constant practice, I learned how to balance the wheelchair on the two large wheels, and roll along the entire length of the ward. As my left arm got stronger, I raced along the corridors as fast as I could go. Once, as I was speeding along the corridor, I passed an intersecting ward just as a doctor stepped in front of me. I gripped the hand brakes as hard as I could, skidded on the polished wooden floor, and clipped the doctor in the legs. He gave me a dirty look and told me to slow down.

Another time, I paid a visit to the second floor by fighting my way up the ramp. After I caught my breath, I turned around and raced down the ramp. When I reached the bottom I was going so fast that I couldn't stop in time without hitting the wall. I released the right brake so the wheelchair could turn and direct me through the doorway. The wheelchair turned sideways but instead of curving through the doorway, the rubber tire pealed off the groove in the wheel. That prevented me from hitting the wall.

An orderly happened by and saw that I needed help. "What happened?"

"I got a flat tire."

The rubber tire was solid and about one inch in diameter. It did not have a tube. I got out of the wheelchair so the orderly could remount the tire in the groove of the wheel. I decided not to try that trick again.

We had wheelchair races when the orderlies were not in the ward. I never won.

Step Two: Crutches

After two months in a wheelchair, I slowly graduated to crutches. The process was not painful, just exhausting, especially as I had to learn how to walk again. At first I had neither strength nor sense of balance. Standing vertical was a new sensation that cannot be imagined by one who has not spent three months on his back and two months in a wheelchair.

At first, an orderly held me up by the armpits while I shuffled across the floor. During the transition stage I wheeled myself around the hospital, then walked short distances in the ward or in the adjacent hallway.

I caught on quickly even though my legs were weak. When I needed to rest, I slumped down onto the crutch arms and absorbed my slowly gaining weight with my armpits. I could rest in this position for only a minute or two before my left shoulder started to ache. Then I stood on my legs again with my knees locked, or I walked a few steps without leaning on the left crutch.

I began to rebuild the strength in my legs. At first, I kind of pole-vaulted by putting my right foot on the floor and lifting my left leg so that it swung through the air. It didn't take too long before I was bearing weight on my left leg. Very little leg.

Heartbreaking Homecoming

While I was still getting around the hospital in a wheelchair, I learned to walk during physical therapy sessions. I practiced on parallel bars by holding my weight on my arms and swinging my legs forward. My broken leg had healed well with some annoying exceptions: despite the weights that had pulled my leg muscles apart during my three months in traction, the femur healed one inch shorter than its original length. Due to the damaged sciatic nerve, not only did I still have bouts of pain, but the nerve damage prevented my leg from regaining its original muscle mass.

Once I demonstrated to the doctors' satisfaction that I could get about on crutches without swooning, falling, or tripping, a great opportunity arose – that of obtaining an off-base pass. This prospect led to a number of problems.

I had no clothes. I had no money. I had no transportation.

My sole possessions were pajama tops and bottoms, and a pair of hospital slippers. And they did not belong to me. They belonged to the Army. As I did with my jungle fatigues in Vietnam, I traded them in for clean pajamas and slippers once a week.

In order for me to leave the hospital, I had to obtain a uniform. Patients were not allowed to wear civies (civilian clothes) on base. This meant that I had to buy a new uniform from the Army. The way the Army system functioned, draftees were given a full set of uniforms upon induction. After the original clothing wore out, soldiers were expected to pay for replacements. My original uniforms (fatigues, summer dress, and winter dress, plus caps and footwear) had been issued to me in basic training. Lifers did not receive replacement clothing for life.

My duffel bag with my uniforms was in a locker in Vietnam. It should have been forwarded to me when I left the country. I never saw it again. I figured that it was stolen along with all my personal belongings.

To buy a uniform, I had to have money. The only cash I had in my wallet was in the form of MPC's (Military Payment Certificates). Stay with me while I explain the situation.

When I arrived in Vietnam, I had to turn in all my American currency (paper bills and coins) to the paymaster. In exchange I received Military Payment Certificates (called MPC's), which were valid only in Vietnam.

The reason for *this* was that American money could be sold on the black market for twice its face value, perhaps even more. And *this* was because American currency could be used by the NVA to purchase arms and ammunition on *another* black market.

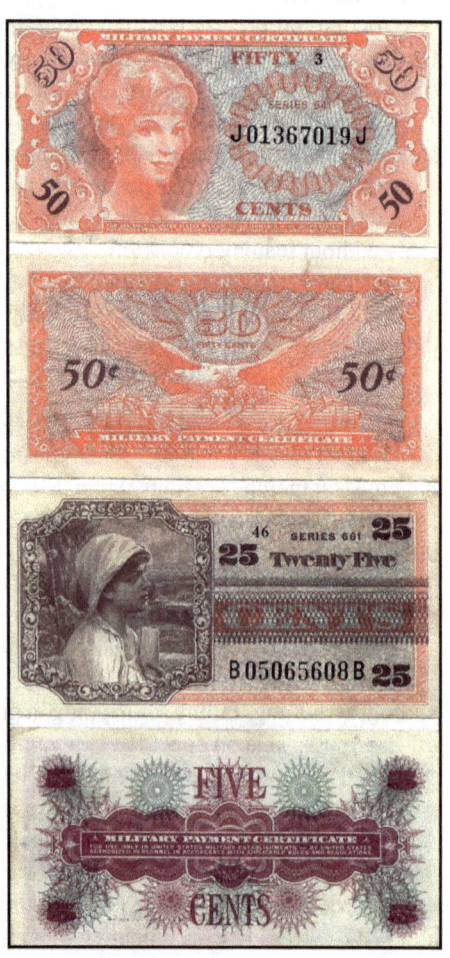

In other words, I could sell an American ten-dollar bill for twenty dollars' worth of MPC's, which I could then spend in the Army PX (post exchange), where common goods such as cigarettes and condoms could be bought for less than they sold for in American markets back home (the States).

Because I was back in the U. S. of A., I could no longer redeem my MPC's. In fact, I had *never* used any of my MPC's in Vietnam. That was because I was sent straight into the bush. I never saw a city or a store or a PX where I could spend my MPC's. And the paymaster at the Valley Forge General Hospital was not authorized to redeem MPC's.

To complicate the issue, my Army records had never caught up with me. They must have been lost or misfiled in the miasma that was Vietnam, gone the way of my duffel bag and personal belongings. My dog tags had been stolen in Fort Dix while I was awaiting an outbound flight. When I tried to have them replaced, I was told that I would have to get them "at your next duty station." My next duty station was the boonies. The only way anyone in Vietnam knew my name and assignment to the 25th Infantry Division was because I answered roll call after landing in country.

(While I'm on the subject, it's no joke that the airfield had to be cleared of water buffalo before landing. I saw them grazing right next to the landing strip, moving closer to the verge as the plane set down on the tarmac.)

You will recall that I was immediately sent to join my division in Pleiku, as per orders. After a week or so, I received a TDA (Temporary Duty Assignment). Perhaps my records went astray when I was temporarily assigned to the 4th Infantry Division, and were never transferred back to the 25th because I didn't return to the 25th. Who knows?

The only way the doctors in Qui Nhon could have known my name was by looking through my wallet, which had been rescued from my upper jacket pocket after it was cut off my body on the operating table. (We all kept our wallets in an upper jacket pocket so it would not get submerged during river crossings.)

In a way I was a ghost. I had medical records from Qui Nhon and Tokyo, but those records appeared not to have been attached to my personal assignment records. Without the continuity, it was as if I had been born in Qui Nhon and sent to Tokyo, thence to Andrews Air Force Base, thence to Fort Meade, thence to Valley Forge.

Without valid records of when I had last been paid, the hospital paymaster couldn't pay me. (This was the same paymaster who couldn't redeem my MPC's.) *But*, said the paymaster, "I know you've been here for two months, so I can give you partial pay for the time spent in this hospital." And that is what he did. He filled out a partial pay voucher, had me sign it, then gave me two thirds of two months' pay. (About $150.)

I may have been a ghost but I was a rich ghost (by 1967 military standards).

Now that I had money, I bought the cheapest uniform that conformed to Army regulations: summer dress despite the cold December weather.

Transportation was the next problem to overcome. My parents were busy; my friends were either working or in college or serving in the military. No public transportation extended to Valley Forge. Fortunately, at the last minute, I met Richie Camburn, a fellow patient who not only lived in northeast Philly but who kept his car on the base. He offered to drive me home and bring me back after the weekend.

Richie had suffered a severe bullet wound in his upper left arm, leaving him with a large indentation and limited joint movement. Because he had served as an MP (Military Police) he was hoping that he could pass the Philadelphia police physical so he could get a job as a patrolman after the army kicked him out of the service when his enlistment time ended.

He let me off on the street at the end of my driveway. I crutched my way to the front door where I had to ring the doorbell because I didn't have a key. (It was lost or stolen along with my duffel bag.)

I said hello to my mother and wife. My father wasn't home from work. I hobbled through the house calling, "Kitty. Kitty. Kitty." My cat had slept with me since I was 10 years old. She always came when I called her. But this time she didn't come. I hobbled to the back door after my mother told me that she had let her outside.

I opened the door and called her name. She didn't come. I called again, louder. She didn't come. She didn't come. She never came. My next-door neighbor found her body in his garden two days later. She had died on the morning of my afternoon arrival. I cried and cried and cried. I am crying now as I type these words.

Jay Enright and his brother Kenny Enright buried her body in the woods next to the house, while I leaned on my crutches and cried some more.

Crutches for Christmas

The world I came back to was not the one I had left. Even today it is difficult for me to understand the dark mood that pervaded the nation during those years known as the Vietnam era. At the time, I naively expected that a lone soldier in uniform who was leaning on crutches would stir some amount of sympathy, yet on subsequent passes when I hitchhiked home, I found it nearly impossible to thumb a ride. I could always get to the turnpike entrance by asking for a ride from another patient, but then I might stand at the toll booth for an hour before a kindly soul would stop for me.

On my second trip home, an ex-Navy officer picked me up and took me all the way to Philly. He gave me the lowdown about the way in which civilians treated soldiers. Soldiers were harassed in airports while waiting for a standby flight. They were jeered on the streets. And worse.

(A standby flight was one that was available only to military personnel. It allowed them pay a reduced fee if they were willing to wait for a plane that was not full by take-off time.)

I experienced the epitome of this mistreatment firsthand when I was going home for Christmas.

Snow fell heavily from a nighttime sky and swirled frigidly around my feet. The thin Army dress shoes offered scant protection from the cold of the winter storm. I leaned heavily on my crutches at a busy intersection only a mile from home, where a Samaritan had dropped me off. As the cars stopped for the traffic light, I held out my thumb, clearly visible in the yellow glow of overhead incandescent lights. It was usual for people in vehicles to look away from someone who was begging for a ride. Now the opposite was the way of life in America.

People saw me. They even stared at me. They looked right into my eyes. And I looked right into theirs. Their faces were blank and expressionless, but their eyes spoke volumes. I saw hatred in those eyes, and loathing.

These people even turned their heads to continue staring at me when the traffic began to move, leaving no doubt about the way they felt. Mine was a fleeting glimpse into the dead soul of the American spirit.

After more than an hour, shivering and half frozen, with snow accumulating on my shoulders, and feeling lonely, dejected, and totally alienated from my fellow man, I hobbled on my way. This was only the beginning, the mere tip of the iceberg, of the treatment I later received from a civilian populace who were more crippled than I was.

It was America's lowest ebb.

Step Three: Cane versus Able

I spent two months on crutches. Nothing untoward happened in the hospital during that time. I no longer had physical therapy, but I was told to walk as much as possible in place of physical therapy. I still had my job sorting mail. And still my primary pastime was reading books. I took a shoulder bag with me to the library so I could carry books back to the ward.

Two months passed slowly as I walked with the use of a cane. This was painful

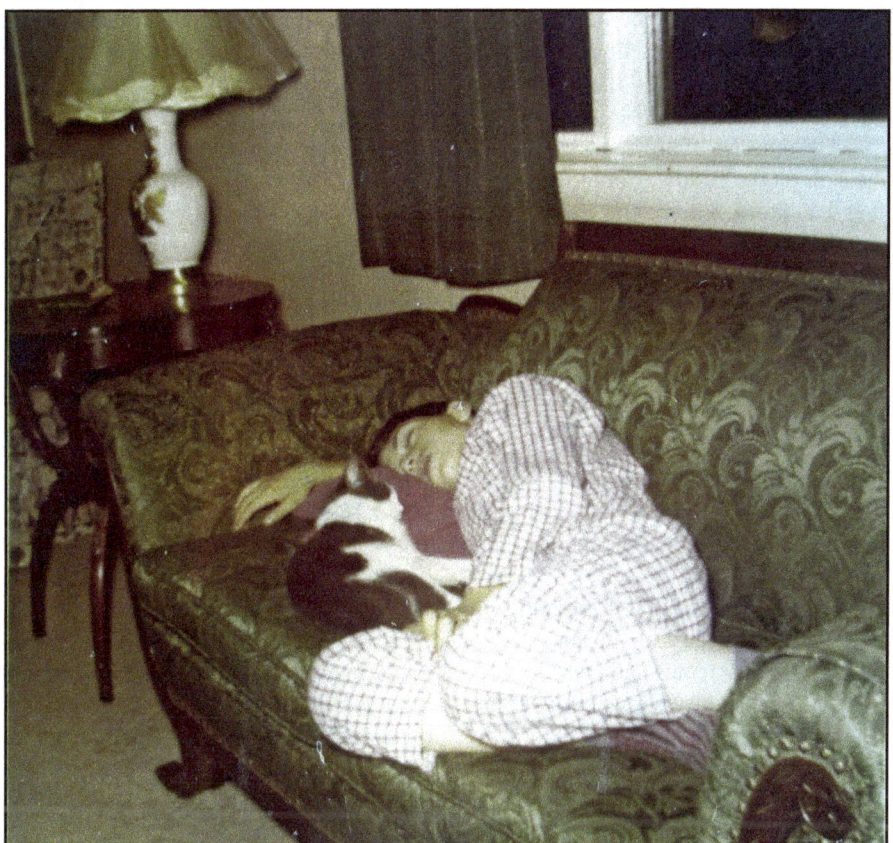

My mother took this photo at Christmas of 1957. Who could possibly have imagined that ten years later would find me sleeping in the same position, but wearing jungle fatigues instead of pajamas, wearing olive drab jungle boots instead of striped colored socks, resting my head on a steel pot instead of a purple pillow, snuggling with a rifle instead of a house cat named Kitty, sleeping in the rain instead of a dry living room? Not I nor my mother.

for me because of my damaged shoulder blade, and atrophied shoulder and lung muscles. I could lean on my left arm for only a short time before fatigue and pain increased to the point at which they became intolerable. I favored both my right arm and leg.

It was difficult to make any longtime friends in the ward. They came and went so quickly. Richie Camburn was released from the hospital after he provided transportation for my first weekend pass. Because he lived in Philly, we got together after my release from the hospital. His wound healed to the extent that he was able to join the Philadelphia police force.

As for other patients, if their physical condition was severe, they were given a medical discharge, and possibly a disability pension. If they were able to conduct useful work for the Army, they completed their enlistment time with stateside elements of their outfit. The eventual discharge was likely to be an honorable discharge instead of a medical discharge. A disability pension was unlikely.

My future was looking better by the time the doctors took away my cane and made me walk on my own two legs.

My bad arm hurt only when I lifted it above my head. The back of the upper arm suffered from two paradoxical conditions: as a result of nerve damage, the skin felt numb when I rubbed my fingers across it; yet it was painfully hypersensitive whenever the skin was pinched. All these conditions were permanent throughout my life, and remain so today.

The muscles of my bad leg did not hurt at all, but the skin below the entry wound, the skin on the inside of my lower leg, and the skin on the top of my foot and on the four small toes, suffered the same paradoxical conditions as the skin on my arm.

The numbness and hypersensitivity of the skin on the top of my foot and on the four small toes gradually faded until, after ten to fifteen years, the skin returned to normal. The skin below the entry wound, plus the skin on the inside of my lower leg, remained impaired throughout my life, and feels the same today.

Step Four: More Surgery

My medical problems were far from over. Months passed, and I should have been well along the road to full recovery and discharge from the Army. But the more weight that I put on my wounded leg, the more my left foot began to ache. At first, I made the obvious correlation that the pain was another aspect of sciatic nerve damage, and said so to the doctor.

Dr. Sergeant thought differently. He observed my gait and detected a limp that appeared unconnected with the gunshot wound. He concluded that despite the heavy traction weight, my femur had healed a little short. X-rays proved him right.

The X-rays also showed that all the ankle ligaments were broken and no longer supported my foot. When he told me this, I remembered the time that I jumped out of the way of that enemy grenade, two days prior to being wounded. I described the incident to him, and told him how the ankle had swelled to double its normal size.

"That would explain it," he said.

Dr. Sergeant told me that I had two choices for treatment. I could wear support hose for the rest of my life, which would furnish only a small measure support. Or I could have an operation that would permanently stabilize the ankle with a great measure of support.

I thought about the options long and hard. After ten months in various hospitals, and learning how to walk again, the thought of undergoing another operation and spending more time in the hospital was abhorrent to me. This is to say nothing about extending my service time. On the other hand, having a permanently weak ankle that would make me a cripple and cause chronic pain was equally as abhorrent.

Undergoing another operation meant that I would have to be hospitalized for another three and a half months, during which time I would have to wear a non-walking cast for the first six weeks. This meant crutches again, followed by a month using a cane, and another month walking with the aid of a steel brace built into my shoe, while the doctor gauged the success of the surgical procedure.

The operation was called a Watson-Jones repair. The procedure consisted of drilling holes in the leg bone, the foot bone, and the ankle bone, then transplanting a living tendon from the leg, weaving the tendon through the three holes, pulling the tendon tight, then tying the loose end of the tendon in a knot around the part of the tendon that remained in place.

(A living tendon was one that was severed only at one end so that the tendon main-

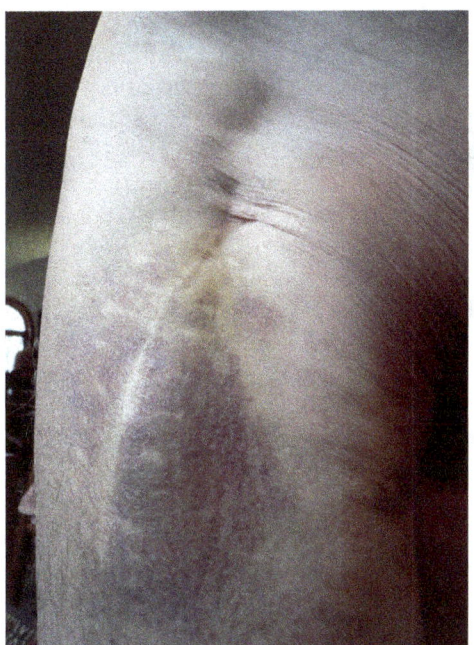

I took this picture of the exit wound on my outer thigh after a hard crash on my mountain bike landed me on a rock. The pain was so excruciating that I couldn't stand up for ten minutes. My leg was paralyzed until I bent it manually at the knee and massaged it. I still had a couple of miles to go. I pushed the bike until I felt well enough to ride.

tained its connection with the body at the other end.)

The result of this procedure would be a permanently stiffened joint that would yet retain some rotary motion. Although I desperately wanted to be released from the hospital, and discharged from the Army, I let reason rule.

Dr. Sergeant performed the operation. I don't know how long the procedure lasted. When I awakened from the anesthesia in the recovery room, I found that my ankle and lower leg were wrapped in a plaster cast. An orderly pushed me in a wheelchair to my ward, helped me onto my bed, and tucked extra blankets around me.

I promptly fell asleep – if in fact I ever awoke for more than a few seconds at a time. I slept soundly throughout the night.

I was hungry when I awoke. I had not eaten the previous day: before the operation due to the doctor's fear that I might vomit during the procedure; after the operation because I had such a strong reaction to anesthesia. The nurses were unable to wake me.

My ankle throbbed with intense pain. An orderly brought a pain pill and poured a glass of water for me. I swallowed the pill. Within minutes I felt much better. When breakfast arrived, I ate every bit of it. I dozed off and on throughout the day. By the next day I was able to stay awake until nighttime. The pain was not as severe as it was the first day.

Gradually the pain diminished until by the end of a week I no longer needed the pills. During my waking hours I passed the time by reading. Of course!

When I felt stable, I took a tour along the ward and back. I had to hold up my left leg so it didn't touch the floor. I felt a little woozy at first, but I quickly acclimated to this previous form of locomotion. By the second week after the operation, I was practically running on three legs like the Martian machines in H. G. Wells' *The War of the Worlds* (the magazine version of 1897, not the film version of 1953).

After Dr. Sergeant's second weekly examination, he authorized an off-base pass so I could spend some time at home.

By this time, I had long been employing a sneaky way of thumbing a ride home: I carried a large civilian shirt and a pair of baggy pants in a small cloth bag with a pair of attached cloth handles which I held like a woman's purse. On Friday afternoons I could always find a patient who would give me a lift to the Turnpike entrance. Hitchhiking was not allowed on the Turnpike, so I had to be dropped off outside the tollbooths. I donned my civvies in the open by pulling them over my uniform. I tucked my Army hat in the bag.

As long as people didn't know that I was a soldier, it wasn't too difficult to hitch a ride. I never told anyone that I was in the military. I usually made up a story such as my car broke down and had been towed to a service station; or my car was a stick shift and I couldn't drive with a cast on my foot. No one questioned either story.

Shortly after surgery, I conned Jay Enright and Kenny Enright into taking me spelunking. I had taken both of them on numerous rides before I received my draft notice, and before I sold my car: a 1960 Ford Galaxie. Now Jay owned a Chevy Nova.

Remember that I was a geology major in college. I was interested in all aspects of the field, one of which was speleology. There were no caves in Philly, so as a preteen, I spent many hours exploring storm drains in the neighborhood. My longest penetration was just over a mile. After I reached driving age and purchased the car that is noted in the previous paragraph, I drove to the Poconos to explore real caves. By that time, I had already bought and read the State geological survey books for the caves of Pennsylvania, Maryland, Virginia, West Virginia, and several other States.

We located the cave from directions that were given in the book. The entrance lay off-road in a forest. I laid a compass course and led the way on crutches. The cave was too narrow for crutches, so I switched to my cane for underground exploration. In the event, most of the passageways required crawling.

The result of this trip and other outdoor activities was excessive wear on the bottom of the cast. By the time I went to the cast department to have the cast removed, the cast was dragging loose plaster and strands of cotton padding that stretched several inches in length. I felt like Boris Karloff playing the 2,000-year-old mummy, Imhotep.

The scowl on the face of the cast remover told me that he was not pleased. After a year in the hospital, I didn't care. After all, what could the Army do to me? Send me to Vietnam? He removed what remained of the cast, then sent me to Dr. Sergeant's office.

The doctor examined the ankle, carefully moved it in various directions, and pronounced the operation a success. He provided me with a cane, told me to take it easy for a couple of weeks, and suggested that I gradually place more and more weight on the foot, as long as it didn't hurt to do so.

A month later, he visited me in the ward along with another orthopedic surgeon. They examined not only my ankle but all my wounds. They conferred about each wound. At one point, I heard Dr. Sergeant say to the other doctor, "He's going to have trouble later on."

I didn't know what he meant. I didn't learn the ugly truth until 43 years later.

Army End, New Beginning

My final week in the Army was a busy one.

My service records from the various commands at which I had served my time (pun intended) were finally located, collated, and forwarded to the hospital. This meant that the paymaster could authorize my back pay in full, minus the partial payments that I had already received.

I also received some hazard pay. According to U.S. labor laws, "Hazard pay means additional pay for performing hazardous duty or work involving physical hardship. Work duty that causes extreme physical discomfort and distress which is not adequately

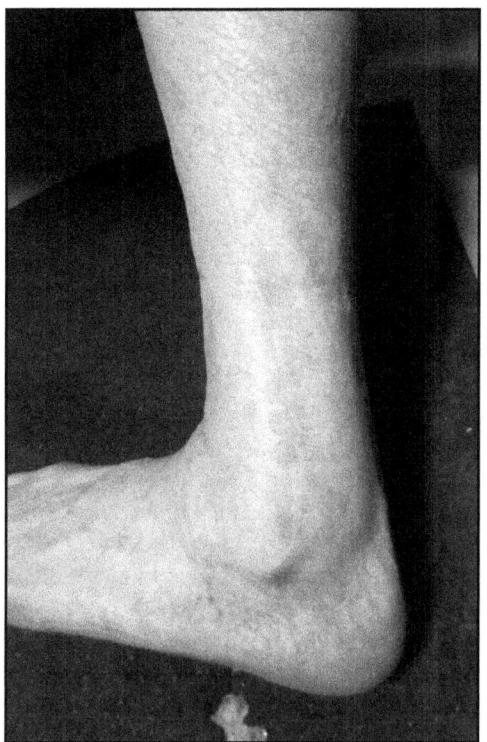

The vertical white line on the outside of my leg is the 4-inch scar which shows the place from which the tendon was transplanted. The bulge on my ankle bone resulted from the knot that was tied after the tendon was woven through the holes that were drilled in the three bones.

alleviated by protective devices is deemed to impose a physical hardship."

Despite this clear-cut official definition, the Army disbursed hazard pay only for the time that I spent on Vietnamese soil, but not for the time that I spent in various hospitals suffering extreme physical pain and hardship. Trust the government to twist the language in order to cheat draftees who didn't want the job in the first place.

Dr. Sergeant provided the results of my final examination to an Army medical board that relied on his suggestions to determine the percentage of disability compensation to which I was entitled. A number of factors were taken into account: the severity of wounds and/or injuries; how those wounds and injuries would affect my ability to work and live; pain; scars; and so on.

(In Army parlance, a wound is different from an injury. A wound is the result of enemy action, such as shrapnel or a bullet. An injury is the result of an accident, such as a fall or a car crash; anything that is not the result of enemy action. Purple Hearts are awarded only for wounds. Thus I was not awarded a Purple Heart for the damage done to my ankle, despite the fact that an enemy grenade was the cause of the damage.

My disability pension was set at 60%.

With more than a year's pay coming to me, including a pittance for hazard pay, I was discharged along with a bundle of cash.

By the time of my discharge, I had spent thirteen months and four days in the hospital, had already served beyond my two-year commitment, and had cost the government an incredible amount of money; in addition to which my body and my career had been irreparably ruined, all for a war that the vast majority of American citizens did not want in the first place.

The army didn't want me; society wanted to forget me. I was given an honorable discharge and a disability pension. I was a civilian again.

I walked out of the hospital on my own two legs.

Many other soldiers never walked again. They lived the rest of their lives as physical or mental cripples,

Too many soldiers were permanently put at rest in peace.

Battle Syndrome Retrospect

Veterans of the Vietnam conflict have been accused of being reticent and uncommunicative about their experiences in the war zone. Psychologists have postulated that this silent circumspection might be a modern form of shell shock or the result of battle fatigue. But the general populace believes that veterans are ashamed of their military conduct, that they are ridden with guilt over what they did in the field of battle, that their consciences are so distressed by their vile and heinous actions that in order to avoid making embarrassing admissions of deed they have refused to talk at all about the conflict or even acknowledge participation. The supposition is that the dark iniquitous secrets and hateful memories have been intentionally repressed because, in light of their reprehensible behavior, that is the only way that they can cope with their actions and live with themselves.

This response to a situation of stress – a form of post-traumatic stress syndrome – has been called the "Vietnam syndrome."

Vietnam vets have been harshly and unjustly censured. The truth is not that veterans were unwilling to share their wartime experiences with the public, but that the people were not willing to listen.

Whereas veterans returning from previous campaigns were feted as many-splendored heroes, Vietnam vets were treated as trash, scum, and baby killers. Veterans were forced to maintain silence in order to avoid persecution. I experienced this pathology firsthand. People became distant when they learned of my veteran status, then wanted nothing more to do with me. I was hounded out of social gatherings. I was openly accosted. I was shunned.

The only way to be accepted by society was not to mention my veteran status. So I quit talking about what people did not want to hear.

What created strife and bitterness among Vietnam vets was not their Vietnam experience, but their subsequent American experience: the "America syndrome." The

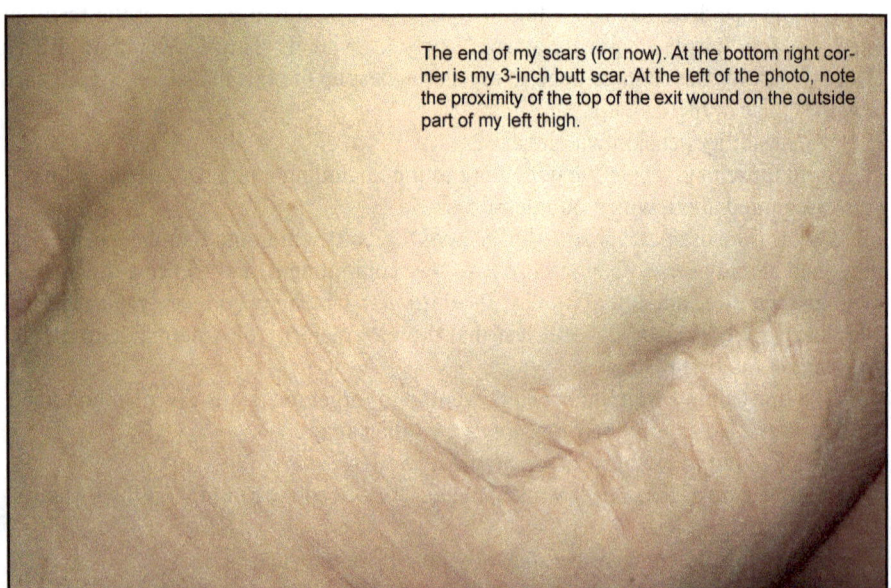

The end of my scars (for now). At the bottom right corner is my 3-inch butt scar. At the left of the photo, note the proximity of the top of the exit wound on the outside part of my left thigh.

American people misplaced the hostility they felt for their elected leaders – those who were responsible for initiating and escalating the war – and castigated the soldiers because they were more reachable.

In many ways, living as an outcast in a homeland full of odious ingrates was more stressful than being constantly under fire.

The War in Perspective

As I look back on my Army episode I realize that I was a failure as a soldier. My commanding officer in basic training branded me as having "a poor attitude toward military service." I can't disagree with him, but I take exception to the implication that such an observation is categorical with respect to the full measure of life. That I react with strong opposition to threats, humiliation, and unreasonable demands, I willingly admit. "Theirs is not to reason why . . ." is a sentiment I can never embrace.

On the contrary, a good soldier must take orders mindlessly and without fear of remorse over the consequences of his actions. He must not exercise emotion or free will. He must be an automaton, an instrument, a tool that is wielded by a superior officer the way a hammer is wielded by an ironsmith. Wars are not won by those who challenge orders, but by those who carry them out, however ruthlessly.

War is anonymous and impersonal.

War is a condition in which immorality has been legitimated.

There is no room in war for charity. You fight to vanquish the enemy – or there's no sense in fighting. Halfway measures don't work. I confess that I lacked the resolve to crush an invisible enemy through the attrition of the civilian population that was forced by threat to support it. But perhaps my greater blindness lay in my inability to recognize that not all the combatants in Vietnam carried weapons, that the enemy was ubiquitous: in every village and hamlet, in every woman and child, in all the hearts and minds.

Corporal Yawn was a good soldier. My platoon sergeant was a good soldier. Each was a successful product of Army indoctrination as prescribed by American acculturation. Each displayed the strength that I lacked and that was needed to achieve political conquest through military aggression. They carried out orders with unquestioning vigor and determination unbothered by guilt. They accepted unflinchingly the martial creed that the rules of conduct in war necessarily oppose the rules of conduct in peace, that war suspends all laws of humanity, and that the end justifies the means. Their behavior in combat was the only way to achieve victory against an entrenched, implacable foe.

Because I couldn't accept such tenets on blind faith, I never developed the resolve to proceed as an effective fighting machine. I was guilty of being misled by an innate sense of righteousness. I saw innocence when I should have seen hostility. I saw good in a background of bad. But my greatest weakness as a combat unit was the belief that I had the right to make moral judgments in a war that I did not understand.

Despite this admission, I suffer no guilt over my conduct in battle. Due to the kind of firefights in which I was engaged, there was too much confusion for kills to be confirmed. When armed soldiers shot at me, I returned fire with a firm intent to kill. Call it self-defense or the will to survive or any other self-serving platitude that fits. If by some chance I failed to take out my target, it was not for lack of trying.

An army of amateur soldiers who think as I did could never win a war like the one that was fought in Vietnam, which found wanting a firm objective beyond pacification by force. This is not to say that amateur soldiers cannot be molded into an effective fighting force, only that they need conviction and a justification for their actions that are more powerful than the threat of criminal discipline. National defense is a far greater calling.

Although I saw the war through myopic eyes, the passage of time has granted me greater vision. I can now look back on events from the perspective of a blind, telepathic being. I can no longer see the uniforms of the men intermingled in battle, but I can read the minds of the opponents, which I find indistinguishable. None are fighting for land, for gain, or for conquest. They are fighting for what they believe in: their perception of freedom. Who is to say that when two of us met on the field of battle, one was right and the other was wrong?

In my defense, and in the defense of my fellow draftees, I was not bred for the brutality of war. Neither were most draftees whose mindsets were similar to mine. I wanted to be a scientist, and therefore had a scientific disposition, just as my fellow draftees were disposed to be an automobile mechanic, or a lawyer, or a plumber, or a store manager, or any occupation that did not require skill with a gun and a longing to be in the Army. Compared to my enemy combatants, I was an amateur.

Like the old saying that you can't make a silk purse out of a sow's ear, putting an automatic rifle in a person's hands does not make that person a soldier.

Nine weeks of jungle warfare training could not possibly compare with the lifetime of training and experience that Vietnamese soldiers possessed. Nor did such training affect the attitudes of draftees. Draftees still wanted to become scientists or mechanics or lawyers or plumbers or store managers.

Winning the war was not my personal goal. In combat, I did what I needed to do in order to stay alive. Even then I barely made the grade.

My new goals were to slip back into society and forget about the traumas of Vietnam: an impossibility in consideration of the issues that now troubled me: multiple wounds, scars, and disabilities.

As I entered the workplace, I quickly realized that I was unprepared to meet the physical challenges that faced me. But face them I did.

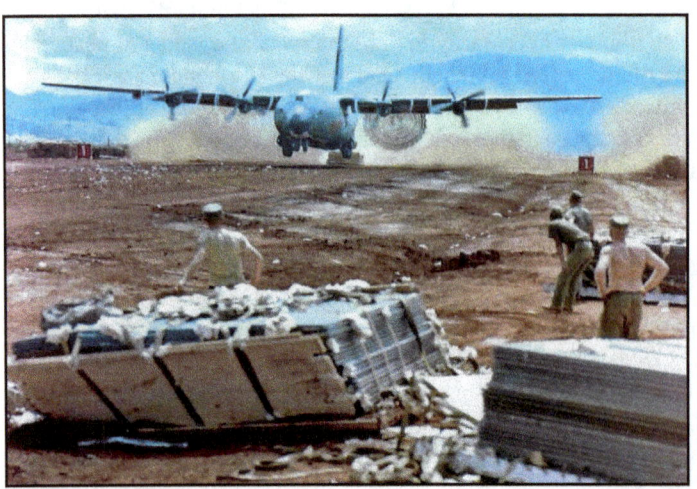

Beleaguered marines receive supplies from aircraft that dare not land, else it will get shot to pieces from enemy soldiers that surround the marine compound. Instead of landing, aircraft performs a touch-and-go by reducing speed to a minimum with the help of a parachute, then pushing crates out of the rear of the cargo compartment.
(Archival photo.)

Part 3
Civilian Life

Although I had a bundle of money, I did not have enough to continue my college education. I had to earn a living, so I went to work as an electrician. I joined Local 98 of the International Brotherhood of Electrical Workers.

I never regained the state of physical fitness that I had before my military induction. Near the end of each workday, I was totally exhausted. I struggled to work the last few hours. I sometimes affected a limp, but as soon as I became aware of it, I put extra effort into my stride so that no one would notice my unnatural gate.

My bad leg ached mildly in the morning. The pain worsened throughout the day. By quitting time, the pain had aggravated to a burning sensation from hip to toes as if my entire leg was on fire.

I tried very hard not to keep up my pace on my way to the el (elevated train). When the train doors opened, I dashed through the crowd in order to grab a seat, preferably a window seat on the left side of the car: that so I could rest my foot on the metal lip that extended along the wall a foot or so above the floor. This bent knee position offered a modicum of relief.

Pregnant women, get out of my way. If I was already seated and a woman was hanging onto a ceiling strap next to me, unlike in my college days when I offered my seat to a lady, now I ignored women altogether. My pain exceeded my chivalry.

At home, I limped into the living room and lay down on the sofa where I placed my leg on the backrest. Within minutes, I felt the pain pouring out of my foot and leg like water pouring out of a tipped-over glass. Ten minutes later I was ready to face the evening. Not only was the severe pain completely gone, but it didn't return until the next day.

I can't explain it; I can only write it the way it occurred.

I suffered this daily pain for the next ten years.

My bad arm was not very strong at the time of my discharge. In order to strengthen it, whenever I had to pick up or carry something heavy, I used my left hand.

Worse than my arm was my shoulder. As long as my arm was hanging down, the pain was hardly noticeable. If I worked with my hands in front of me – say, installing a switch or receptacle – the pain was minimal. But when I lifted my arm more than 90 degrees, after several minutes my shoulder started to ache.

I could endure this ache for no longer than a minute or two before I had to drop my arm along my side and rest it for a while. If I was working on the floor, I moved to the nearest doorway where I could lean over and press the muscle between my shoulder blade and my neck against the edge of a door jamb. This pressure helped to alleviate the pain in a few seconds, although I did not get total relief for half a minute.

If I was working on a ladder, I let my arm dangle freely and used the forefinger and thumb of my right hand to squeeze (not massage) the aching muscle.

The most painful jobs I had were hanging overhead fixtures and making splices in ceiling junction boxes.

One time, while I was an apprentice on a 38-story office building in downtown Philly, I was running EMT (electrical metallic tubing) across a concrete ceiling that

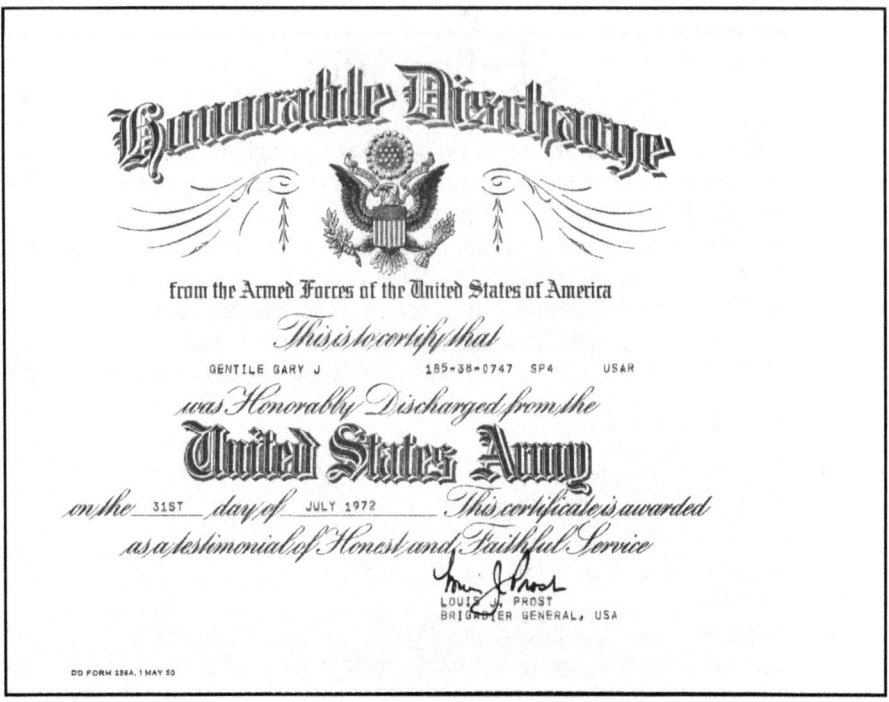

My personal emancipation proclamation. Note that I was promoted from rank E3 (Private first class) to rank E4 (either Corporal or Specialist) shortly prior to my release from prison, er, Army (same thing). Note, too, that my discharge certificate was dated July 31, 1972. I was freed from the Army hospital on August 5, 1968. I suspect that July 31 referred to the date on which my discharge certificate was signed. If you read the fine print, the true term of service was 6 years, not 2. The full term of service called for 2 years of active duty, followed by 4 years of inactive duty. This means that I was not permanently discharged in 1968, but only pardoned (placed on inactive duty). I could be called back to active duty at any time on a moment's notice until July 31, 1972. During inactive duty, a soldier remained in "reserve." Reserve status required a reservist to attend monthly meetings, and to serve 2 weeks of active duty every year until the terminal date of service . . . except that (in the finer print) he could be recalled to active duty in times of (declared?) war. The only true time at which a reservist may no longer be recalled to active duty under any circumstances was DOD (date of death), better known as RIP. As you can see, despite my scars, disabilities, and loss of height, I have not lost my sense of humor.

had been sprayed with water-soaked asbestos. EMT is like pipe except that the metal wall was thinner and the ends were not threaded; one length was connected to the next one with a slip-on metal tube that was secured by a pair of bolts. The first job that I had to do was to chop or scrape off the asbestos that was now dried to a powder. I constantly inhaled the floating asbestos dust. I made a track through the asbestos where the EMT had to be secured.

A metal strap was used to secure a length of EMT to a wall or ceiling. The strap was shaped like a question mark. The curved part of the strap fitted halfway around the EMT, and a heavy-duty nail was hammered through a hole in the flat part of the strap, and into the wall or ceiling.

I secured the straps by using a Hilti gun. A Hilti gun was an electric tool that used a .22 cartridge (without a bullet) to shoot a nail into concrete. This system enabled me to hold the strap onto the EMT for only a few seconds before I shot the nail in place. The job was moving along quickly with relatively little pain in my shoulder until the shop steward wandered by and saw what I was doing.

The shop steward was a pain in the neck – or some other body part that was halfway down his body – who made sure that union rules and regulations were being followed to a T. He watched me shoot a strap, then told me to get down off the ladder. He told me that apprentices were not allowed to use a Hilti gun. What ensued was an argument that eventually involved the boss (of more than a hundred electricians) and my pusher. (In the electrical union, a pusher was a sub-boss (similar to a squad leader) who was in charge of a small group of electricians, say, six to ten. Not to be confused with a drug pusher.)

A heated argument ensued. In my defense, I told them that I was trained to shoot everything from handguns to automatic rifles to machine guns to grenade launchers to anti-tank weapons. I had never fired a weapon whose bullet was as small as .22 caliber. And I had fired more rounds in the Army than everyone else on the job had fired in a lifetime. I was way overqualified to handle a Hilti gun.

Nonetheless, the bosses ceded the argument and the shop steward got his way.

Now I had to secure the strap by chiseling a hole in the concrete by hand, using a star drill and a hammer, then hammering a threaded lead cinch into the hole, and then screwing a quarter-twenty bolt through the hole in the strap.

I had to do all this work with my arms stretched upward, stopping occasionally to let the pain drain from my bad shoulder.

It took me ten minutes of laborious hammering to do what a mechanic could do in five seconds by picking up a Hilti gun and squeezing the trigger. How absurd.

I had nothing against hard work. In fact, I liked hard work. I just didn't like painful work.

A hard-headed shop steward and overhead working conditions were not all that I had to endure. Read on.

The Civilian War

Getting back to civilian life meant more than going to work and earning a living. It meant dealing with people who blamed veterans for the conduct of the war. At least now I could wear civilian clothing in order to avoid the stigma of the Army uniform. Civies protected my identity as a Vietnam veteran.

Parading as a sheep in wolf's clothing did not afford total anonymity. Neighborhood people knew who I was, as did friends of my friends who were strangers to me. Thus word got around that a baby killer was on the loose. This American attitude toward Vietnam veterans led to a certain amount of emotional distancing.

I was not impervious to the vocalizations of college students that I saw on television but I did not take it personally, because I was not being confronted in person. They and their opinions were remote, like movie characters.

What did bother me were the sneers of passing persons, especially those who muttered unintelligibly under their breath – as if they were afraid of offending me out loud for fear that I might retaliate. I never did. Well, almost.

On occasion I did hear the words that they were uttering, but those individuals were careful not to be looking in my direction when they spoke – as if they were children counting coup on their parents.

And I did get spit *at* but never *on*. Again, these expectorations were never made in my direction. Many veterans whom I met throughout the years have been subjected to situations that were similar to mine. Some were worse.

Now for the almost.

By and large, construction workers did not hold veterans responsible for the Vietnam conflict. This is not to say that they supported the war. It means that they knew that draftees were not responsible for being drafted, and that there was no need to blame them for the conduct of the war.

During my ten years in construction, I had trouble with only one construction worker: a fellow electrician. To be fair, this particular trouble was not motivated by my status as a veteran, but by his thoughtlessness of my situation with regard to the draft.

I was a third-year apprentice when this altercation occurred. Several of us were in a room where electrical panels were being installed. The journeymen (mechanics) were discussing placement of the panels when one of them took over by telling the others the best way to proceed. In the course of the conversation, he said, "We'll get the kid to" do something I don't remember.

This guy was three inches taller and thirty pounds heavier than I was. At quitting time, I approached him as he was getting into his car. I don't remember my exact words, but it went something like this. "You should know that I'm older than you. The only reason you're a journeyman and I'm still an apprentice is because you joined the union right out of high school, while I went to college, got drafted, and was sent to Vietnam. So while you were getting coffee for the mechanics, I was fighting with guns and grenades in the jungle."

I didn't raise my voice or speak aggressively. But I was firm. "So don't ever call me 'kid' again."

He could have knocked me down, but didn't. He could have yelled at me, but didn't. He could have apologized, but didn't. But he never called me 'kid' again.

The Worst Cut of All

My wife liked to be the center of attention. I was quiet and retiring. At parties she liked to hog the dance floor. I didn't dance. She liked to ridicule me in public. I stood up for it but only to a point.

The consuming Vietnam conflict was a common topic at the time. Two guys in my gang were serving in Vietnam. Others were in fear of being drafted. One of my cousins had gone into hiding in Canada. And I was still limping from my combat wounds.

This next revelation may be difficult for my readers to believe, but at one party she stood up in the middle of the crowd and shouted, "Here's Gary." She waved her arms over her head. "Shoot me! Shoot me! So I can go home."

She was the only one who thought it was funny. Yet despite my telling her how much her performance hurt me, she continued to give it at other parties and get-togethers. She didn't seem to care about how much pain I had suffered, as if the hospital was a military spa where soldiers went to celebrate and have a good time.

She continued to express her uncaring attitude until I filed for divorce. By then it was too late to make amends.

Concealment

My status as a Vietnam veteran, especially while the war was still ongoing, led to me being shunned when people learned about my monstrous past. I didn't understand this attitude. I still don't. Eventually I just learned to live with it.

I kept my seedy past a secret. So well did I maintain this secrecy – as well as other Vietnam veterans did the same – that only until a few months ago did I learn that a man I have known for more than thirty years was also a Vietnam veteran. Nor did George Place know that I was a Vietnam veteran until I made a Facebook posting about the poor medical treatment that I received from the Wilkes-Barre VA Medical Center. (More on that later. Much more.)

Even more secretive than I was about my military past was how reticent I was about my pain and disabilities. I did not mention these debilitating conditions to anyone, because to do so would lead to questions about how I obtained them. Even some people who knew about my Vietnam veteran status did not know about my wounds; or if they did, they did not know how extensive my were wounds.

I kept a low profile about all my military involvement. It was the only way to avoid castigation.

Pain in General

I don't want my readers to think that I was in chronic or extraordinary pain. Pain came and went, depending upon circumstances. For example, if I had a job that was largely indoors where I was splicing wires all day in electrical panels, I might come home in extreme pain. Yet if it had a job bending and installing heavy-duty four-inch conduit outside during inclement weather, I might feel fine when I got home.

The difference was not how demanding the work was, but whether I did the job standing still or walking back and forth.

Similarly, I could backpack from dawn till dusk carrying a fifty-pound load on my back, and feel fine by the time I was ready to pitch the tent. Yet shopping for food in a supermarket for an hour would cause incredible pain in my bad leg, such that I would have to lie down with my leg elevated when I got home.

The difference was between standing still or walking slowly in what I called "shopping mode," in which I had to browse for items and determine which brand to buy, instead of walking at a normal but steady pace.

Make sense?

I don't think so, but that's the way it was.

Flashbacks

I started having flashbacks about two years after leaving the hospital. My initial flashbacks were not like any kind of flashback that I ever read about or heard discussed. I distinctly remember the first one.

I was talking with a co-worker after leaving work when an image flashed before my eyes. I don't remember the image other than that it was a picture of combat. The image lasted for only a moment, a fraction of a second. It was like a subliminal image of popcorn that psychologists claimed could be flashed to movie viewers for one frame – a sixteenth of a second – that would make them hunger for popcorn.

I continued the conversation as if I had never seen the image.

This kind of split-second flashback recurred every week or so, or twice a week, or every other week. Its occurrence was erratic.

The strange thing about it was that the flashback did not interrupt my conversation.

If it happened while someone was talking to me, I heard every word he said. If it happened while I was talking, I never missed a beat, but kept on talking as if the image had never appeared. In that sense, the flashback was not even an annoyance. It was just a happening of no consequence.

These flashbacks continued for several years: perhaps three to four. I don't even know when they stopped. I just suddenly thought about them one time, and realized that they must have stopped happening sometime in the past.

* * * * *

I had a rather upsetting flashback that was different from the "micro" flashbacks that I described above. I was hiking alone through the woods in the Poconos of Pennsylvania when I spotted a strand of wire stretching from one tree to another. Such strands like this one were not uncommon.

It has been said there are only one or two original stands of trees in the entire Commonwealth. In other words, Pennsylvania is now populated almost exclusively by second growth; or third. I've seen postcard pictures that show mountains which were completely denuded of vegetation: not only trees were missing but also the groundcover. Some of this denudation was due to strip mining, much was to do with clearing patches of farmland, but the vast majority of it was due to clear-cutting for lumber.

There is hardly any place in the woods where I now live – Jim Thorpe, a borough that was named after the early twentieth-century Olympic champion – that doesn't have stone fences; that is, long piles of rock that were removed from the ground to make it available for tilling, then stacked to create fences that enclosed farm fields. These stone fences were a couple of centuries old. Later farms used wire to make fences.

It was in one of these latter areas in which I was hiking when I spotted what looked to me like a trip wire. This thought struck me so suddenly and strongly that I came to a full stop and found myself paralyzed. My heart immediately started thumping so hard that it hurt my chest.

One part of me saw a trip wire in a jungle while the other part of me saw the remains of an ordinary wire fence on an overgrown farm field. The latter part of my mind was telling me that there were no trip wires in the woods of Pennsylvania. But the former part of my mind was staring right at it. I could not separate the two visions.

My eyesight split vertically down the middle, as if I were watching two television screens that stood side by side. I saw jungle on the left, deciduous forest on the right.

Almost a full minute later I started to breathe again. Slowly, deliberately, I bent my knees and finally knelt on the ground. Gradually I lowered myself to all fours. I crawled toward the wire. The split screen would not go away. Part of me still thought that I was back in Vietnam.

Not until I saw the thickness of the wire did I begin to accept the fact that the trip wire was an illusion. Farm fence wire was as thick as the wire used to make coat hangers, whereas trip wire was so thin that its presence was difficult to perceive.

When I looked at the trees on either side of me, I realized that they had overgrown the wire by more than an inch; that the wire was embedded in the wood. This common feature meant that many years must have passed since the wire had been nailed to the tree.

Like the hallucination that had overwhelmed me in Tokyo, when the doctor had prescribed codeine to ease my pain, reality gradually took the place of mirage. Only this time, instead of the false imagery morphing into reality, the side-by-side images

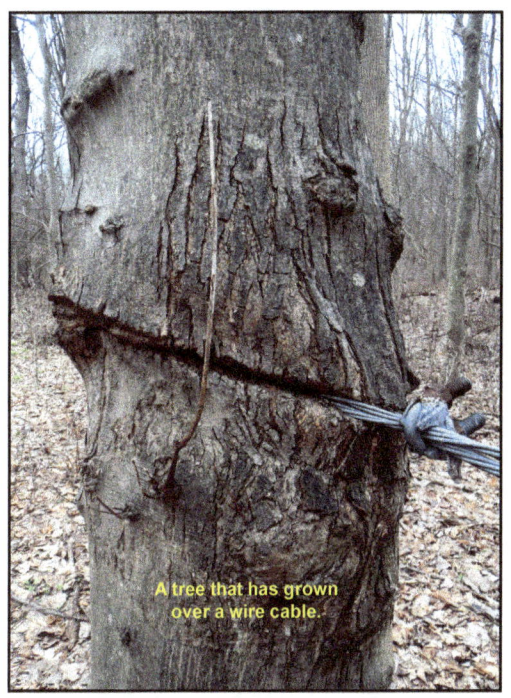
A tree that has grown over a wire cable.

gradually merged, with the real image moving over the false image until only the true image remained.

Not that I needed reminiscence, but this flashback served to remind my conscious mind that the chilling moments that I suffered in Vietnam still lurked in my subconscious memory.

Since that occasion, I've seen many wires overgrown by trees. I have photographed them often. Thankfully, I've never had another flashback like the one I have just described. At least, not yet. Better yet, when I saw an old fence wire, I recognized it for what it was without recalling that singular incident when I believed that it was trip wire. That image no longer lingers in memory.

*   *   *   *   *

Another kind of flashback has unfortunately stayed with me all my life. It started about five years after my long hospital stay.

I would go to bed after a normal day at work or any kind of activity. The trigger was pain in my bad leg. After I lay my head on the pillow in preparation for sleep, pain triggered the obvious association: memory of the reason for having the pain.

In the first scene, I perceived the muzzle flash of the bullet as it left the barrel of the AK-47. In my daydream I could see the speeding bullet as I frantically pulled the trigger of my M-16. I felt the icy penetration as the enemy bullet struck my chest; I saw it pass through my body; I watched the blood and bone exploding as the bullet exited my back . . .

In the second scene I saw the muzzle flash of the bullet as it left the barrel of the AK-47. In my daydream I could see the speeding bullet as I frantically pulled the trigger of my M-16. I felt the icy penetration as the enemy bullet struck my chest; I saw it pass through my body; I watched the blood and bone exploding as the bullet exited my back . . .

In the third scene I saw the muzzle flash . . . over and over and over for two to three hours as I constantly changed the position of my pillow and my body.

Sometimes the daydream shifted to other scenes of combat. But the first scene always returned first. Then it looped over and over until eventually I fell asleep, drained from the emotionally exhausting reruns of my near death experience.

These horrendous flashbacks have haunted me three to four times per year after year after year, ad nauseam.

Because I got so little sleep when these flashbacks occurred, I was always groggy on the morning after, and tired and sluggish throughout the following day.

Status Quo

As time passed after my hospitalization, I began to regain my strength and endurance. Electrical work helped me to overcome my handicaps, but only to a certain extent. I accepted the fact that my bad leg would always be weaker than my good leg, and that my left arm would always be weaker than my good arm. These physical disabilities manifested themselves through my various outdoor activities: hiking, biking, backpacking, canoeing, climbing, skiing, and scuba diving.

For instance, while hiking and backpacking, I always favored my right leg. As a result, my right leg grew stronger than my left leg. This difference was not as noticeable while biking. But it was more noticeable while climbing because difficult maneuvers relied on the strength and mobility of my right leg. This sometimes forced me to cross my legs in order to push up from one ledge to another.

I never became an expert skier. Whenever I jumped over a mogul, I always landed with the majority of my weight on my right leg, while my left leg barely touched the snow, thus allowing my left ski to swing from side to side above the snow. Sometimes my left ski slipped over my right ski; this led to catastrophe.

The combination of a bad ankle, a shortened left leg, and weakened left leg muscles contrived to throw me off balance.

With regard to scuba diving, climbing up the boat's ladder in rough seas always presented a problem. As the dive boat rolled or wallowed in a trough, the motion tended to throw me to the side and break my grip. It was difficult to hang onto the ladder's railing because my entire left side lacked strength. My bad ankle did not help in keeping my fins on the ladder rungs.

Ninety Foot Bridge overlooking the right-bank horse trail and Pennypack Creek. That's my Chevy Blazer in the parking lot. I used to fish in this stream when I was a kid. It was a 2-mile walk from my house, but I usually rode my bike. As an adult, the trail became my favorite jogging route.

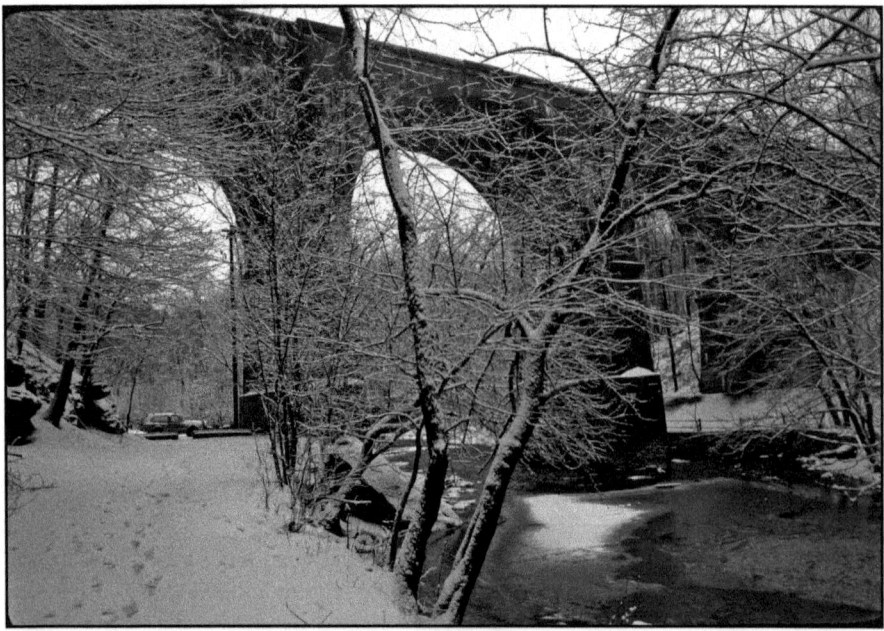

If I was doing underwater photography, I had to switch the heavy camera housing and connected strobe from my left hand to my right, then hand the camera rig to a crewmember before I attempted to climb the ladder. I had to do this because of my bad shoulder, I could not lift the weight of the camera rig above my head and out of the water, where it lost the support of buoyancy.

Lest I sound like a whiner, I had nothing but admiration for one of my dive buddies who lost one leg and part of another in Vietnam, and had to perambulate on crutches. Yet despite having worse handicaps than I had, this stalwart ex-marine still managed to scuba dive from a boat. Semper fidelis (Always faithful)! He never complained, and neither did I. We both overcame our disabilities as best we could.

Jogging Episodes

When I first got out of the Army hospital, I could not run up a flight of steps without getting out of breath. I had to pace myself even when walking fast. If I tried to hold my breath, I could not do so for more than half a minute. My damaged lung was at fault.

To overcome this handicap, I started jogging at Pennypack Park, which was located about two miles from my house. At first, I could not jog more than a hundred yards before being forced to stop due to shortness of breath. By that time I was gasping. I then walked for a hundred yards, then jogged, then walked, and so on for a mile or so.

It took a full year of jogging twice a week before I could jog for half a mile without stopping to catch my breath. And then I suffered a sharp pain in my lower left abdomen.

By the end of two years I could jog a full mile, albeit somewhat slowly.

At the end of three years I could jog for two miles by walking a mile in the middle of a three-mile route. I also lost the pain in my lower left abdomen.

At the end of three years I could jog the full three-mile route through the woods without stopping. Half of my route was on a paved bike trail; the other half was on a dirt horse path. I gave horses the right of way.

My limiting factors were twofold: loss of lung capacity because the upper left lobe consisted primarily of scar tissue, and nerve damage that resulted in atrophy of the diaphragm: the primary muscle that compressed the lung.

Despite these disabilities, I gradually worked my distance up to six-and-a-half continuous miles. This distance was predicated upon the length of the loop that brought me back to my vehicle in the parking lot on Krewstown Road. The loop started at Ninety Foot Bridge: an active railroad crossing over Pennypack Creek. I learned to scamper up the steep dirt slope, then dash across the bridge when no trains were in evidence. I did not run between the rails because the space was filled with loose rocks which caused my ankle to bend and twist. Instead, I ran along the concrete verge where I planted my feet less than a foot away from the drop-off, while looking down at the water that flowed 90 feet below. A stumble could be fatal.

Then came two miles of horse trail followed by a mile or so of paved bike trail to my turnaround, where I jogged across the bridge on Pine Road, then continued for three more miles on a single-track horse trail back to Ninety Foot Bridge.

Not only was this route physically challenging, but it was mentally therapeutic by enabling my mind to wander about ongoing events. After I changed occupations, my mind usually wandered about the writing projects that I was presently creating. I wrote

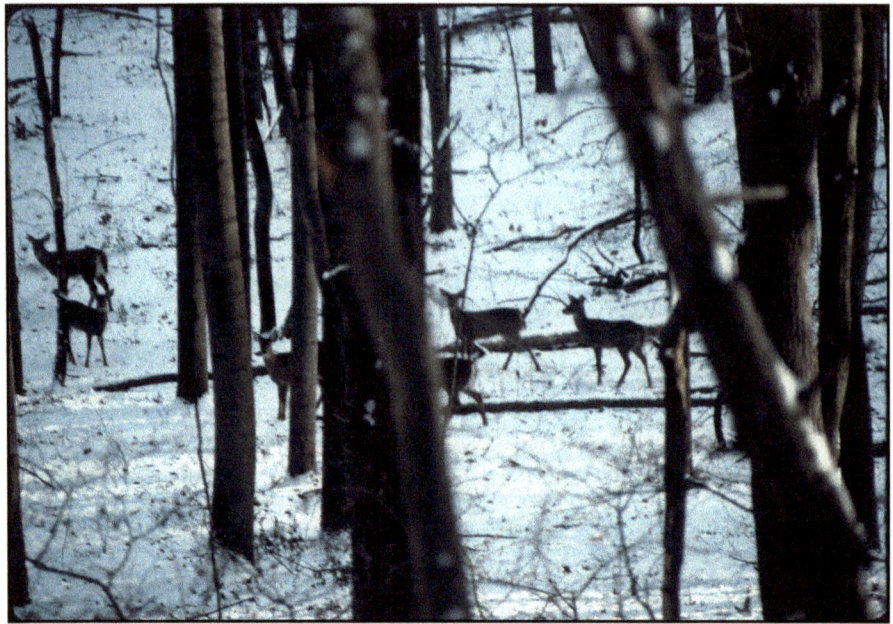

Pennypack Park had its own herds of white-tail deer. They were protected by Philadelphia's ordinance against the discharge of firearms within city limits. After winter snowstorms, I often spotted deer while cross-country skiing in the park. I knew where they congregated - away from trails where they wouldn't be bothered by humans. When I skied toward the herd, they stood up and danced away. I kept skiing after them; they kept moving. They knew Penn's Woods so well that they described a 2-mile circle that brought them back to their sleeping grounds, where I parted ways and skiied back to my Blazer. I called this routine "taking the deer for a walk."

entire paragraphs in my head which, as soon as I got home, I transcribed onto a note pad or typed on a sheet of paper.

One time I "woke up" on the trail without knowing where I was. I wasn't actually lost because I was still on the trail, but I didn't know where on the trail I was jogging at that moment.

My top speed was seven minutes per mile. This was shameful in comparison with Olympic runners, who ran a mile in 4 minutes, and maintained a pace 5 minutes per mile for 26 miles! I was humbled.

Nonetheless, I felt invigorated by my six-and-a-half-mile loop through the woods. It exercised not only the diaphragm, but it exercised the damaged muscles in my bad leg.

Now for the downside. While this weekly exercise was helpful for my state of health, in consideration of my combat wounds and resulting disabilities, there were also problems associated with my jogging regimen (plus my bike riding interludes). This may be a little offtrack, but come along for the ride. Jogging has built-in hazards.

Sometimes, rather than drive to Pennypack Park, I elected to jog to and through the park and come back to my house by a different route. This was especially true during the first few weeks of fishing season, and on nice summer weekends when families enjoyed picnicking: both of which were legitimate uses of the park. But they did create a parking problem.

Philly streets were warzones for walkers, joggers, and bikers. At least a dozen times in my life I've been nearly run down by vehicles on streets that did not have sidewalks. Some drivers liked to scare people by seeing how close they could get to them without actually hitting them.

Before you blame teenagers for playing this deadly game of near missing pedestrians, know that although teenagers did sometimes shout and wave their hands as their car passed by me, never did they come close enough to put me in danger. They were just having joyous times. Adults were the ones who came the closest to knocking me down – and this after making eye contact. Their intentions were definitely criminal.

One time, a carful of four female senior citizens crossed two lanes of traffic in an attempt to do me bodily harm. I stepped over the curb and onto the grass before they reached me. This was why I always jogged while facing traffic: so I could see those drivers who wanted to play touch football, or tackle, or worse.

Once while riding my bike in a sudden thunderstorm, I decided that it would be less dangerous to get off the wet and slippery road onto the empty sidewalk. No sooner did I reach the so-called safety of the sidewalk than a woman turned off the street in front of me and nearly ran me down as she bounced her car over the curb and sidewalk, then sped away across a parking lot and out the other side.

Twice on my bike I have been struck by a car and knocked completely over the curb and onto the ground. Both times the car then accelerated to get away without stopping to see if I was hurt.

Another time I was on a weekend paddling trip down the Delaware River with a large group from the Mohawk Canoe Club, of which I was a member. We camped on shore overnight. I arose early on Sunday morning and decided to go for a jog before breakfast. Only one other person was awake; because her husband was still cuddled cozily in his sleeping bag, she elected to come along with me. A dirt path led through a grove of trees to a rural paved road with single family dwellings on either side.

No vehicles were in motion. As we passed one house we heard barking, followed by a 40-pound dog that was charging full-speed toward us. We each reacted instinctively. (I apologize in advance for sounding sexist, but this is exactly the way the incident proceeded.) She dashed behind me for protection while I stepped in front of her as her guard.

The dog leaped into the air, aiming its gaping mouth straight at my throat. At the last moment, I swung my fist upward and smacked the dog on the chin. The dog did a full gainer, turning 360 degrees backward in the air. As it slammed into the hardtop, I lifted my right leg in preparation for a kick. The dog shook its head, struggled up onto its paws, then turned and limped away.

On our return along the road, as we passed the same house, the dog came racing across the lawn, saw who we were, screeched to a halt like a cartoon character, whimpered, and, lesson learned, trotted back to the house.

My worst incident occurred on a cold winter night after a freak snowstorm dropped twenty inches of snow on the ground and Philly streets. The sidewalks were piled with drifts that were too deep to negotiate. I jogged on streets that had been swept clean by snowplows. When a plow pushed snow off the street, it couldn't help but to leave a strip of snow between lanes.

As I jogged on one street on which cars were parked on both sides next to the curb, the beams of a pair of headlights swept across me from behind when a car turned onto the street from the intersection that I had just passed. I was jogging in the lane next to the park cars. The car was in the adjacent lane.

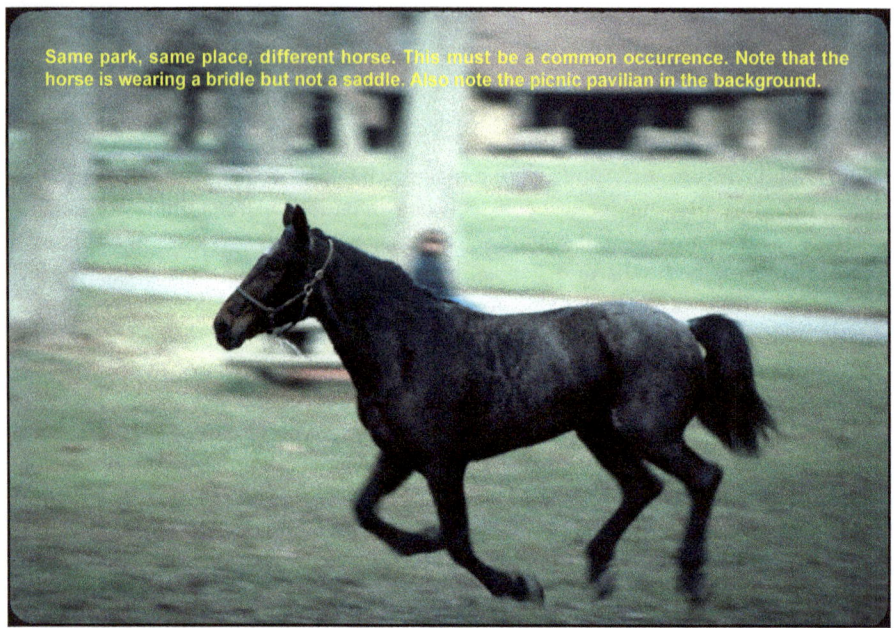

Same park, same place, different horse. This must be a common occurrence. Note that the horse is wearing a bridle but not a saddle. Also note the picnic pavilian in the background.

    I was always on the alert for all sights and sounds. As the car approached me quietly from behind, I heard the telltale crunch of snow as the tires rode over the strip of unplowed snow between lanes. I have fast reflexes and reaction time. I glanced over my shoulder and swiveled my hip as the car crashed into me. The hip-swivel saved me from getting my pelvis and previously broken femur shattered by the headlight.

    The fender struck the scar where my femur had been broken, and knocked me sideways. Although the snow-bound cars were parked bumper to bumper, I was thrust aside at the only place on the block where there was a three-foot gap between cars. Had I been knocked against the side of a car, my body would have rebounded to the car that hit me, where I would likely have been run over by the rear tire.

    As it was, I was thrown to the side where I landed on the curb. I jumped up and ran after the perpetrator, but he or she drove through the red light at the end of the street and accelerated away from me.

    After the adrenaline wore off, the pain set in. I leaned against a parked car until the pain became endurable, then limped the rest of the way home.

    Jogging on the Pennypack Park trails was relatively safe. I tripped a few times on rocks or roots, but my college judo training kicked in so fast that I always hit the ground on my shoulder and rolled with the momentum. I had only two minor incidents from the hundreds of times that I jogged along those trails.

    The first one occurred when I saw a woman get thrown off her horse at the picnic pavilion next to Verree Road. She hit the ground hard. Unencumbered, the horse bolted for the barn. It ran to the trail, then turned in my direction as if it knew the way to go – which I am certain it did. I stopped on the other side of a bridge that crossed a small tributary. The horse ran full speed straight toward me.

    A woman with whom I used to ride horseback once told me that horses will always try to get out of the way of a person because they did not like to step on them. Either she was mistaken or this charging horse had not read the same book about polite equestrianism. I stood in the horse's way and waved my arms frantically. Just before it ran me down, I stepped aside and tried to grab the bridle or the reins. Fortunately I missed the grab; if I had succeeded with the grab, I would have been lifted off my feet and dragged along the trail until I either disentangled myself or was scraped into oblivion. This horse must have had nothing but oats on its mind; I never saw it slow down.

The equestrienne brushed dirt off her clothing. She told me angrily that she was unhurt. The barn was several miles away. There was nothing that I could do to help her, so I continued on my way.

Another time at the same picnic area, on a summer day that was exceptionally hot, instead of staying on the trail, I veered toward the stream where families were picnicking. I whipped off my sleeveless T-shirt, slapped it into the water, then donned it without slowing down or missing a step. My purpose was to beat the heat through evaporative cooling.

As I passed by the picnickers, I saw a flock of Canada geese that was perched lazily on the ground, and one hobnosed goose that was honking and chasing people. Children were running and screaming while mothers and fathers did their best to protect them from the aggressive goose.

A few days later I repeated my routine of soaking my T-shirt at the picnic grounds. No sooner did I don the shirt than the goose ran straight toward me, squawking aloud. It was hunched over in its typical harassment posture: neck stretched forward and wings fluttering. Its snapping beak was aimed at my crotch. Without missing a beat, I swung my hand upward and slapped the goose so hard in the throat that its head was knocked backward and slammed into its tail feathers. I kept jogging.

Another few days later I again repeated my T-shirt routine. The hobnosed goose squawked as it ran toward me . . . only this time it must have recognized me, because

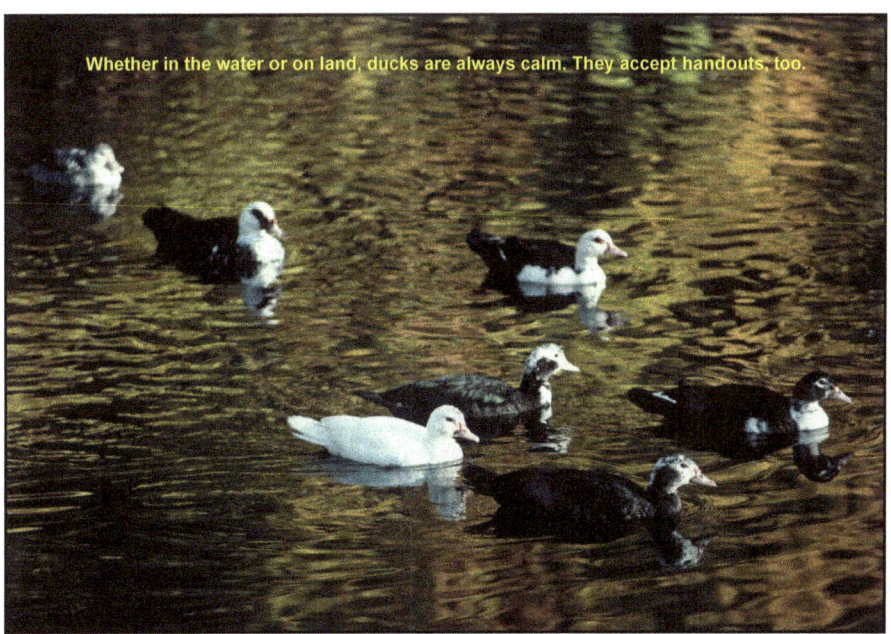
Whether in the water or on land, ducks are always calm. They accept handouts, too.

it skidded to a stop, quit squawking, and watched me pass.

Yet another few days later, the picnic area was mysteriously quiet. Children were running and playing, adults were sitting on blankets, Canada geese paid no nevermind, and the hobnosed goose was sitting by itself. As I jogged past the latter goose, it opened its mouth, whispered a plaintive quack that sounded more like a peep, did not even rise from its perch.

In just those few encounters, I had changed the goose's entire behavior pattern. It never caused any trouble ever again. It was tamed.

Kayaking, Not

I started canoeing in 1969, when I was a first-year apprentice. On one of my jobs I worked with a mechanic named Ronnie. (I don't recall his surname.) He introduced me to Joe Volk, an experienced canoeist who belonged to the Mohawk Canoe Club. Joe gave me my first instructions on how to paddle a canoe. He and I became lifetime friends.

After ten years of canoeing, I wanted to try kayaking so I could paddle whitewater and more challenging waves than I was able to paddle in an open boat.

My Mohawk Canoe Club friend Walt Daub was a kayak instructor. Along with several other club members, I took his training course so as to learn and perfect the Eskimo roll. We had a mixed class of men and women. In order to roll a kayak, a paddler must press his or her knees against the inside of the hull while stretching his or her feet against the pedals. This outward pressure locked the paddler in the cockpit so that swinging the hips moved the boat from side to side.

We practiced in a swimming pool. One person gyrated the boat while another person acted as safety in case the boater got stuck upside down in the water and was unable to find the ball that pulled off the skirt, which enabled the boater to escape from the boat.

We all felt proficient by the end of the course. Walt's students organized a kayaking trip down the Lehigh River, which all of us had already paddled many times by canoe.

The trip started well in comparatively smooth water. The farther we paddled downstream, the larger the waves became. Stretches of rapids grew longer and longer. This was when I learned that when I had to spread my legs against the hull while pressing my feet against the pedals, for a long period of time, my left leg started to ache.

Soon the pain got so bad that I was forced to remove my left leg from the pedal and let it hang limp inside the boat. These rest periods allowed the pain to subside until the next set of rapids. Even under these severe circumstances, when I got knocked over by a large standing wave, I was able to roll the kayak upright on my very first try.

After each stretch of whitewater I was in agony. Shooting pains engulfed my bad leg from hip to toes. My entire leg felt as if it were on fire. The pain increased with each passage through pounding waves until finally the river did not offer enough flatwater stretches to rest my leg and reduce the pain to a manageable level before I entered the next rapid.

To make matters worse, my bad shoulder started aching. This seldom happened when I canoed. Canoeing was different from kayaking in that a canoeist wields a single-bladed paddle, whereas a kayaker uses a double-bladed paddle.

A canoeist paddled from a kneeling position in which one arm was low while the

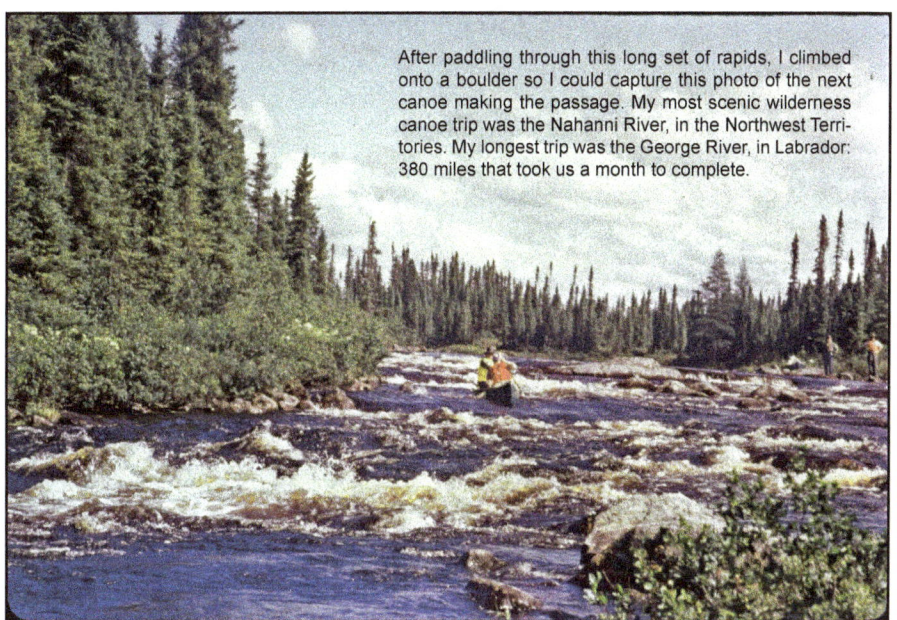

After paddling through this long set of rapids, I climbed onto a boulder so I could capture this photo of the next canoe making the passage. My most scenic wilderness canoe trip was the Nahanni River, in the Northwest Territories. My longest trip was the George River, in Labrador: 380 miles that took us a month to complete.

other arm was high. Because of my shoulder wound, I always paddled "left;" that is, with my paddle on the left side of the canoe where my left arm hung down. In that position I could paddle for hours – indeed, all day, on multiweek wilderness trips. Also, in a kneeling position, my bad leg usually did not reach the point where it started to ache; and if it did ache, I could change the position of my legs, how they were bent, and how I sat.

This 25-mile-long trip became one of unbearable torture.

Near the end came the Rock Garden: a mile and a half stretch of solid whitewater with only one rest stop along the way. The Upper Rock Garden measured half a mile in length. Then the river turned sharply to the left. At this point there was a calm eddy on the right. I sat there and stretched my leg until all my fellow paddlers had passed me.

I don't know how I made it through the mile-long-stretch without fainting from the pain. There was no rest stop in the Lower Rock Garden. Once I entered the rapids there was no turning back, and no place to pull over. An expert kayaker could make a hard turn behind a boulder in order to rest in the eddy. But I was no expert.

I had to ignore the burning pain and concentrate on paddling through the biggest boulder field on the entire river. If I flipped over and was dumped out of the boat, I would have had sto swim the rest of the way through mounds of mountainous whitewater.

Somehow, I managed to paddle through the horrendous rapids without rolling over. The group was waiting for me at the bottom of the rapids. After a short respite, during which time the pain slowly diminished as I caught my gasping breath, I paddled the last couple of miles to the take-out in Jim Thorpe.

That solitary trip convinced me that, due to my disabilities, kayaking was not for me. I sold my kayak and went back to canoeing.

Job Change

I was no longer an apprentice. In 1973, I graduated from apprentice school and became a full mechanic.

Construction workers of all trades constantly worked themselves out of a job. When a job was completed, a union member visited the union hall in order to seek other employment. If jobs were available, he could choose any job he wanted. If jobs were not available, he got at the end of the line, behind the other unemployed members.

In the 1970's, new construction in Philadelphia reached its lowest ebb in decades. Nearly half the union members were "on the bench" (unemployed), with little hope of improvement in the foreseeable future. In 1976, I joined the long line of bench warmers.

But I had a plan. I had decided to become an author. This notion originated in eleventh grade, when my English teacher told the class that if anyone wanted extra credit, and wrote a short story or article or poem, he would increase his or her report card grade by one full letter. For example, on my midterm report card I received a B; if I wrote something, he would give me an A.

I wrote a short science fiction story that I called "The Nothing." It was 47 double-spaced pages long (16,000 words). I think the teacher was as astonished by the length as he was about the story. I got my A.

During summer vacation I wrote a pastiche of Jules Vernes' *A Journey to the Center of the Earth*. My version was 76,000 words in length, against Vernes' 86,000 words. In my version, the explorers actually reached the center of the Earth. In Vernes' version, they never got deeper than a hundred miles.

While I still had a fulltime job, I bought an electric typewriter and a how-to-type book, and practiced every night after work.

For the next three years, I alternately worked as an electrician when a job was available, or practiced writing while I eked out a living on unemployment benefits. In 1979, I started working fulltime as an author. The volume that you are holding in your hands is my 70th book.

Life Gets Better

I started my writing career by sitting on a chair in front of a typewriter on a table. I soon learned that this position became painful after a short while of writing. The problem was twofold.

Anytime I sat on a chair – any chair, anytime – I could not assume a normal posture for very long. This was because when the back side of my bad leg rested on the front edge of the seat, the weight of my leg pressed against the damaged sciatic nerve. In addition to that, the weight of my upper body pressed the scar on my left buttock on the cushion.

The only way I could sit comfortably was to slouch. I did this by sitting on my spine and leaning my body to the right, so that my left buttock was slightly off the cushion. This may sound uncomfortable to you but for me it was normal. This peculiar posture was mostly hidden by my clothes so that observers didn't notice it.

If I was going to write for a long time, I would have to elevate my leg. I accomplished this by resting the heel of my foot on a bookshelf so that my foot was higher than my hip. Then I twisted my body 45 degrees to the left so I could face the typewriter. This unusual posture became my standard working carriage for the rest of my life.

Try it! You might like it.

Every author has his style of writing. A number of well-known authors wrote while standing. I was forced to adapt my writing posture to accommodate my combat wounds and scars.

But the best was yet to come. The chronic pain in my bad leg gradually diminished until it became tolerable. I still had twinges, and certain ways of walking still aggravated my aches and pains, but by and large my leg pain was nearly gone. This was because I didn't have to stand still most of the day as I did when I worked as an electrician.

This unanticipated benefit enabled me to concentrate on my writing instead of being distracted by constant discomfort. Add to this the strengthening of my muscles, and I literally became a new man. Not as good as one whose body wasn't riddled with bullet wounds, but a whole lot better than I had been for a decade and a half of torture.

Strange as it might sound, on long drives I still had to rest my left leg on the dashboard. But as soon as I reached my destination, and stood up and walked, the pain diminished to its normal state of annoyance.

I still hugged my bad leg to my chest when I sat, not necessarily because it relieved any pain, but because it made my leg feel better. If this sounds like a contradiction, think of it as a form of stretching. When people stretch after they get out of bed in the morning, it doesn't mean that they were in pain; yet they feel better after stretching. Comprende?

Fifteen Years Later

I got out of bed early on a cool April morning in 1985, eager to go diving off the New Jersey coast. On the way to the shore, I stopped at a doughnut shop to buy coffee and a doughnut. The shop was on the opposite side of the highway. When there was a break in the traffic, I leaped over the concrete barrier that separated the eastbound lanes from the westbound lanes.

What followed was nearly a repetition of that day in Vietnam when I jumped out of the way of an enemy grenade. I landed wrong on my left ankle and fell flat onto the macadam. This scenario was nearly as deadly as a grenade. Before I could be hit by a speeding vehicle, I quickly jumped up and ran – or rather, limped – toward the shoulder of the road.

I knew exactly what had happened: I had broken the tendon that had been transplanted from my leg to my ankle. The pain was considerable.

I bought my coffee and doughnut, then continued to the shore. My fellow divers assisted me in loading my tanks and gear onto the boat. During the ride offshore, I examined my ankle and saw that it was badly swollen.

Once on site and in the water, the pain increased with every kick: pushing myself through the water made the fin on the bad ankle twist and turn. It was agony.

Doctors always say to put ice on a sprain. The water temperature was 48 degrees; it didn't ease the pain at all. The worst pain came when I had to climb aboard the boat by putting my weight on the ladder rungs.

By the time I got home, the pain had increased considerably. Aspirin didn't help. Neither did acetaminophen. They were the only pain killers that I had in the medicine cabinet. I slept okay, and the next morning I was not in much pain . . . until I started walking. Then the ankle ached somewhat, but not so bad that I couldn't endure it.

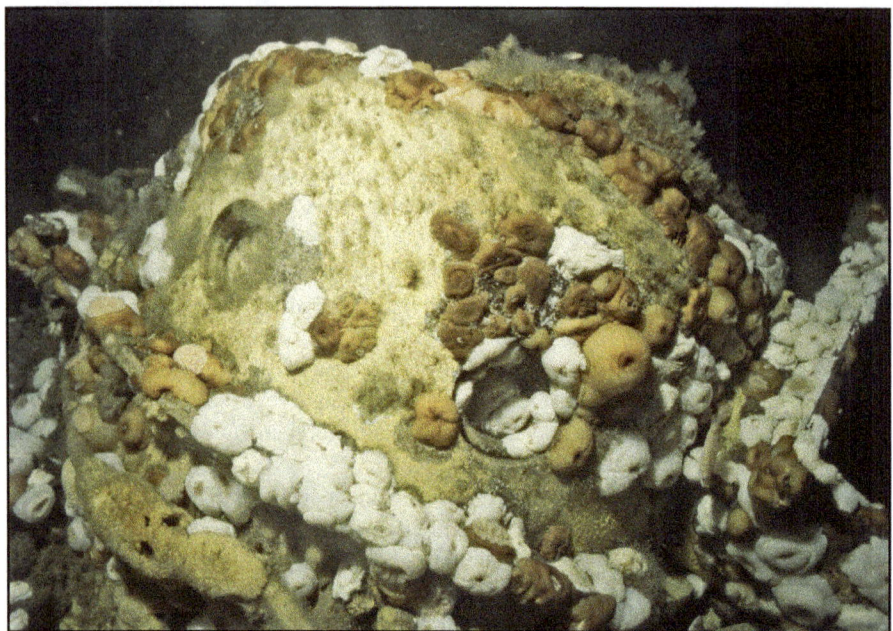

The dive that I made that day was worth the effort and pain. It was my first dive on the recently discovered *S-5*, an American submarine that sank in 1920. Above is a photo of the conning tower. Note the windows. When I was a kid, my father used to tell me that before he joined the Army, he was in the Navy and served on submarines. But he got thrown out because he slept with the windows open. The *S-5*'s conning tower was not enclosed as it is in modern submarines. The aft end was so that the conning tower flooded upon submergence; thus the *S-5*'s conning tower was actually a spray shield.

Because I now worked sitting, I was able to process words as if nothing had happened to my ankle. By the following day the pain was pretty much gone. I treaded lightly on the floor.

This was my first underwater excursion of the diving season. Although I knew that my ankle needed medical attention, I ignored that fact. By the end of the week I was ready to go diving again. Diving was no longer a hobby for me. Because I was writing a series of shipwreck guides, it was part of my occupation. I needed to survey shipwrecks in the summer so I could write about them in the winter.

Throughout the summer I suffered a number of falls when my ankle gave way and I was unable to save myself. The only time the ankle hurt badly was when it twisted. Otherwise, I was not too discomforted.

Because the injury to my ankle was one of my Vietnam casualties, I figured that I could have it treated by the local Veterans Hospital, in Philadelphia, on the opposite side of the city from where I lived. In October, near the conclusion of the dive season, I called the hospital and described the issue with my bad ankle.

The gal who answered the phone said, "Come on in any time. We've got your records on file."

I arrived at the hospital at 9 o'clock the following morning. I gave my name to the receptionist. She gave me a single-page form to fill out. Half an hour later, a doctor entered the lobby and called my name. I raised my hand. He escorted me to his office where he asked me to explain my condition.

After I told him how my ankle had been damaged initially, and about the Watson-

Jones repair, he gently flexed my ankle. He could feel the looseness of the joint. The first thing he said was that he needed to obtain an X-ray of the ankle. Then he added that as long as I was in the hospital, why not do a full workup and take X-rays of my other wounds as well. I agreed.

The doctor escorted me to another floor where the X-ray lab was located. Lab assistants helped me get into various positions for an assortment of X-rays. Afterward, they showed the X-rays to me. The doctor indicated the places where holes had been drilled through the bones for the Watson-Jones repair.

What interested me more was the chest X-ray. A black smudge about the size of my palm covered the upper left part of my ribcage: scar tissue in the place where the enemy bullet had penetrated my lung. No wonder I had trouble breathing.

After various other tests – temperature, blood pressure, and so on – the doctor made an appointment for several weeks later. In the meantime, he planned to go over my medical records and the new X-rays, and determine the best course of treatment. He told me definitively, no jogging.

I returned a few weeks later. In his office, the doctor told me what he had learned about ankle operations. No matter which method was used, the healing time would be six months: two months in a non-walking plaster cast, two months wearing a steel brace which would be secured to the outside of a shoe, and two months wearing an inflatable brace around my ankle but inside a shoe.

There was a new procedure in which the ankle could be stabilized by means of threading a synthetic plastic string through the existing holes in the bones around my ankle. The downside of this procedure was that the lifespan of the string was only one year. This meant that I would need a new operation every year, followed by six months enduring the healing process.

The doctor was quick to add that he did not recommend this procedure. Both of us laughed.

Although my outside tendon had already been used in the Watson-Jones repair, there was still a way to utilize a living tendon transplant by using a tendon from the inside of my leg. This would require drilling another hole through the leg bone in order to thread the tendon to the inside of my leg, then through the other existing holes. This was his ideal suggestion.

But, this procedure might not be possible because the inside tendon was not always thick enough to provide the strength that was needed to stabilize the ankle. The thickness of that tendon varied among individuals.

If the inside tendon were not thick enough, then it would require utilizing a free-floating tendon from my upper leg. The disadvantage of removing a tendon from elsewhere was that the tendon would no longer be alive; that is, as I understood the situation, whereas a living tendon was "fed" by the body from the end that was still attached, a free-floating tendon was basically a "dead" tendon, which might not last as long as a tendon that was kept alive by being attached at one end.

As long as the tendon was one of my own, whether it was dead or alive, there was no issue with respect to organic rejection.

There was no way to know in advance how to proceed until the surgeon cut into my leg and examined the inside tendon. He had to be prepared for all eventualities in case he had to conduct the operation "on the fly."

I didn't mind working on the fly as an electrician, but I can't say that I was all that enthusiastic about having a surgeon work on the fly on my body. Nonetheless, the doctor and I agreed on a date in December, about two weeks before Christmas. I trod lightly until then.

Operation Gary

On Monday of the operation, I took public transportation to the Philly VA hospital: first by bus, then by el, and finally by subway. I checked in with the receptionist, then sat in the lobby and read a book. The doctor arrived a few minutes later. He told me that everything was on schedule. Well, not everything.

The receptionist would not let the doctor take me away until she received the paperwork to officially admit me to the hospital. This took *hours*. The doctor kept checking with me and the receptionist, but the paperwork was lost somewhere in VA officialdom. Noon came and went, yet my admission papers were still on hold.

The doctor was frantic. There were pre-operation tests that had to be performed before the labs closed for the day, such as blood work and X-rays. If these tests were not completed, the operation had to be postponed and rescheduled. I was getting antsy because I was famished. I missed lunch.

Finally, about midafternoon, I was released to the doctor's care. He rushed me to the various labs where I was pricked, poked, prodded, and X-rayed. The sun had set by the time all the tests were done. He took me to the ward where I was to spend the night and the rest of the week. I shared the room with three other patients. A nutritionist was barely able to provide me with dinner before the kitchen closed.

Bright and early the next morning, the anesthesiologist arrived at my bedside to transfer me to a gurney and deliver me to the preparation room, where he readied a needle to give me a pre-operation drowsy shot.

I said, "I don't need that. I'm already sleepy because I stayed up all night reading *Coma*."

He did a double take. "Well, you're in a good humor."

That was the last thing I remember until I awoke in the post-op room. I was shivering from the cold. I already had two blankets on me, but I asked for a third. The next time I awoke I was in my own hospital bed. I have no recollection of how I got there. I was still shivering.

I didn't fully awaken until dinner was served. I was so hungry that I barely chewed my food before I swallowed it. Later, a nurse appeared in order to give me pain medication. I slept peacefully throughout the night.

It wasn't until morning that I realized that I had a cast on my foot. I devoured breakfast, then read until the doctor arrived to tell me about the operation. In addition to the doctor who performed the operation, several interns from the nearby hospital of the University of Pennsylvania were in attendance.

The operation was a complete success. There was only one hitch the git along. Because there was no guarantee that the inside tendon of my left leg was thick enough for its purpose, the doctor had to be certain that he could quickly choose one of the free-floating alternatives. His first backup choice was a tendon from my left thigh. This because he preferred to take a tendon from the leg on which the operation was conducted, rather than to have both legs out of service. Otherwise, I would not be able to walk even with crutches.

The doctor's second backup choice was a tendon from the right lower leg, either inside or outside the ankle. The third backup choice was a tendon from the right thigh.

The doctor then explained that he could not stop in the middle of the operation to have the next chosen tendon area shaved. All the tendon areas had to be prepped in advance. This meant that . . .

I threw off the blankets and found that both legs had been shaved from hip to ankles. With my usual levity, I screamed, "I came in for a haircut, not a full body defoliation!"

He smiled. He knew that I was just making jest. "The hair will grow back."

He gave me a bottle of pain pills to take as needed. There were enough pills to last at least ten days.

I spent the rest of the week reading in bed. On day five (Friday), a nurse arrived with a pair of crutches. I stood on one foot while she adjusted the handholds. She then waltzed me around the ward and along the outer corridor in order to teach me how to walk with one leg in the air. I still remembered from seventeen years ago, but my balance was a little off, so I was glad that she was holding onto one shoulder.

After work, Drew Maser, one of my closest friends, arrived in his car to collect me from the VA hospital and take me home. He lived only two blocks away from me.

It was good to be home. The only problem I had was navigating up and down the stairs. I lived in a two-story house. The first floor held the living room, dining room, and kitchen; the second floor held two bedrooms, a bathroom, and my study.

I didn't dare try to climb the stairs on crutches. I felt way too wobbly. For the next two months, I crawled up and down the staircase, clutching my crutches in one hand and using my other hand to, for example, place a mug of coffee on a higher step until I crawled past it, then reached back and grabbed it and placed it on a yet higher step. I reversed the process for going down the staircase, by crawling backward.

One of my dive buddies lived in New Jersey but worked in Philadelphia. She stopped by my house one afternoon to give me a small pail (with a bale) that I used from that time onward to carry items between floors. This pail proved to be indispensable. It was certainly more convenient than my prior routine, especially for transporting multiple items. Spilled coffee stayed inside the pail.

The Holidays

I spent a quiet Christmas at home. Come New Year's Eve, Drew insisted that I go out to dinner with him and his family: wife Linda, daughters Laura and Marie. Laura was two and a half years old; Marie was eighteen months. I was Laura's godfather.

Fitting my crutches into the car between the baby seats was quite a challenge.

At the restaurant, a waitress served water while we pondered over the menu. Linda started to feel unwell. She excused herself and went to the ladies' room. A few minutes later she returned looking pale, and declared that she had just passed a clot. She needed to go to the hospital.

Drew apologized to the waitress that we had a medical emergency. He carried Marie while Linda held Laura's hand. I crutched myself between crowded tables and out the door that Drew held open. He drove us home – the Maser residence – where Linda put out food for me and the girls. I stayed behind to babysit while he drove Linda to the hospital. They expected to be gone no longer than an hour or two.

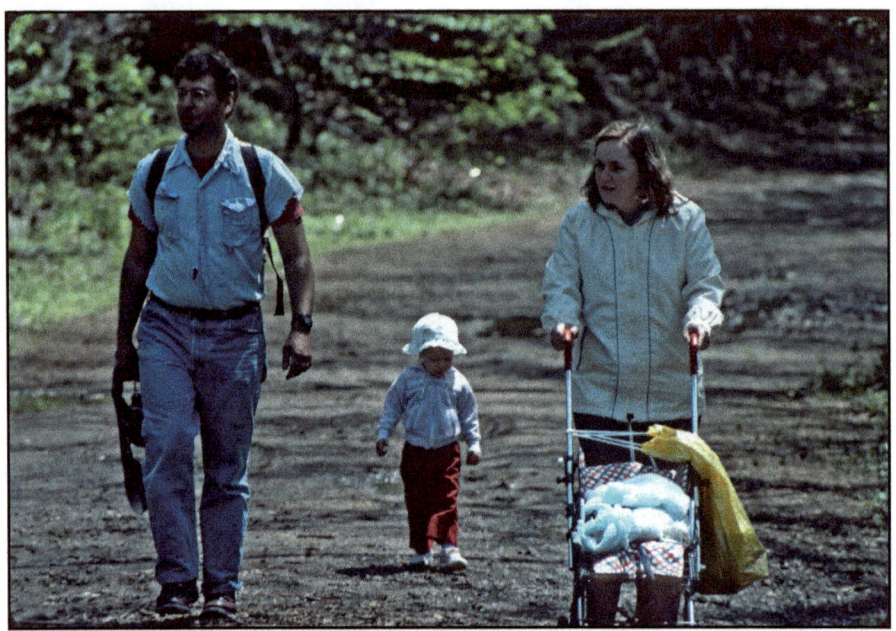
Left to right: Drew, Laura, Linda, and Marie (under the blankets in the stroller) at Pennypack Park.

Babysitting the girls was no big deal. They were comfortable with me because I always played with them whenever I visited their household – which was often, as they lived only two blocks away from me. They nibbled contentedly while I got off my crutches and sat in a comfortable chair.

When they were done eating, they wanted to play. They had toys but because I was there, they wanted to play with me. I got off the chair and lay down on my back for our favorite game. They jumped on my chest and held on tight while I squirmed to the top of the staircase. The apartment was split level, so the staircase was half the height of a full-story staircase. I back-crawled over the landing and slid down the stairs, bumping over every step, while the girls screamed and squealed.

The girls rolled off my chest and scampered up the steps: Laura running and Marie crawling on knees at nearly the same speed. I followed them and we slid down again. After a few more slides the girls played keep away. Catching them was like herding a litter of kittens. Laura was a speed demon, and Marie could crawl faster than I could. I chased them all over the living room and around the table and chairs as if we were re-enacting a military escape-and-evasion course. They won.

When I finally caught up with Marie, I made an unsavory discovery. Her diaper was wet. I had not expected this situation when I accepted the babysitting job. Now I was stuck with it. Laura was a big help because she knew where the supplies were located.

It had been a long time since I last changed a diaper. How hard could it be? I fussed around Marie's hips but couldn't find the pins. Finally, Laura showed me how modern diapers were secured, with a Velcro tab. Silly me. I pulled off the tabs and the diaper unfolded itself. I lifted Marie off floor, pulled off the wet diaper, and set her down. I grabbed a dry diaper, lifted Marie off the floor again, slid the diaper underneath her, set her down, and pulled the tabs until they were firmly in place but not too tight. Tada!

Laura called out from the bathroom, "Come do me."

I didn't know what "do me" meant, but I had a bad feeling about it. When I glanced down the hallway, I saw her standing outside the bathroom without her pants. My bad feeling got worse.

I rolled Marie out of the way and put her on her knees. I crawled along the hallway to the bathroom door. I looked inside. Laura was bent over the side of the tub with her naked butt facing me. By now, part of me was wishing that I had stayed home, eaten a frozen TV dinner, and read a book. I took the matter in hand, wiped her clean, and helped her to pull up her shorts.

The girls were finally running out of steam. They gradually settled down. Their eyelids got heavy. Eventually they fell asleep.

It was nearly midnight by the time Drew and Linda returned home. Linda looked tired and weak. The obstetrician had confirmed that she had suffered a natural abortion. We were still eating pizza when the New Year arrived. Drew wouldn't let me walk home on crutches in the dark. He drove me to my house just two blocks away.

Recuperation

I cannot state that I had any major difficulties during the recuperation process. Working at home as an author meant that I did not lose my job. I obtained a small folding table for my study. This enabled me to rest my bad leg on a leaf while I typed. My position was somewhat awkward but as long as my leg was raised, I did not suffer exorbitant pain. In fact, after my pills ran out, I no longer taking any medicine for pain.

Hobbling on crutches was an inconvenience, but one that I could live with (as if I had a choice).

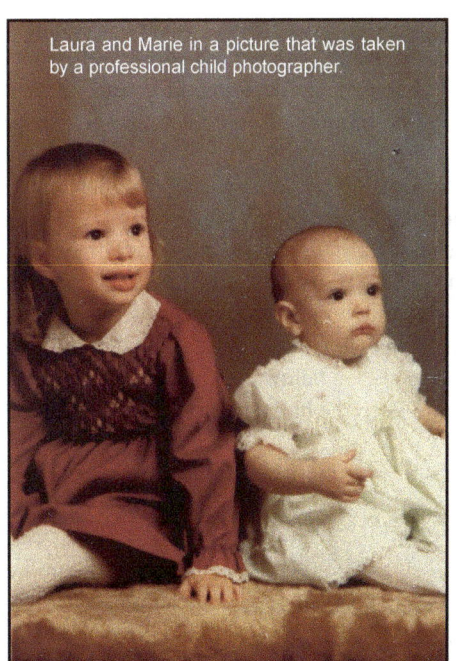
Laura and Marie in a picture that was taken by a professional child photographer.

Another advantage of being an author was that I had gotten into the habit of writing mostly during the winter, and using the warmer seasons to travel and conduct research for my books and magazine articles. Thus I pounded the keys the same as I did the previous winter.

At the end of February 1986, I visited the Philly VA hospital so that my cast could be removed. At the same time, I provided my doctor with an old pair of shoes that I no longer wore. He in turn gave the left shoe to the orthopedic department where a steel brace was built into it. This was done by removing the heel, securing the bottom of the brace to the shoe, then restoring the heel.

The brace was shaped like a U, with the two vertical extensions rising to a position between the top of my calf and the bottom of the knee. A padded Velcro

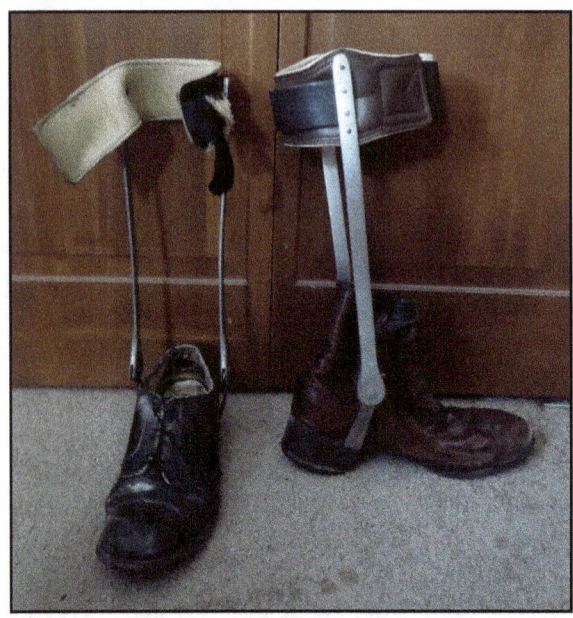

Ankle braces
These are the steel braces that were inserted in my shoes after my tendon transplants. The black Army shoe on the left was the brace from 1968. The brown shoe on the right was from the second transplant in 1987 (although I didn't wear it until 1988. I kept them in case I had later issues with my ankle.

strap was used to secure the strap to my leg. This brace enabled my foot to pivot up and down without allowing my ankle to twist or bend from side to side.

I nearly gagged when I saw how much muscle mass I had lost from my left leg during the two months that I bore all my weight on my right leg. Yet it was astonishing how fast my left leg muscles regenerated to their former mass – which was still far less than the mass of my right leg, which as always bore most of my weight.

I wore the brace constantly from morning till night, even as I walked around the house: basically, whenever I was not in bed. Naturally I wore it outside as well.

Toward the end of the two months that I had to spend wearing the brace, I started jogging again. I quickly learned that the rubbing motion of the tight strap against my leg caused scraping of the skin. Therefore, I left the leg strap slightly loose so that the brace could rise and fall unencumbered along my leg without causing abrasion

Then I spent two months wearing an inflatable brace. This brace was affixed with a band that passed under my heel inside the shoe; any shoe. Where the steel brace possessed steel risers, this brace was fitted with plastic balloons inside a thin canvas coating for abrasion protection. A plastic tube that was much like a flexible straw enabled me to inflate the balloons orally until they were tight against my ankle. The balloons were connected at the top with a Velcro strap around my leg below the knee. I carried the inflator hose with me when I traveled so I could keep the balloons firm. I could also jog while wearing the inflatable brace.

I visited the hospital at the end of June for my final checkup. As I soon learned, this new tendon transplant provided better stability than the first transplant. Not once has my ankle ever given out on me.

Now I was as good as new. I mean, as well as I could ever be in light of my more severe bullet wounds and chronic leg pain. I still had to sit in weird positions that made me look like a reject from a posture class; I sat on the bottom of my spine instead of on my buttock. I kept my left leg raised whenever possible. And I occasionally drove my van with my left foot on the dashboard. The only pain killers I had in my medicine cabinet were aspirin and acetaminophen: aspirin for mild headaches, acetaminophen for more painful headaches. These drugs had no effect on the pain from my bullet wounds. My ankle did not hurt.

Another Fifteen Years Later

In 2001, I experienced a pain explosion that felt like concussion bombs detonating inside my bad leg.

It happened on an ordinary day at home. I was working at my desk as I sipped on my second cup of coffee, when I felt a strange discomfort in my left leg. I always had pain in that leg but this felt stronger than usual. I moved my leg into a different position so that the back of my thigh was not resting on the edge of the chair. The move did not help.

I stretched my leg as I shifted my body so that all my weight lay on my right thigh. Not only did the strange discomfort remain, but the odd sensation intensified. Over the course of the next ten minutes the annoyance became such a strong pounding pain that I could no longer concentrate on my work.

When I stood up and tried to walk, my leg buckled under me. I had to lean against the wall to prevent me from falling onto the floor. I dragged myself into the adjoining bedroom where I threw myself on the bed. By now the pain was full blown, as if my leg were being beaten with a meat softener. The pain extended between my hip and my knee. The throbbing was so agonizing that I could do nothing but lie on my back, tuck my knee under my chin, and groan as I rolled from side to side, trying to find a moment's respite but failing miserably to do so.

Eventually I arose and went to the bathroom where I took two acetaminophens from the medicine cabinet, and swallowed them with tap water. For all the relief they afforded, I might as well have just drunk the water.

The abominable pain lasted throughout the day. Other than an occasional visit to the toilet, I stayed in bed and hugged my leg while I tried but failed to find a comfortable position in which I could relax without suffering such torture. I skipped lunch and dinner. Toward midnight I felt enough relief to doze.

When I awoke in the morning, I felt the same as I did on any other day. Although I felt sluggish, I was able to go back to work.

My diagnosis was that I had had an attack of sciatica.

Five Years Later

In 2006, I suffered another traumatic event like the one in 2001 – except that the pain was doubly excruciating and the attack lasted for two days. I had no food during the first day, and no good sleep that night. By the second morning, I was so exhausted from the previous day's tremors that I didn't get out of bed until noon.

Because I don't drink alcoholic beverages, I don't know what a hangover feels like, but if it felt anything like the way I felt that second afternoon, I wonder why people drink themselves into oblivion just to face a morning of agony.

I managed to nibble on some snacks that did not require cooking. I microwaved coffee that was left over from the day before. I began to feel almost human by dinner time. I ate a little food by nuking leftovers that I found in the refrigerator.

The aching in my leg subsided somewhat by bedtime. I slept only because after two days of groveling in pain, I was too weak to stay awake. I had a fitful night.

I figured that this was another attack of sciatica.

The Next Five Years

The attack itself was gone but not the sciatica. The next five years was a roller coaster ride of ups and down that seriously affected my life. I never knew when an attack would occur, nor how severe it would be.

I knew enough about sciatica to understand the mechanism. Swelling against the sciatic nerve caused pain in the upper leg. Ibuprofen was an anti-inflammatory; it helped to reduce swelling. That was as far as my medical knowledge would take me. I stocked up on ibuprofen because in most cases it helped to alleviate the pain. It didn't always stop the pain, but it made it easier for me to bear the pain.

I might go for months without feeling the increased nerve pain in my leg. Or I might suffer the pain for weeks at a time, after which the pain went away to return … I never know when. There was no way to predict when I would have another bout of leg pain.

I remember one time when I was climbing up a boat ladder, Gene Peterson was standing at the top of the ladder. He had issues with lower back pain. After I doffed my tanks and other dive gear, he handed me two ibuprofens. He said, "I could see the pain in your eyes."

I did not go anywhere without a bottle of ibuprofen on my person or in my van or on the boat. I kept it handy in my onboard parts kit.

The Lost Weekend, er, Month

Ibuprofen was only a stopgap medication that did not always work. One summer I experienced another attack that crept up on me daily until it reached the point at which ibuprofen did not provide the relief that I needed. My leg hurt so much that I lay in bed at night unable to get to sleep.

I changed the position of my leg until the pain was somewhat reduced, but a minute or so later the pain returned in full. So I moved again until I found a different comfortable position. This one might last two to three minutes, enough to almost fall asleep. I might doze for a minute or so, but never any longer. This restlessness kept me in intermediate pain all night long – and throughout the next day.

This situation lasted for more than a month – a month that I spent at Cheryl's house. My memory of that month is a little hazy. She remembers that she gave me codeine pills for my pain. Here's the background story.

Cheryl had a lifelong history of migraine headaches. She knew when one such headache was forthcoming because the initial symptom was the sight of an aura. She was able to obtain a prescription for codeine from her family doctor, but the prescription was expensive. However, a pill with the same amount of codeine was sold over the counter in Canada at a fraction of the price it sold for in the United States.

For many years, I organized annual week-long dive trips to Halifax, Nova Scotia, Canada, to dive on local shipwrecks. When she told me what she was taking, I said that I would buy some for her on my next trip. Thus every year I made a stop at a Haligonian pharmacy.

Cheryl remembers that she gave me some of her migraine pills during that month. One weekend there was an outdoor craft show thirty miles from her house. She expected me to stay home. Instead, I went with her because the severity of my pain was the same whether I was lying in bed or walking our dog, Teeny, through the show.

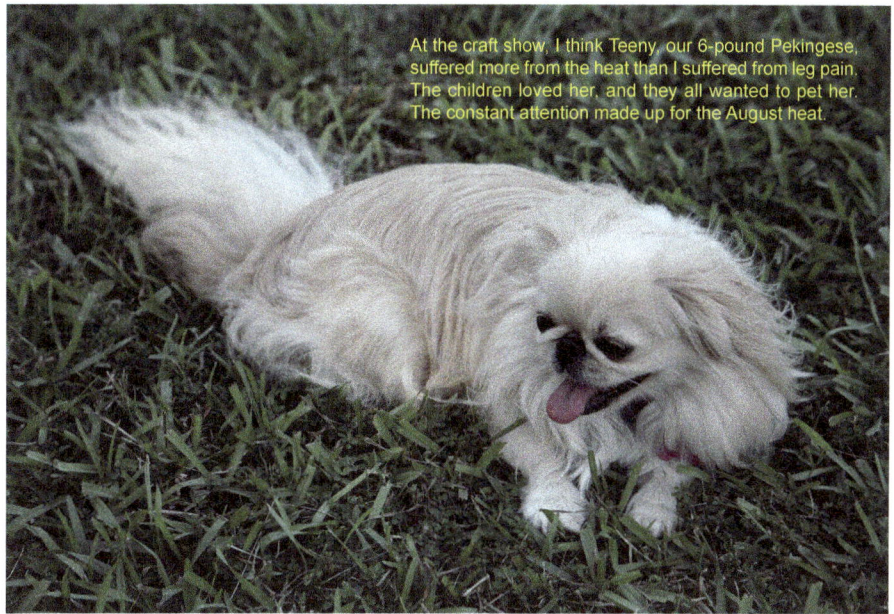

At the craft show, I think Teeny, our 6-pound Pekingese, suffered more from the heat than I suffered from leg pain. The children loved her, and they all wanted to pet her. The constant attention made up for the August heat.

Toward the third week I began to recuperate somewhat, enough to get some sleep without waking constantly throughout the night. By the fourth week I could feel some comfort. I tried to jog but I got only half a mile from the house before I had to stop and walk back. Thus I stayed housebound for the entire month. I managed to work a bit during the day, but whatever I wrote needed some strong editing after the distracting pain finally went away.

As information, the codeine that I obtained from Canada was not pure codeine. It was a mixture of acetaminophen (300 milligrams) and codeine (60 milligrams). In the States, this percentage of codeine was sold under the brand name Tylenol 3.

Medicine and Diving Don't Mix

On one multiday dive trip to explore shipwrecks that lay in 250 feet of water, I was struck with a bout of leg pain while I was driving to the marina. Upon arrival, I mentioned this to one of my dive buddies. He said, try some of these. Because he had chronic lower back pain, he always carried hydrocodone with him. One of these pills took all the pain away, almost immediately.

The problem with hydrocodone was that I could not obtain it on my own because it was a prescription medicine. He gave me enough to last through the trip. But I perceived a potential side effect that might occur under water.

At extreme depths, the nitrogen in compressed air was likely to cause narcosis, which could manifest itself in a number of ways, depending upon the individual's tolerance. This was equivalent to the kind of tolerance that affected people who imbibed too much alcohol. Some people could be adversely affected after two martinis, while others could drink all evening without experiencing loss of motor skills.

Scuba divers were always warned never to drink alcohol before going under water. Keep in mind that the human body is a chemical factory, one in which a balance of chemicals was crucial for maintaining steady operational efficiency. Add the disabling effect of alcohol on the brain with unknown side effects of a strong pain killer like hydrocodone, and that could be a recipe for disaster. The loss of mental acuity at depth might leave a diver unable to handle an emergency situation on the bottom, where time was limited by the amount of air in his or her tanks.

Once at sea, I took the hydrocodone to enable me to sleep at night. When I emerged from my sleeping bag in the morning, in pain, I was afraid to take hydrocodone before the dive. I took ibuprofen, then suffered with the pain as best I could. Ironically, after I submerged and descended the down-line to the working depth, I didn't notice any pain until I surfaced a couple of hours later.

I pondered about whether this painlessness was a psychological effect, in which I was too distracted by the excitement of exploration to feel the nerve pain, or whether the pressure of the water and/or the compressed air that I was breathing was responsible for impeding the pain.

The pain returned as soon as I climbed up the ladder and onto the boat. Yet I still would not take hydrocodone because after four to five hours I planned to make a second dive. I took ibuprofen between dives, and suffered abominably. Not until the second dive was over did I take the hydrocodone, and felt the wonderful relief that I had craved since breakfast. I took another one at bedtime.

No one knew how hydrocodone affected the human body under pressure. Medications were not tested for such an extreme environment. I was unwilling to learn by experience what effect hydrocodone had under water; it might prove to be fatal.

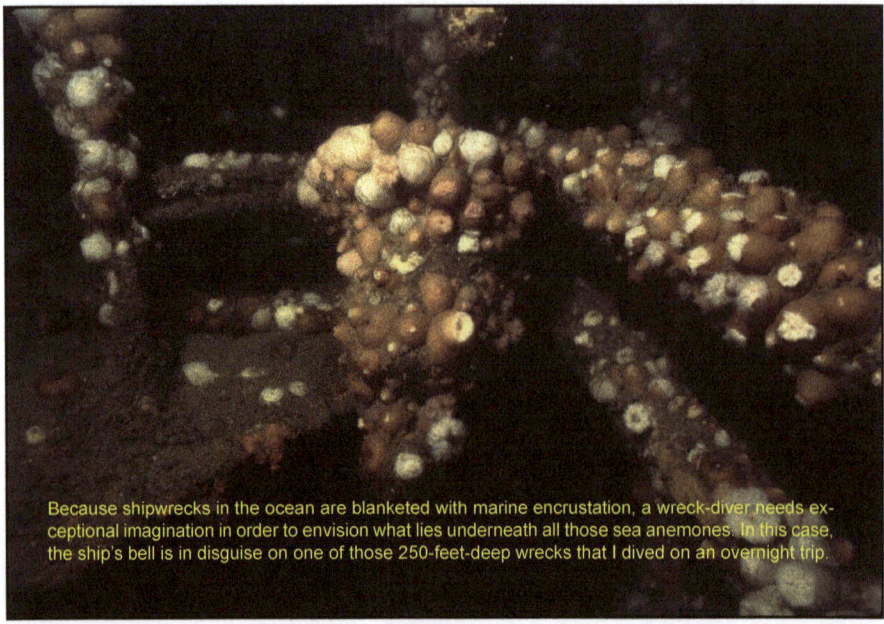

Because shipwrecks in the ocean are blanketed with marine encrustation, a wreck-diver needs exceptional imagination in order to envision what lies underneath all those sea anemones. In this case, the ship's bell is in disguise on one of those 250-feet-deep wrecks that I dived on an overnight trip.

Worsening Pain, Increasing Frequency

Toward the end of this five-year span, especially in the fifth year, my sciatic condition worsened in both pain level and duration. Weeks might pass during which I needed no medication at all. Then the pain would flare up for a day or two, or three, or four, or more. I was sometimes away from home when these bouts occurred.

Part of my occupation as an author was writing books about shipwrecks. In order to do my job, I had to survey the shipwrecks that I was writing about. I also had to do historical research about these shipwrecks. By daily account, I have spent more than three years at sea, and more than a year in archives and museums. Many of my dive trips were multi-day excursions; sometimes lasting for two to three weeks.

I went on one dive trip on which foul weather kept us off the ocean for a week. This was not as unusual as it may sound. For example, on a different trip I was holed up in a motel for three days, then went home without ever getting into the water. On another trip, my buddy and I spent nine days waiting out a storm that kept getting worse. Eight-foot seas on the first day grew to fifteen-foot seas by the ninth day, after which we packed our gear and went home, again without ever getting to dive.

To save on travel expenses, I outfitted my van so I could sleep in it. On some trips I roughed it in a tent. Many times I slept on the boat. Sometimes I stayed at the house of the boat owner or one of my dive buddies. I think I slept in more places than George Washington ever did.

I always carried my electric typewriter or, later, my computer on multiple-day trips, so I could work when the weather turned foul and I was staying in a motel or someone's house, where I had access to electricity.

Then I bought an inverter which I could plug into the cigarette lighter of my van, and utilize the output of full-wave alternating current, with high enough wattage to power my computer. Because I did not smoke, this was the only use to which my lighter was ever put.

The inverter was particularly handy when I was staying at the home of my girlfriend, Cheryl Novak, during a hurricane in which there was a power outage for nine days. I parked my van under her house (which stood on stilts), and ran an extension cord up the back staircase. During daytime, I used the inverter to operate my computer. At dinnertime, Cheryl used it to power the microwave oven. After she cooked the meal, we used the inverter to run the videotape machine so we could watch a movie. The inverter was a handy little device for both work and pleasure.

An Involuntary Medical Experiment

During a dive trip that was scheduled for the last year of the five-year span of this section, I was staying at the home of the boat owner when a northeasterly storm struck the area. The flags at the marina called for gale-force winds. Coincidentally, when I got out of bed the next morning, I had the worst sciatic attack that I had ever experienced. I felt fine under the covers, but as soon as I straightened my leg to stand alongside the bed, my entire leg from hip to toe erupted like a volcano into burning, throbbing, unbearable pain. I flopped back onto the bed.

I wanted to scream. It was all I could do to breathe through gritted teeth. I had not experienced pain of such severity since the time that I was wounded. I lay unmoving for five minutes or so. The pain did not ebb.

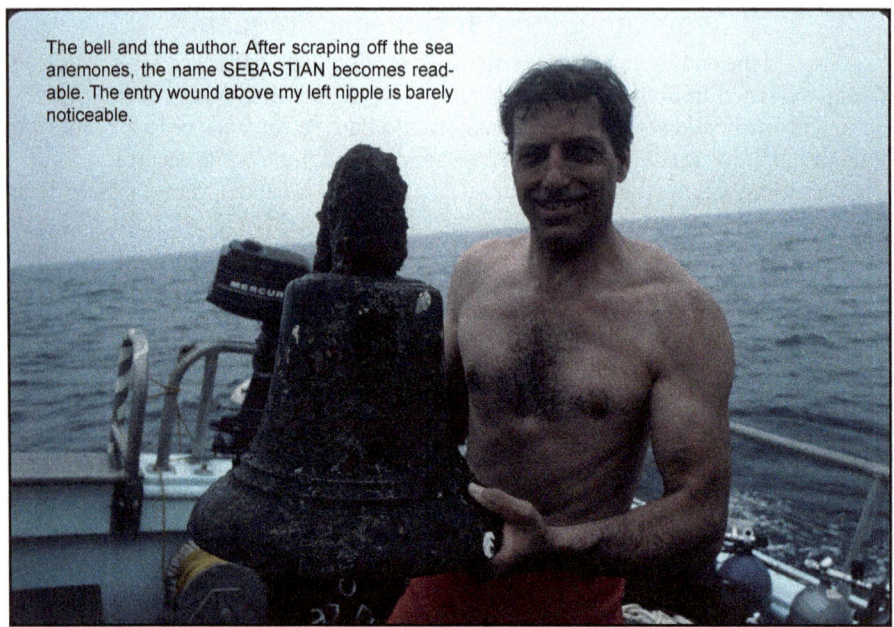

The bell and the author. After scraping off the sea anemones, the name SEBASTIAN becomes readable. The entry wound above my left nipple is barely noticeable.

I knew that the skipper had severe back pain. I forced myself to stand up, then, stiff-legged, and leaning against furniture and the wall, I dragged my bad leg across the hall to the opposite bedroom, and shoved open the door. I screamed for the location of the meds, got directions to a cabinet inside the bathroom, and hobbled into the bathroom (which was between the two bedrooms.

I found the bottle that matched the description. Using sink water, I washed a single pill down my throat. I hobbled back to bed as best I could. I felt the pain evaporating in only two to three minutes. After four minutes I was comfortable. By five minutes I was completely pain free.

What a miraculous recovery!

I felt good enough to walk normally, so I went downstairs and prepared the coffee pot. Then I was in for a surprise.

Because the weather precluded diving, I plugged in my computer and went to work. I was able to process words normally, but soon my body began to feel "funny." By "funny" I mean odd. This feeling did not affect my ability to think or type, yet I felt as if I were sitting two inches above the seat of the chair. I felt as if I should not drive a car or operate heavy equipment. I felt slow, or sluggish, as if my mind and my body were floating somewhere in the clouds.

As a result of these adverse feelings, I walked slowly through the house, and held onto the handrails when I traversed the staircase. These feelings persisted until 5 o'clock in the afternoon. The feelings wore off unnoticeably so that I did not immediately become aware of their absence. Suddenly I felt normal, without my head in the clouds. If this feeling of cloudiness was what junkies described as a "high," it wasn't for me.

Despite the so-called high, I managed to write a full day's work, the same as I would have done on any other day. Plus, after the 5 o'clock return to normality, the pain did not return.

The name of this wonder drug was oxycodone. Research informed me that it was twice as strong as hydrocodone. In my opinion, oxycodone did its job too well. I loved the way it relieved my pain lickety-split. I just did not care for the side effect. On the latter basis, I sincerely hope that my pain level never reaches the height at which only oxycodone can offer relief. Some people might call the side effect "mind expanding." I called it "mindless evanescence."

But the story is not over. The next morning, as soon as I stepped out of bed, my wounded leg exploded with agonizing pain, as bad as it had been on the previous morning. I gritted my teeth, stumbled to the bathroom, and grabbed another oxycodone.

I noticed that the pill was scored along the middle. I broke it in two by pressing the center with my thumbs, and swallowed one half. The pill worked exactly the way it had worked the day before. Within five minutes I was completely pain free. Soon I began to feel that floating feeling between my butt and the chair seat. I was still able to work effectively. But this time the side effect wore off at noon.

Not to sound repetitive, but the following day was much the same except that I used a butter knife to cut the remaining half pill in half. This time the floating feeling evaporated at 10 o'clock. Ditto for day four.

On day five, when I put my foot on the floor in the morning, I felt a slight ache in my thigh muscles. I took two ibuprofens and the pain went away. The next day I needed nothing for the pain because it was essentially nonexistent. I needed nothing but ibuprofen for the next several months. Then . . .

This is the End

July of 2011 found me on a multiday offshore dive trip to the *Andrea Doria*, an Italian passenger liner that sank after a collision with the Swedish liner Stockholm, 55 miles south of Nantucket. On the last day of the trip, I jumped into the water to make what for me was a milestone dive: my 200th dive on the *Andrea Doria*.

As luck would have it, I found an opening in the hull which enabled me to swim along a corridor that led to the wine closet. Because the door had rusted away, I was able to collect three full bottles of wine that was nicely aged. The collision had occurred on July 25, 1956. The corks were still in place. This meant that I could celebrate my dive with 55-year-old wine (which I did not normally drink).

After a 15-minute dive to 219 feet, I dragged my booty to the anchor line for 57 minutes of decompression. I broke the surface of the sea, swam to the stern of the boat, and handed my net bag to the mate so that the bottles would not get broken as I climbed up the steel ladder.

I watched the waves, waited for the best time to grab the handrails, pulled myself up to the bottom rung, and rested my weight plus 150 pounds of tanks and scuba gear on my right foot, as I always did. I took a higher grip with my hands, placed my left foot on the next rung, pulled up with my arms, pushed up with my left leg . . . and burst into a leg spasm of unutterable pain. I screamed for help.

The mate was right there, ready to help. "What's wrong?"

My leg was paralyzed. I couldn't move it, and I couldn't put weight on it in order to push up with my other leg. "It's my leg. It's in pain. But I'm not bent."

The latter statement was intended to inform the mate that I was not suffering from decompression injury, alias DSI or bends. I was trapped on the ladder. I don't know what happened next. My eyes were clamped shut.

Between gritted teeth, "I can't move my leg."

I felt arms grabbing me under the armpits. The mate could not lift me onto the deck by himself. The total weight of me and my gear was more than 300 pounds. He must have had help, but I don't know who helped him. All I knew was that I was lifted onto the deck and dragged away from the ladder. Frantic faces peered down at me.

"I'm not bent. Help me get my gear off."

Hands flashed over my body, loosening straps, unclipping carabiners, unsnapping snap hooks, removing my weight belt, pulling off my fins, slipping off my face mask, unstrapping my dive knife.

Another diver was climbing up the ladder. I was dragged to the side and then forward along the port railing to make room for other divers. I screamed the whole time.

I couldn't do anything to help myself. Someone pulled down the zipper of my drysuit. Several others worked my arms out of the sleeves, yanked off my two hoods, pulled the drysuit opening over my head, then slid the legs of the drysuit off my lower body. Now I was clothed only in my insulated undergarments.

I was helped to my feet. I couldn't walk because my leg was still paralyzed. I assured everyone that I was not bent. When I said that the problem was my bad leg, no one knew what I meant. They were unaware of my combat history and associated wounds. I had to explain about sciatica and nerve damage.

I asked if anyone had any pain medication. In this case I was lucky. Three people had hydrocodone for lower back pain. Someone gave me a pill while someone else gave me a glass of water. The pain was so bad that I was oblivious to who was helping me. I was focused strictly on the pain.

I expected the hydrocodone to alleviate the pain in no more than five minutes. But due to the severity of the pain, I did not feel any relief for fifteen minutes. It took twenty minutes before the pain was mostly gone. Mostly.

I lay down on a sofa in the main cabin. Friends, acquaintances, and people I didn't know, commiserated with me as I explained about the sciatic attacks that I had been having for the past several years.

An hour passed before I felt hardy enough to go below in order to get my shoes and jacket from my cramped cubicle, so I could walk onto the wet deck, gather my equipment, and organize it in my gear box before the boat got underway. Everyone aboard had made his or her final dive of the trip.

The overnight ride to the marina in Montauk was 123 miles away. We didn't arrive until after sunrise the next morning. Now was the time to unload our tanks and equipment from the boat, load it into our vehicles, say our fond fairwells. I was still feeling weak, so I had help with offloading my heavy double-tank rigs. I also received another hydrocodone for the 5-hour drive home.

Home, by the way, was no longer in Philadelphia. In 2009, I moved north to Jim Thorpe. When I got home, Cheryl was waiting for me. After two decades of a long-distance relationship – I in Philly, she in Columbia, North Carolina – she retired from her job as a school counseler and moved in with me.

After I limped into the house and sat down on the sofa in pain, I told her about the trip, and about the painful bout with sciatica that I was still experiencing. I was in too much pain to unload and rinse my dive gear.

I had some trouble getting to sleep that night, I supposed because that morning's dose of pain killer was wearing off; or had already worn off.

The next morning I awoke to a brand new life: Cheryl was by my side. But as soon as I stretched my bad leg and put my foot on the floor, I was gripped with pain that was at least as severe as it was when I climbed up the ladder. I rolled back into bed, howling in agony.

If Cheryl had not been awake, she certainly was awake now. I buried my head in my pillow, and rolled back and forth in a lame attempt to find a comfortable position. I grabbed my shin and tucked it hard against my chest and under my chin. Cheryl appeared with a glass of water and a bottle of pills. Neither one of us can remember whether she gave me ibuprofen or codeine. Whatever she gave me didn't help.

I could not stop the tears from rolling off my cheeks onto the pillow case, but I did my best not to scream. As far as I could tell, I succeeded. I continued to roll and hug my agonizing leg in the mistaken belief that those actions helped to reduce the pain. Lying still did not make me feel any better. The leg continued to burn in pain no matter what I did or how I moved or what position I adopted.

If you want to know what Hell is like, I can tell you. It's chronic unbearable pain.

I felt a hand on my shoulder. I rolled onto my back and looked up into Cheryl's worried face.

"Take these."

She gave me two pills and a glass of water. I swallowed the pills as instructed. Within a few minutes I felt much better. I was even able to sit up. A few minutes later I stretched my bad leg – slowly – but the pain did not return.

When I asked her what she had given to me, she said, "Hydrocodone."

Here is another backstory.

I was born and raised in Philly. After my marriage, I used my back pay from the Army to buy a house in Philly. At my divorce, my ex took the house and nearly all my personal belongings. I had to sue her to get my belongings back. I escaped with my books and my Chevy Blazer. As an apprentice electrician, I worked hard to support my son by doing side jobs on weekends and driving a delivery truck on some evenings . I lived in an apartment with no furniture. I removed the back seat from the Blazer so I would have some place to sit. I slept on the floor with the roaches. At least the floor was carpeted.

Eventually I bought another house in Philly. I lived in that house for 36 years. In 2009, I bought a house in Jim Thorpe. A year before Cheryl was slated to retire, I bought her a GPS that was powered by a cord that plugged into the cigarette lighter.

She said, "What am I supposed to do with this?"

She knew nothing about Jim Thorpe or the surrounding counties. I told her to practice using it. "After you retire and move to Jim Thorpe, whenever you go anywhere and need to find your way home, all you have to do is push the 'Home' button, then follow the directions."

It was the next best thing to closing her eyes and clicking the heels of a pair of magic red shoes, which I failed to find in any antique shoppes. Only in Oz.

She had been to the new house several times, during holidays when school was closed for a week. But she knew nothing about the area. Nonetheless, she was quite resourceful.

She had never seen me cry from pain (although she saw me cry terribly when our dog passed away). Seeing me in such agony prompted her to take action. She searched the phone book for nearby doctors. Then she got into her car and visited the closest one. When she pulled into the parking lot, she saw that he was a nephrologist: a specialist in kidney functions.

She didn't think that he could take patients, so she went to another doctor. The office was tiny, with a waiting room that held only three chairs. She explained the situation to the receptionist. The receptionist gave her a form to fill out, but did not seem overly eager to accept a new patient. Cheryl accepted the form, but instead of filling in the blanks, she left and returned to the first doctor.

There she was greeted with a smile and a hope that the doctor could help. Cheryl spoke with the doctor and explained the situation. Instead of brushing her off, he listened closely to her story. He agreed to prescribe three days of hydrocodone under two conditions: one, that he talk with me on the phone that afternoon, and two, that I make an appointment to see him in three days (which was based on the doctor's availablity). The doctor was being cautious. Cheryl agreed to both conditions.

The doctor called the prescription to a pharmacy. Cheryl picked up the pills on the way home. Then she gave two of them to me. In accordance with the doctor's instructions, I was to take six pills per day: two in the morning, two in the afternoon, and two at night.

The doctor called me in midafternoon. I gave him the background of this issue of recurring pain. I told him how long I had been dealing with the pain. I explained where the pain was located and how the pain struck when I stretched my leg in the morning. He asked several questions which I readily answered. Finally, he made an appointment for me for three days hence, by which time the present dose of medication would expire.

Cheryl accompanied me to the doctor's office on the appointed date and time. When the doctor examined my leg, he asked me about the very evident scars. I told him about my wounds from Vietnam. He told us that before he could make any determination about how to treat my symptoms, he needed more information about my condition. Specifically, he needed an X-ray, an MRI, and a neurological examination of my leg.

The way the hospital system was organized (or disorganized, as the case may be), the doctor could order an X-ray but not an MRI nor a neurological test. An orthopedic doctor had to order an MRI. After examining the MRI, the orthopedic doctor would send the results to the doctor. If the results did not satisfy the doctor, he could make an appointment for me to have a neurological test.

It seemed like a cumbersome and time-consuming process, but that was the way it was. The doctor ordered a refill of hydrocodone. He arranged for me to have the X-ray done immediately, as there was an X-ray laboratory across the street. He also made an appointment for me to see an orthopedic doctor in two weeks' time (the orthopedic doctor's earliest availability. We stopped at the X-ray lab on the way home. We also picked up the hydrocodone from the pharmacy.

In the meantime, my physical condition played yo-yo by first seeming to heal and by then worsening. The next day, I got out of bed carefully, limped into the bathroom without straightening my leg, swallowed two hydrocodone pills, then went back to bed until the medicine had time to activate. A few minutes later, I waltzed into the kitchen and switched on the coffee maker. I felt pain free and vigorous.

In fact, I felt so pain-free that I even went shopping with Cheryl in order to purchase a medicine cabinet for the master bathroom. I was able to walk normally. After we returned home, I used toggle bolts to hang the cabinet on the wall next to the toilet.

I was able to work on my current book project throughout the afternoon. It was like having a new lease on life.

A few days later I lost the lease. My leg was pain free until I donned my pants. Then I nearly screamed because I thought that my leg was on fire. In actuality, my *leg* did not hurt; it was the skin on my leg that caused such agony. As long as nothing was touching the skin on my thigh, I felt normal. But if I touched my skin with my finger, or brushed it against some object, even the bed sheet, the burning sensation became intolerable.

The only way I could sleep at night was by hanging my leg off the side of the bed. This was an awkward way to sleep but I had no choice in the matter. This condition also left me impotent for the following month.

At first I could walk normally as long as I was not wearing long-legged pants. For house wear, I donned jogging shorts instead of my usual sweatpants. But a day or two later, walking became painful when the fiery hypersensitivity spread to my lower leg and foot. Even hydrocodone did not remove this skin pain. To add to my uncomfortable sleeping position, I had to hang my leg in such a way that my foot did not touch the floor.

I suffered this pain long enough to climb up the pull-down ladder that led to the attic, in order to retrieve the crutches from my 1985 ankle operation. After 36 years, the rubber pads for the armpits, hand grips, and toe tips were hardened and slightly cracked, but the wooden crutches were still functional. I used these crutches for the next month and a half.

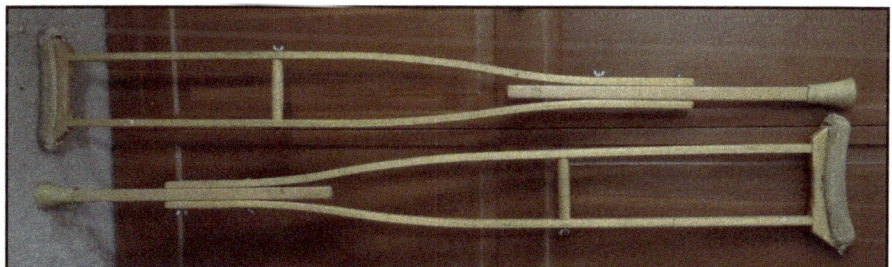

Cheryl had to drive me to my upcoming doctors' appointments. We had company who wanted to see the historic town in which we lived, and which was now named after the famous Olympic champion. I hobbled along the sidewalks wearing jogging shorts. My left foot was bare.

My visit with the orthopedic doctor was disappointing but ultimately productive. I limped into his office on crutches, sat on a gurney, and awaited his appearance. When he finally arrived, he told me up front that he didn't know if he could help me. He said that if I had a broken leg, he could set the bone. But he didn't know much about pinched nerves. He made an appointment for an MRI, which was not available for a couple of weeks. He told me to call his office after I had the MRI procedure, and make another appointment.

The MRI procedure was scheduled for 7:30 in the evening. The hospital had an open-ended unit so that my head reached outside the top opening while the magnetic resonance imaging machine was diagnosing my body from the top of my spine to the bottom of my upper leg: essentially everywhere that a nerve could be pinched in such a way that it could cause the pain in my leg. All I had to do was to lie still for 45 minutes.

The soonest appointment that I could then obtain with the orthopedic doctor was two weeks away. After I hobbled into his office, still on crutches, he examined the MRI. He found no compression of the discs in the spine, and nowhere that a nerve appeared to be pinched. Therefore, he placed an order for a neurological examination in two weeks' time.

He told me to make an appointment to see him after the neurological examination was conducted. I never did. In my opinion he was useless to me. I would be wasting my money to see a doctor who had already informed me that my problem was not his area of expertise.

Instead, I visited the first doctor: the one who had treated me initially. He couldn't diagnose my condition until I had the neurological exam. By this time the skin pain was receding enough that I was able to walk into his office without crutches. I was wearing sweatpants. In short, my condition was improving all by itself, without any medical intervention.

But as I have already shown, this condition has been coming and going for a decade. Just because my pain was decreasing on that day was not confirmation that it would not increase the next day. It was imperative that the doctor and I knew the underlying cause of the pain.

Due to my decrease in pain, Doc changed my pain medication from 6 hydrocodone pills per day, to 4 per day – morning and night – with 2 tramadol pills at midday. He suggested that I should try to reduce the hydrocodone to 2 pills per day – at bedtime – and 4 pills per day in the morning and afternoon.

Not only did I follow his directions immediately, but within a week, on my own, I switched to tramadol in the morning instead of hydrocodone.

When I arrived at the neurologist's office, I learned that the examination was a two-part process. One neurologist would conduct the examination; a different neurologist would interpret the results. Keep in mind that the neurologists had access to the previous tests, both X-ray and MRI. This access was crucial to the conduct of the neurological test by informing them what was *not* wrong with me.

The first neurologist wasted no time on examining my spine. He homed in on my leg because that was where he expected to find the cause of my pain. This test consisted of attaching electrodes to the bottom of my bad leg, above the ankle, and to the top of my leg, below the hip: in other words, my entire leg. Then he sent high-voltage shocks through my leg from one electrode to the other. This procedure was supposed to determine how effectively the nerves were functioning.

As an ex-electrician, I know all about shocks. I have been shocked on numerous occasions throughout my career in the field. To me, the electrical shock that was sent through my leg felt like a 480-volt shock. In other words, extremely painful. Although I neglected to ask the neurologist how much voltage he was injecting, I suspect objectively that it was more likely to be less than half that amount. It just felt like more.

What made the jolts feel worse than they were was that he shocked me again and again and again, in the same spot, then repeated the process at a nearby spot. This went on for close to half an hour. I felt like Frankenstein's monster being subjected to lightning jolts.

I returned to the neurologists' office a fortnight later. This time the first neurologist's partner did a physical examination. When he wanted me to walk toward him in a straight line, he castigated me for limping. I told him that I couldn't help it because my foot was in so much pain.

Over the months that were required to reach this stage in my affliction, the pain had been constantly reducing itself, not only in severity but in area. After a month or so the pain no longer persisted in my upper leg. My lower leg hurt all over except for the inside between the shin bone and one quarter of the way around the inside of my calf. Indeed, that part of my leg had never felt nerve pain. But I still couldn't walk without limping.

By the time of this examination – more than two months after the onset of my condition – the skin pain was gone and only my foot and toes hurt. The sole of my foot hurt just from feeling cold in the air. Yet I couldn't wear a sock because the material pressing against my foot caused pain. Cheryl found special socks that were made for diabetics; the fabric was thin and loose, so that it did not press against the skin. Because the sole of my foot felt cold even under a sheet and a blanket, I had to wear socks at night. I still do.

Anyway, the neurologist conducted a physical examination that included tests for reflexes and motor skills. He then explained the situation. I did not have sciatica. "The nerves in your leg were so badly damaged by the bullet that nothing can be done but to treat the pain." This pure and simple statement left no room for doubt about my physical condition: it was permanent.

This was a gigantic revelation. I spent a thousand dollars of my own money for medical services that I could have had treated by the Veterans Administration!

He suggested that I keep taking tramadol and hydrocodone, as needed.

Another two weeks passed before I got to see the person who I now looked upon as my family doctor. At this point I should advise my readers that the time delays between the various visitations were not exactly fourteen days. For ease in scanning, I used the phrase "two weeks" as an approximation. The actual difference between onset and final visit was three months, during which time I was basically homebound, almost never leaving the house except for doctor visits. Half of that time I was on crutches.

Nonetheless, it had occurred to me that the current civilian hospital system operated in such a way that if I had caught something that was eventually lethal, I could have died long before the tests had been completed.

Reviewing the test results, my family doctor understood that my condition could not be cured because my sciatic nerve had been irrevocably damaged by the rifle bullet that shattered my left femur. Even though the present condition of my pain had ameliorated, there was no way to predict when it would flare up again. In short, I just had to live with it. Which I had been doing for nearly all my adult life.

By this time, I had voluntarily quit taking hydrocodone altogether. I had eleven pills remaining, which I saved for a "rainy day." That is, an event like the one that I had experienced while climbing up the boat ladder after my dive on the *Andrea Doria*, or the way I felt on the morning when Cheryl found me in tears. So far, I have not had a repetition of those serious events.

I was now taking ibuprofen in the morning and afternoon, and taking tramadol only at bedtime.

The Doc put me on another medication, called gabapentin. This was not a pain reliever as such; it was primarily a nerve desensitizer that was usually prescribed to prevent seizures. Gabapentin helped to reduce pain by treating the cause instead of the symptom. The way I understood the chemistry, in a greatly simplified manner, was that gabapentin "deadened" the nerve endings that received and transmitted false information that the brain interpreted as pain.

I suffered two side effects: constipation and temporary loss of balance. Cheryl cured the constipation problem by purchasing an over-the-counter stool softener.

I was stuck with the balance issue. At home, I was forever bumping into furniture and walls, and crashing against door jambs as I passed from one room to another. For the first time in my life, I started using a hiking pole on day hikes. Because I could no longer ski – neither downhill nor cross-country – I converted my ski poles to hiking poles by shortening them to the appropriate length. For me, the appropriate length was one that placed my left hand slightly lower than my elbow. Any longer than that caused pain in my bad shoulder. I felt pain in my shoulder any time it was elevated, much like it was during my electrician days.

I sure miss skiing.

As for hiking on mountain trails, I approached cliffs and drop-offs by sidling with the right side of my body heading forward. This was because whenever I lost my balance, I fell backwards and to my left: 235 degrees by the compass.

I've had some pretty bad falls. The worst one occurred when I crouched to take a close-up picture on a rocky coast in Maine. I landed on a pile of jagged rocks that caused deep cuts and abrasions.

About four months after this long episode of constant pain, I phased out the tramadol altogether. I took ibuprofen when necessary.

Then I decided to quit taking gabapentin. According to the directions, abruptly quitting gabapentin could cause a seizure. The directions recommended that weaning off gabapentin should be done gradually. I was then taking 3 pills per day: morning, afternoon, and night. For the first few days, I cut my intake of gabapentin to 2 pills per day: morning and night. After 3 days I cut my intake to 1 pill per day. After another 3 days, I quit altogether.

The only aftereffects that I noticed from *not* taking gabapentin were that I was no longer constipated, and the temporary loss of balance no longer occurred. I stopped bumping into walls and door jambs. I was more sure-footed in the woods.

My body returned to normal – that is, what was normal for me: sore shoulder, sore leg, uncomfortable sitting positions, and walking with a barely noticeable limp which I did my best to disguise.

The pain in my foot gradually shrank until only the sole hurt. The pain soon left my heel, then left my arch. But the ball remained painful and hurts yet today. I still had to wear a sock at night, because exposure to cold air remained an annoying ache.

What I called "cold exposure" applied to my entire sole. I could not walk barefoot across a tile or linoleum floor without feeling extreme pain from the cold that those flooring materials imparted to the bottom of my foot. To do so felt like having an ice cube pressed against my skin for several minutes. A sock didn't help. I needed to have a shoe on my foot in order to prevent the cold feeling from penetrating lightweight materials. I could bear to walk barefoot across the bathroom or kitchen only by touching the floor with the back of my heel: an awkward way to walk. This condition was permanent so I was still plagued with it.

The top of my foot and the four small toes were numb, the way they had been throughout the 1970's. As of this writing, the feeling has not returned.

Never in my life had I needed to use bathroom spray air freshener. Now I couldn't live without it.

Never as an adult have I had to pee in the middle of the night. Now I couldn't go through a night of sleep without having to pee 2 or 3 times.

My body temperature changed constantly. Ever since the "episode," as I refer to the 3-month aftereffects of the sudden pain that ended my dive career, I have gotten what I call "cold spells." These spells struck unannounced. One minute I was comfortable, and the next minute I was shivering. I often had to don a sweater or sweatshirt even in the middle of summer. Each spell lasted an hour or more.

I also had another issue with temperature. This one was chronic. For me, so-called "room temperature" was no longer 72 degrees. At 72 degrees, I had to wear a full sweatsuit plus a winter vest overtop the sweatshirt – always. Even as I type these words I am wearing sweatpants, sweatshirt, and vest.

Cheryl and I could be sitting next to each other during dinner. She would be wearing a pair of shorts and a sleeveless top, while I would be wearing my standard sweatsuit and vest. The cold spells were over and above the chronic cold.

I adopted a limp when I got out of bed in the morning because I felt pain in the exit wound of my thigh. The hurt was neither sharp nor excessive, but it was a warning that if I straightened my leg, I might feel extraordinary stabbing pains along my entire leg. Therefore, I kept my knee slightly bent for half an hour or so to give my morning dose of tramadol time to become effective.

Tramadol was the weakest of all the opioid painkillers. It relieved mild pain if taken before the pain was felt. If taken after the pain was felt, the pain grew worse before the pain-relieving component activated enough to overcome the worsening cause of the pain. In other words, tramadol then must play catchup before it started to alleviate any pain. This means that it was important to adhere to a strict 8-hour schedule for 3 times a day: morning, afternoon, and bedtime.

I could no longer jog. For physical workouts, and to obtain much-needed cardiovascular exercise, I started mountain biking. At first I had to place my left heel on the pedal. As the pain ebbed, I was able to pedal with my arch on the pedal. Because the pain in the ball was chronic, I could not pedal the way a biker was supposed to pedal. I make do with what I can do.

I was forced to quit diving. That 200th dive on the *Andrea Doria* turned out to be the final dive of my career: number 2,596. After 40 years of underwater adventures, I miss diving more than anyone can imagine.

In short, my entire life and lifestyle have been irrevocably altered as a result of combat wounds that I received under fire in Vietnam in 1967.

Bullet wounds in real life differ from those that are depicted in the movies. An actor faking a gunshot wound might exhibit pain for no longer than a minute, then ignore it for the rest of the movie. Nor does it come back to haunt him. Once gone it is forgotten. As actors are wont to say on stage, "The play must go on."

But the good news is that, for those who survive the initial wound, life does go on, however painful it might be from time to time.

Wounds are forever.

Part 4

During this period of near normalcy with regard to pain, I never lost sight of the fact that a lot of Vietnam veterans were suffering, either physically or emotionally, or both. After all, a vet who had his leg or arm blown off could never be one hundred percent normal again, and could never hope to lead a perfectly normal life, no matter how much he or she tried. I was quite conscious of the fact that my troubles were minor when compared to the incurable amputees of many of my fellow vets.

What I didn't know was that my situation was about to get worse. Much worse.

I was about to become embroiled in an administrative system that had my worst interests at heart; that many Vietnam veterans were already trapped in an unsympathetic system in which I was about to be embroiled: a system that did not truly care about the forgotten veterans of a forgotten war.

I was soon to learn that I was about to be shoveled into an administrative and medical trash bin.

Ankle Pain

I horded my leftover pills in case any of my conditions returned. Except for the cold exposure of my left foot, I was pretty much pain-free. I took ibuprofen now and again whenever I felt pain that could be attributed to swelling.

The next summer I caught Lyme disease. I recognized the large red splotch on the inner side of my right thigh, and wasted not a minute before calling my family doctor. The nurse made an appointment for me for the following morning.

I wore shorts to the doctor's office so he could easily see the giveaway symptom. He took one look at the bright red splotch and said, "*That* is Lyme disease. I'll still have tests done for confirmation, but I will start you on antibiotics without waiting for results."

As expected, blood tests proved that I had Lyme disease.

The ten-day, twice-a-day course of antibiotics cured me. The antibiotics were so powerful that three times I vomited within an hour of taking a pill. Better that than Lyme disease.

The following year I started to feel pain in my left ankle: pain that did not go away. I suspected that I must need another tendon transplant. I did not look forward to a third operation and six months of recovery time. I increased my intake of ibuprofen, which provided partial relief. The ankle hurt only when I was walking or hiking. It did not ache or throb if I were sitting or biking.

When I walked or hiked, especially in the woods, my ankle was constantly being bent or twisted. When I was biking, although I had to pedal with the arch of my left foot on the pedal, my ankle never bent or twisted. My foot didn't move at all; it remained on a flat and level surface that was maintained by the rotation of the pedal.

As in 1985, I endured the worsening pain throughout the summer, until I could no longer stand it. By that time, I was also suffering a recurrence of nerve pain in my leg. I did not take either the hydrocodone or the tramadol that I was saving because the pain was not yet severe enough to require strong medication. But the pain was getting worse.

I decided that, because this was a combat related injury, I could go to the closest Veterans Hospital as I did in 1985. I now lived in Jim Thorpe, Pennsylvania. I secured a list of nearby cities that had a Veterans Hospital. My two closest choices were Allentown and Wilkes-Barre. I chose Wilkes-Barre because it was likely to have less traffic.

I called ahead and spoke with a receptionist on the phone. After I explained the situation, she said, "Come on in. We'd love to see you."

NOTE: From this point onward, my recollections are somewhat fuzzy – not about the incidents but about the dates and the chronology of events. I have done my best to keep the timeline in order.

I gathered all the paperwork that I had collected about on my two-year-old spell with the pinched sciatic nerve in my leg. I photocopied everything and put it into a briefcase. Then Cheryl and I drove to the Wilkes-Barre VA Medical Center, as it was called. I had to be processed and given a cardboard identification card. Then I was sent to a doctor who was called a "Primary Care Provider," or PCP. The VA PCP was equivalent to a civilian family doctor, like the one I had seen for my initial pinched nerve attack, and later for Lyme disease treatment. Or so I thought.

Whereas the family doctor had been extremely helpful and had exerted every effort in treating my health issues, the PCP was more like a brick wall that prevented me from receiving the treatment that I so desperately needed. I learned this on my very first visit.

The first step in meeting with a PCP was to speak with one of his nurses. The nurse started by asking questions that any doctor's nurse would ask, primarily my name, age, and whether I had any current health issues. But after that came some questions that were surprising to me, and that could be considered "questionable questions," such as whether I smoked, and if not, had I ever smoked; whether I drank alcohol, and if so, how much, and if not, had I ever drunk alcohol; was I taking recreational drugs, and if so, how much and how often, and if not, had I ever taken recreational drugs.

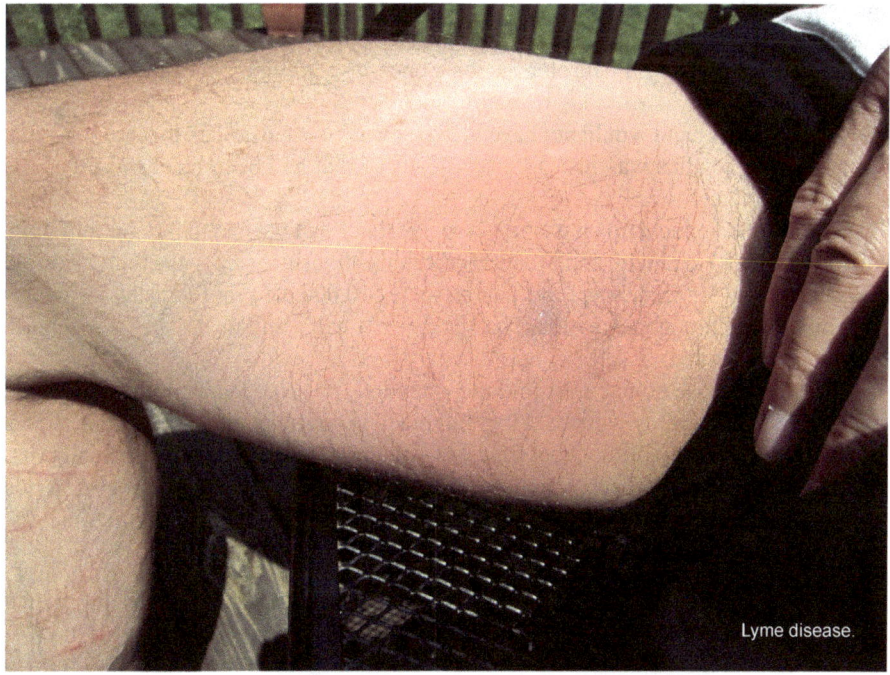

Lyme disease.

I suspect that many people would be offended by having to answer such private questions as a requirement for seeing a VA doctor. I answered them all because I had never smoked, had never drunk alcohol, and had never taken recreational drugs. I had nothing to hide. Afterward, I realized that my lifestyle choices were irrelevant to the issue at hand. The real issue that I had overlooked was that the VA had no right to ask such questions. The answers related to personal matters that were not the business of the VA.

As I was to learn, I was asked these very same questions prior to every subsequent PCP visit, even though the nurse had recorded my answers on the computer.

Revelation!

The question that was the most significant – although now moot – was whether I had a service-connected disability, and if so, how much.

When I told him 60%, he said, "In that case you have full coverage."

"What does that mean?

He spoke as if it were common knowledge. "It means that you can get treatment at any VA hospital for any reason, whether it's service connected or not."

My heart skipped a beat.

The nurse continued to ask questions, and I continued to answer them methodically. Meanwhile, my mind was in turmoil about the implications of his off-the-cuff statement. If what he said was true, then I could go to a VA hospital for an annual flu shot instead of paying $10 to the local pharmacy. It meant that I could have saved $50 to have my eye treated for what turned out to be a simple case of an "inflamed pinguecula," plus the cost of a bottle of Visine. It could have save me the charges of two opthalmologist to treat a severe case of conjunctivitis (pink eye). It meant that I would not have had to pay an emergency room doctor to stitch my thumb after I cut it on a sharp piece of metal. It meant that I would not have had to pay, first a hospital, then six months of treatment by a neurologist, for a once-in-a-lifetime case of idiopathic seizure.

It also meant that I would not have had to pay a thousand dollars to learn that what I thought was sciatica was instead a sciatic nerve that had been damaged by a rifle bullet in Vietnam.

And worse – much, much worse – it meant that I had not had to pay for a lifetime of Blue Cross, Blue Shield, and Major Medical health insurance. By the time I was old enough to apply for Medicare, I was paying some $10,000 per year for health insurance. That meant that throughout my life, I had paid nearly half a million dollars for insurance that I had not needed.

All this because no one ever told me when I was discharged from the Army that, due to the severity of my wounds, I had full medical coverage for the rest of my life: a benefit that had been willfully kept from me – not because I hadn't read the small print, but because I had never been given *any* print, just a curt goodbye and not even a ride to the Turnpike entrance from which I could thumb a ride home. The Army had disowned me as soon as I left the hospital parking lot.

Worse was yet to come. I just didn't know it yet.

PCP in Reality.

My visit with the PCP was short and, rather than to the point, almost pointless. I told him the reasons why I was in need of a doctor's care: my sore ankle and the damaged nerve in my leg. As requested, I showed my wounds to him, including the scars from the two tendon transplants. After looking at the scars, he listened to my heart.

One at a time, I brought out the paperwork that related to the examinations of the damaged nerve: my family doctor's, the orthopedic doctor's, and the neurologist's. One at a time, he glanced at the top page, then smirked as he handed it back to me without bothering to look at it. He also refused to add them to my newly formed file.

I had tried to obtain copies of the X-rays, MRI, and neurology examination, but I was refused on all three items. Only a doctor could obtain that data. Instead, I had typed the phone numbers of all three doctors on a sheet of paper. He refused to take the paper, and shook his head as he handed it back to me.

I had also brought with me the leftover prescription containers. I handed the plastic bottles to him. Each one had my name and the prescription printed on the label. He glanced at them, then handed them back to me without recording them.

It seemed to me that as far as the VA was concerned, I was a newborn babe with no background and no history, and no need for either. A decade later, the VA would use this lack of background and history as an excuse for the Chronic Pain Clinic to refuse to treat my ailments. Thus began a long and fruitless relationship with the VA.

When I mentioned how much my foot hurt from both nerve damage and ankle damage, especially when the ball touched linoleum, he neither spoke nor shrugged. He did nothing but stare at me.

Despite this somewhat shaky beginning, there were some positive points about this visit. The PCP let me have a limited dose of tramadol (three per day, or half the original dose that was printed on the label of the pill bottle), and three gabapentin pills per day (again, half the original amount). He also made an appointment for me with the VA orthopedic doctor, and sent me directly to the X-ray lab.

There is another kind of PCP. It stands for phenylcyclohexyl piperidine: a hallucinogenic drug that is better known as "angle dust." I think that the VA made a mistake and gave me the latter kind.

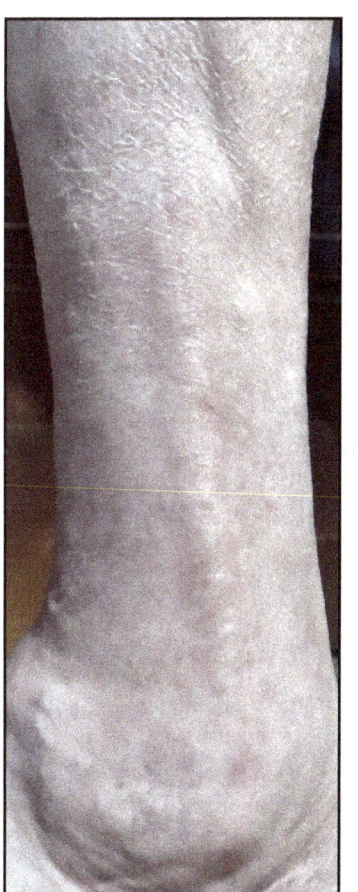

The 6-inch tendon transplant scar on the outside of my left leg to below the ankle. The ankle is bulged because of the knot that was tied after the living tendon was threaded through the bone holes.

A Difference of Opinion

A couple of weeks later, I visited the VA medical center for my appointment with the orthopedic doctor. I checked-in at the front desk. As I sat in the waiting room, a doctor entered and called someone's name. When no one answered, he called the name again. Still no one answered. The doctor left the room. When he returned a few minutes later, he called my name.

I stood up and said, "Here."

He asked me to follow him. My impression was that when he called the first name to which no one answered, he was confused and had called for the wrong patient. This was not a good start.

In his office, he showed me an X-ray and pointed to a small circular hole in my leg bone. He asked me if I knew what it was. I told him that it was a hole that had been drilled through the bone during my initial tendon transplant, an operation that was called a Watson-Jones repair. He did not want to examine the scars from the two operations.

He told me that he had never heard of a Watson-Jones repair. He also told me that the pain I felt was caused by post-traumatic arthritis. He explained that when a bone was damaged, it had a tendency to contract arthritis at the site of the damage.

I felt relief because this meant that I did not need another operation on my ankle.

When I asked him what I should do to relieve the pain, he told me to take ibuprofen, which would help to reduce the swelling. When I asked him for a prescription that I could collect at the pharmacy downstairs on my way out of the hospital, he told me to contact my PCP.

His advice did not help much because at that time I did not know that the hospital had such a thing as an internal email system. Nor did I have the PCP's hospital phone number (if he even had one). In fact, I knew nothing about the way the hospital functioned because none of the staff had explained anything to me. In my ignorance, I wound up buying ibuprofen at my local pharmacy, when according to the nurse's explanation, it should have been administered to me without paying for it.

Don't think that I was getting medication for free. I was not. Instead, think of medication as having been prepaid for life when I was wounded in Vietnam.

Later that summer, while I was hiking in the woods, I felt my ankle pain increasing to the point that tramadol and ibuprofen did not alleviate the pain. While I was pondering what I should do about it, Cheryl suggested that I go to the VA medical center's emergency room. That is what we did.

There I was examined by a physician's assistant (PA for short). I gave her my ankle history, including the fact that I had had an ankle X-ray recently. After reviewing my folder and the previous X-rays, she ordered another set of X-rays to be taken from different angles. She escorted me to the X-ray lab.

Afterward, in the emergency room, she examined the new X-rays. She thought that an ankle support would help to keep my ankle from twisting and bending sideways, thereby reducing the level of pain that I was feeling. She procured a generic brace from the prosthetic department. At the same time, she made an appointment for me with the prosthetic department, where I could be measured for a brace that was better fitted to my ankle.

I left the hospital with a brace on my ankle. The brace consisted of two plastic

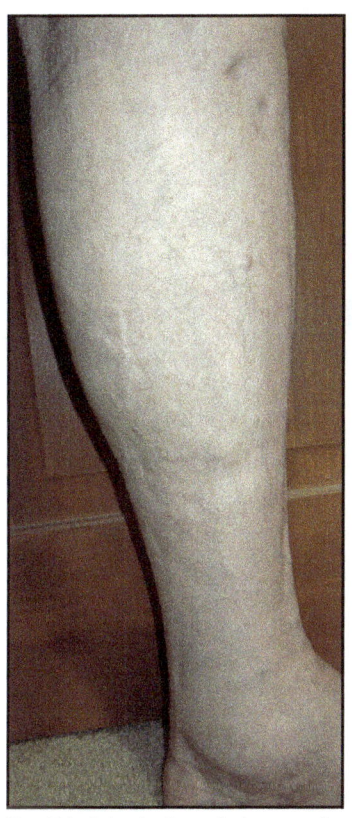

The 11-inch tendon transplant scar on the inside of my left leg to below the ankle. The new knot created another bulge. Note the two divots on my leg in the upper right corner. They are traction assembly scars from the pins that were driven through my shin.

sidewalls that stood vertically alongside my leg for about ten inches, and that were held together by top and bottom straps that were connected by means of Velcro. I did not wear the brace in the house because the floor was flat and level, and there were no tripping hazards. But I wore the brace whenever I stepped outside of the house. The brace was the most useful whenever I was hiking or biking in the woods, where I constantly had to hike on sloped and uneven ground, and where I had to hike in order to lift the bike over rocks, roots, and deadfall. Not only did I feel safer, but I felt less pain.

A few weeks later, I visited the prosthetic department where a prosthetic specialist found the correct size brace for me. He told me that he didn't know how long it would last under the conditions that I encountered during my outdoor activities, but that I was allowed to order a new one every three months by sending a request to my PCP. What is more important is that he told me how to do this by introducing me to the hospital email system, and how to use the system.

I did not again see my PCP until the following year. By "year" I do not mean exactly twelve months. I do not claim to understand how the VA hospital system operated its schedule, but like the precession of the equinoxes, my annual PCP visits occurred approximately every eleven months. This meant that every year I saw my PCP a month earlier in the year than I saw him the previous year.

The protocol for a PCP visit was a stop at the hospital laboratory where blood samples were drawn for various tests, followed by a fifteen-minute quiz with the nurse, ending with fifteen minutes with the PCP (if I was lucky). It was all cut and dried. The blood tests were completed and added to my folder so the PCP could examine them during our person-to-person visit. The laboratory people were extremely reliable. In the event that the blood work was not completed in time, the results were sent to me via the postal service several days later.

Before my next visit, I received a postal service notification that the VA was switching to a computerized check-in system that required each patient to have a plastic identification card on which my photograph was depicted. I was told to visit the check-in office on my next visit. Also, if I were a Purple Heart recipient, that fact could be annotated on the face of the card. As proof, I needed to bring my discharge document.

If the hospital had been functioning as it should, the PCP would have accepted my list of phone numbers on which the Philadelphia VA hospital was listed, and had my records forwarded to the Wilkes-Barre hospital. As I have already noted, the PCP refused to accept my list of phone numbers, or to request my military records.

I arrived early for my next visit with my PCP, and went straight to the personnel office on the first floor. For personal information, I handed my business card to the clerk. Then I had my photograph taken. While the image was being processed, I was directed to the waiting room where I would be called to see a personnel clerk who would confirm my Purple Heart authorization. I was told to return to the photo ID department afterward, in order to collect the validated VA identification card.

The personnel office was an open room with benches on one side and exposed cubicles on the other. Every person in the room was visible to every other person.

The personnel clerk asked for my contact information. Then he asked for my discharge certificate. After I gave the certificate to him, he told me that the discharge certificate had the wrong designation number for Purple Heart authorization. I told him that it was the only discharge certificate that was issued to me when I was discharged from the Army hospital. In that case, he told me, he could not authorize my Purple Heart.

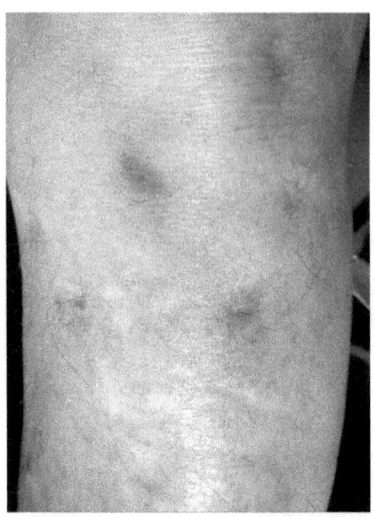

The scars from the traction assembly pins. The first traction assembly was not fitted for weights. The doctors in Tokyo rigged me with a traction assembly that was fitted for weights, the purpose of which was to pull the segments of the femur apart, thus forcing the bone to "reach" for the other segment before knitting, thereby reducing the loss of the bone's length.

For your information, according to the Department of the Army Individual Service Review Board:

> (2) DD Form 256A (Honorable Discharge Certificate), per AR 635–200.
> *b.* A pay grade is needed only when the individual was killed or received service-related injuries or disease during the equivalent military service period. It is needed to obtain VA benefits.

Ironically, I was not asked to produce my Honorable Discharge Certificate when I checked into the Philadelphia VA hospital for ankle surgery, presumably because the Army had already forwarded my records to that hospital upon my discharge, based on the fact that I lived in Philly. Even more ironic is the fact that the Wilkes-Barre VA Medical Center did not ask me to produce that Certificate when I checked into its hospital the previous year. Apparently, the Wilkes-Barre hospital simply took my word that I was an Army veteran. What kind of slipshod hospital was this? You'll find out.

I had come prepared. I had also brought with me my original Purple Heart certificate. I pulled it from my briefcase and handed it to him. He glanced at it, handed it right back to me, and accused me of Photoshopping it.

I said, "Then call my doctor. He'll tell you about my wounds."

The clerk wouldn't budge. The only certificate that he would accept was an Honorable Discharge with the correct number in the lower left corner.

Now I was angry. "All right. I'll show you my scars." I stood up, unbuckled my belt, pulled down my pants, and . . .

He started screaming. Everyone in the open office area looked at us. He waved his hands and started yelling, "No no no. Don't do that." He repeated that he had to see an Honorable Discharge certificate with the correct number.

I got redressed, grabbed my paperwork, and stormed out of the room. Everyone watched me go.

I duly collected my VA identification card but without the Purple Heart certification.

(Years later, I received a free lifetime fishing license from the Commonwealth of Pennsylvania, because it was being offered to veterans who were at least 60 % disabled. My application was accepted without question. That was likely because my name had already been entered into the Pennsylvania veteran system upon my discharge. The Commonwealth gave $25 per month to veterans for every month they served in Vietnam.)

After getting screwed over by the VA clerk, I went upstairs for my near-annual appointment with my PCP. The nurse asked me the same boring questions that I had answered the previous year and that were already on record.

When I saw the doctor in the adjacent room, he looked at my folder on the computer, listened to my heart, then asked if I had anything to add. I told him that I was suffering from two side effects of gabapentin – the same two side effects that I had suffered three years earlier: constipation and temporary loss of balance.

He said, "You can't have those side effects because they are not in the literature." Case closed!

I didn't know about the so-called literature, but I knew that those same side effects returned as soon as I started taking gabapentin again. Furthermore, I had two friends who were also taking gabapentin. Charlie Ogletree had constipation, Pete Manchee had balance issues; I had lengthy conversations about these side effects with both of them. They were real.

Furtherest (my nonce word) more, consider this irony. When doctors of my friend Sophie Long prescribed gabapentin for her neuropathy, they warned her about these potential side effects. She did not succumb to either one of them.

I said, "But – "

Without uttering a word, my PCP interrupted me by jumping out of his chair, opening the office door, and motioning for me to leave. Just like that, my office visit was terminated.

He did not investigate the possibility that those side effects could have been due to a different cause. A harmful cause. A deadly cause. He simply dismissed them – and me – without further investigation.

I suffered increasing pain for another year. Once again, Cheryl came to my rescue by purchasing an over-the-counter medicine to counter constipation. I am still stuck with temporary bouts of loss of balance. I use a hiking pole for gambols in the woods.

Next year's exam was just as bad. I was in the nurse's office when the PCP burst into the room and insisted that he had someplace to go, and that he couldn't wait for the nurse to finish my pre-examination. The PCP told me to follow him to his office. He did a quick exam which did not offer me time to ask any questions about my condition. At five minutes to noon, he wrapped up my so-called medical examination and ran out of the office. I thought that he must have been very hungry.

I returned to the nurse's office in order to continue the first part of the annual exam.

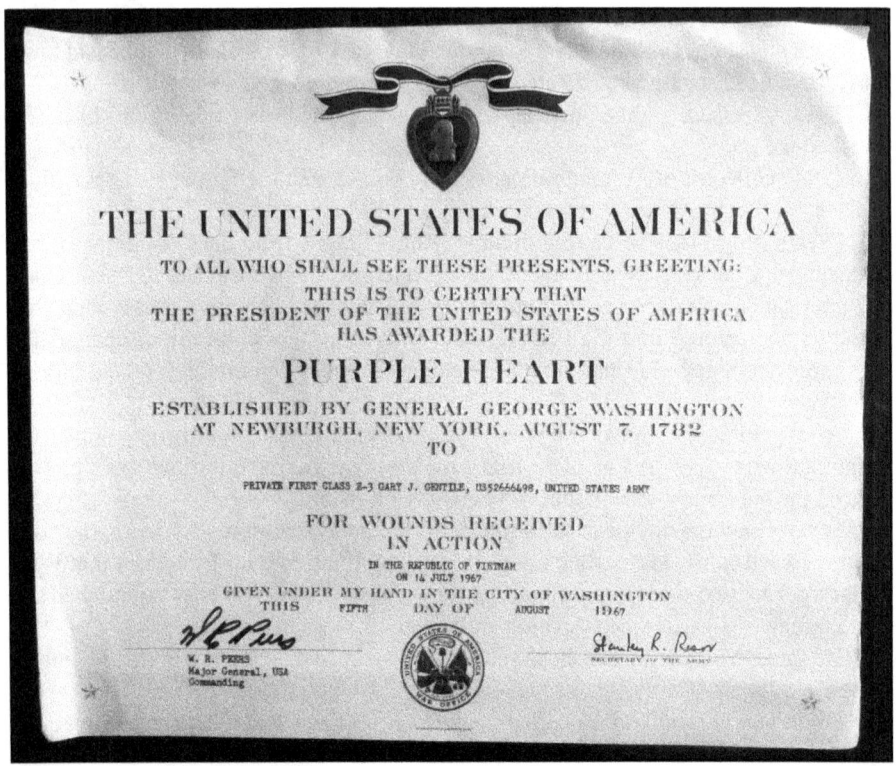

Ironically, because this certificate was too large to fit on my scanner, I had to take a photograph of it with a camera, then crop the image by using Adobe Photoshop. However, although the image was Photoshopped, I swear that the certificate is real! Because the certificate has been bent and warped throughout the years, due to its extraordinary size, I have let the black background show instead of cropping off the edges.

All this time, the aggravating pain in my ankle was my paramount issue. The brace was doing its job of holding my ankle firmly, so I had no complaints in that regard. The rough treatment from hiking and biking caused the straps to tear loose or the Velcro to peel off the vertical plastic supports. By using the in-house email system, I was able to order a replacement and receive it within a week. The problem was that the post-traumatic arthritic pain kept getting worse. The pcp refused to do anything about it.

Next year's visit with the pcp was a repetition of an earlier visit. As soon as I mentioned the word "pain," he opened the office door and motioned for me to leave. He would neither provide any treatment nor make an appointment for me to see an orthopedic doctor. Nor did he listen to my heart. Once I mentioned the word "pain," he terminated the examination.

Yet I had pain in my ankle. That was the primary reason that I went to the VA hospital in the first place. I wanted to be treated for pain that was the result of a combat injury that I sustained while I was in Vietnam. I had a right to receive treatment.

Now I wanted to have a new X-ray taken, and I wanted another examination by an orthopedic doctor, because the condition of my ankle was worsening and was causing more intense pain. But the PCP did nothing to help me. So this year passed without the VA providing me with any treatment for my injuries and wounds.

The next year's appointment was different. A week or two before my scheduled appointment with the PCP, I received a message from the Wilkes-Barre VA Medical Center, informing me that my annual examination had been canceled because my PCP was unavailable.

Note that my visit was not postponed; it was cancelled. Along with that, the blood tests and nurse's quiz were also canceled. As the PCP had thrown me out of his office the previous year, this meant that I must go another year without an annual medical exam: three years in all.

After thinking about this for a few weeks, I decided to take advantage of the situation. I sent either a memo or a letter to the director of the hospital, asking for a permanent transfer to a different PCP. After three months passed without a response, I sent another request. And another. I never heard from him.

The following year I had my so-called annual visit with the PCP. When I reminded him that I had not seen him the previous year because my visit had been canceled, he asked me for the date. After I gave him the date, he said, "I was in India at that time."

This time he was somewhat conciliatory. When I mentioned the pain in my ankle, he made an appointment for me with a VA orthopedic doctor – *years* after I first asked for it. And I used to think that two-week waits in the civilian world were long.

It was three to four weeks before I got to see the orthopedic doctor. He was a different doctor from the one I had seen before. I told him about my ankle pain, and about the new pain that I was having in my bad shoulder: so bad that I could not put away dishes in cabinet shelves that were located above the countertop without enduring extraordinary pain or dropping the dishes. He sent me to the X-ray lab where I had both my left ankle and left shoulder X-rayed.

Back in his office, he acknowledged the post-traumatic arthritis in my ankle but did nothing about it. The shoulder was a different story. He gave me a steroid injection which helped greatly in reducing the pain. For the next eight to ten months I could raise my shoulder above my head, and reach behind my back without enduring sharp pain. By the time of my next annual visit with the PCP, I was ready for another shot.

I kept complaining of increasing pain in my ankle, to no avail. Neither the PCP nor the orthopedic doctor would do anything about it.

I also raised another issue, this one about pain in bullet wound number three, the one on my butt. The deep scar was getting progressively more sensitive to the point at which I had to adopt new ways of sitting. On an ordinary chair that did not have arms – such as the dining room chair or the adjustable chair on rollers in my study – I sat with my left butt hanging off the edge of the seat. On a sofa or on a seat in a car, I twisted in such a way that my left buttock was raised in the air while all my weight lay on the outer side of my right buttock.

The PCP offered no suggestions. Cheryl solved the problem by buying special (and expensive) seat cushions that were made of honeycombed elastic gel that stood an inch and a half high. The relief that these cushions offered was immense. I wonder why my PCP didn't make such a recommendation.

Covid 19

Few people on planet Earth are unaware of the worldwide pandemic that was known officially as "coronavirus disease 2019." The so-called "Wuhan pneumonia" first made its appearance in China in December 2019. Due to global aircraft travel, "the virus quickly spread around the world. So far, the human death toll has risen to approximately seven (7) million people, and still counting due to variant viruses as the original specimen mutated. More than one (1) million Americans have died of the disease due to physiological complications."

One complication that could result in death was respiratory failure; another was kidney disfunction. These complications were more likely to result in death among older people, especially senior citizens. At that time, Cheryl and I were 74 years old. Worse, we were at additional risk due to pre-existing medical conditions.

When Cheryl was ten years old, she slammed into a tree while sledding. One kidney was so badly damaged that it had to be removed. She was now being treated by a nephrologist (a kidney specialist) who closely monitored the function, intake, and output of her remaining kidney.

In Vietnam, I was close enough to my second assailant to see that he was shooting an AK-47. This was good for me. A bullet from an AK-47 generally maintained a relatively straight flight path through the human body, whereas a bullet from an M-16 commenced to tumble as soon as it made contact.

During Jungle Warfare Training, I watched a demonstration in which a sergeant fired a round from an AK-47 through a #10 can of stewed tomatoes. The diameter of the entry hole was the size of the bullet; the size of the exit hole was slightly larger and somewhat jagged.

The sergeant performed the same test with an M-16. When the bullet hit the can of stewed tomatoes, the entire back of the can exploded, with the metal peeled outward. The backboard was splattered with tomato sauce that measured the size of a basketball. At the same time, the sergeant demonstrated the recoil of the M-16 by holding the butt against his testicles. There was virtually no recoil.

The point of all this is that had I been shot in the chest with a bullet from an M-16, the bullet would have expanded enough to blow out half my back. When I had my ankle operation in 1985, the doctor had my chest X-rayed. He showed me the image. A black smear about the size of my fist covered the upper lobe of my left lung: scar tissue that no longer functioned or transported hemoglobin.

Nerve damage caused the lung compression muscles to atrophy: a condition that has gotten worse with age. Between lung damage and muscular deterioration, I would be in serious trouble if I caught covid and had to be put on a ventilator to keep me breathing. I doubt if I would have survived for very long, as many people who did not have a damaged lung died anyway.

When the first vaccine was developed and was available at the Wilkes-Barre VA Medical Center, it was made available only to staff, residents, and "high risk patients over 75 years of age." By this time I was only five months shy of the allowable age.

I sent a memo to my PCP in which I reminded him of my damaged lung, and asked him to make an exception in my case. He refused to do so. Answer: "You will be notified when vaccine is available to you." His lack of regard for my health sounded to me like a death knell.

Cheryl and I made enormous efforts to avoid human contact with family members, friends, neighbors, and especially strangers we met on the no longer "happy trails to you." We immediately quit hiking on popular trails and explored places that were seldom visited, due largely to the rugged terrain. On the rare occasions when we did meet someone, we kept a discrete distance as we waved or chatted.

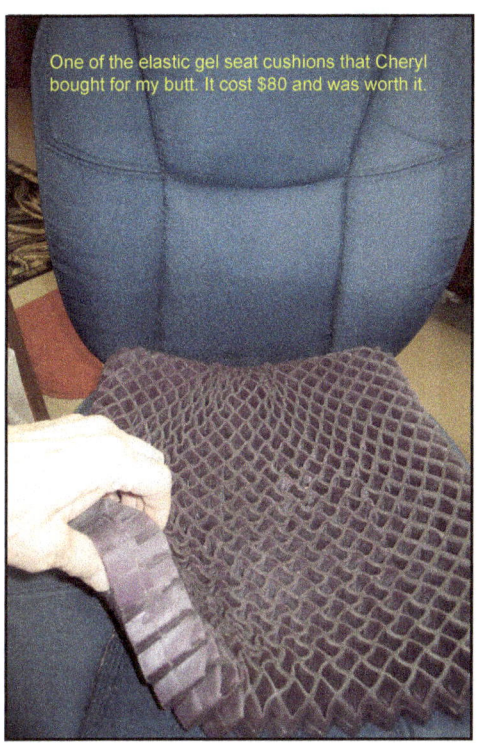
One of the elastic gel seat cushions that Cheryl bought for my butt. It cost $80 and was worth it.

A couple of months later, I received a memo from the PCP in which he allowed that "I can schedule you for the covid vaccine." By that time the issue was moot because I had already gotten the vaccine from my local pharmacy (as did Cheryl).

The Cold Shoulder

My PCP would neither have me tested nor treated for anything unless I prompted him to do so. My visits with him ended as soon as I mentioned the "p" word. I thought that the only way I could obtain treatment for pain was to circumvent the PCP and go directly to the orthopedic doctor. However, according to VA hospital rules and regulations, he or she was not permitted to prescribe medicine to his or her patients. Only the PCP could do that. Thus the system did not allow me to obtain pain relief from any other internal source.

In essence, a VA PCP was a medicinal god with totalitarian authority.

The pain in my shoulder was getting worse. My only recourse was the orthopedic doctor – the same one who refused to do anything about my ankle pain other than to suggest a brace. The brace was preventing my ankle from bending sideways, but it did little to nothing for the pain. What I needed was stronger pain medication, but my PCP continued to refuse to either increase the dosage of tramadol or prescribe a stronger medicine. I was at a dead end.

Could I expect any better treatment for my shoulder? All I could do was to hope. Thus I demanded an appointment with the orthopedic doctor, preceded by an X-ray, in the hope that I could obtain a steroid injection.

A miracle occurred!

After examining the X-ray, the doctor thought that another steroid injection might help. Not cure, you understand, but alleviate the pain. And it did. Not one hundred percent, but pretty close. He offhandedly mentioned that I could have steroid shots every six months: something that he had neglected to tell me the first time. I was flabbergasted by his casual attitude and lack of information that was so important to my condition.

Whenever I had to push my bike, I had to do so by standing on the left side so that my elbow was bent as I held onto the handlebars. The irony was that I had to dismount on the right side because of my bad left leg, for two reasons: my left leg was an inch shorter than my right, so if I tried to dismount on the left side, I had trouble getting my right leg over the seat; and because of the pain and instability of my left ankle, if I put all my weight on that ankle I usually lost my balance and fell over with the bike on top of me. Therefore, I dismounted on the right side of the bike, then held it upright by gripping the rear tire as I stepped around the bike.

Cumbersome? Yes. Annoying? Yes. But I had spent a lifetime adapting to my disabilities in the least painful and most effective manner. This maneuver was hardly worth a shrug.

Temper Tantrum

Then came the year when the incredible happened, when the extraordinary happened: an event so bizarre that you might not believe the truth of what I must now relate to you; an event that was a once in a lifetime event. No, it was a *never* in a lifetime event; an event that may never have happened in the history of medical science, and likely will never happen again.

I won't blame anyone who hesitates to accept the validity of the event that I will now describe. Yet the consequences of that event speak for the truth of my description, because the rest of this Part of the book would never have happened had this singular event not occurred. Here goes.

My meeting with the nurse went as usual. My meeting with the PCP started normally. He read the results of the blood tests. He listened to my heart. Then came the departure. He asked how I was doing.

I removed my shoe and sock, and showed him how one toe pressed against the adjacent toe. In jogging shoes and dress shoes the pressure was unnoticeable. But in hiking boots, which I wore whenever I hiked and biked, the rigidity of the toecap that was made of hard leather forced the two toes to bunch, and caused strong discomfort that was getting worse. He told me that I needed an operation.

After a while he suggested that I wad a tissue and pack it between my toes to prevent them from rubbing together.

Then I complained about the worsening – indeed, unbearable – pain in my ankle. I could hardly walk, not only from the post-traumatic arthritis on the left side of the ankle, but from the bottom of the ankle where each step felt like an icepick was being driven into the sole of my foot.

The so-called doctor exploded like a bundle of dynamite. He leaped out of his chair, jumped to my side with his lips only inches away from my ear, and started screaming at the top of his voice. This went on for a full minute. Because of his harsh accent, I could not understand most of what he said. The only words that I clearly comprehended were, "You're a drug addict."

Then he threw open the office door, stormed into the hallway, and vanished from my view. He was gone. He did not return. I never saw him again. Ever.

I did not know it then, but his fantastic action turned out to be good riddance.

Topsy Turvy

My PCP knew better than anyone that I was not a drug addict. Every year the VA had me tested for recreational drugs by ordering a urinalysis and specific blood examinations. I had never failed the test. By this I mean that no drugs that had not been prescribed by my PCP were ever found in my system. Ever. Yet he had the temerity to call me a drug addict.

Like everyone else in the world, I *was* an addict. I was addicted to the absence of

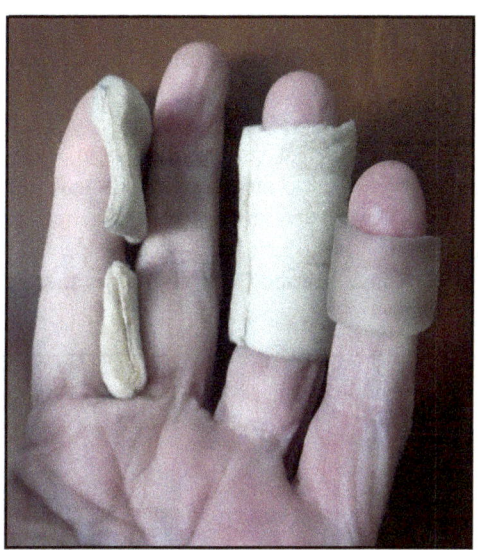

Cheryl found several types of toe spacers with several ways to employ them. My PCP told me to wad a tissue between digits. Perhaps they should exchange occupations.

pain. The fact that I could not satisfy that addiction was due to a PCP who maliciously withheld from me the very medicine that I needed: either a high dosage of tramadol or a return to hydrocodone, which had already proven to free me completely from pain. He refused to give me the treatment that I needed.

A few days later, Cheryl returned from the local pharmacy with a box of padded toe separators. Why didn't my PCP know about these simple devices?

If you are beginning to see a pattern here, that's because there is one. I found it ironic that Cheryl had given me more relief from pain than my so-called doctor. Her college degrees were in art history and guidance counseling, not in medicine.

Yet she was the one who suggested gel insoles that relieved the nerve pain in my foot; she found medicine for constipation which the PCP told me I did not have; she shopped for gel seat cushions that alleviated the contact pain in my buttock; she took me to the emergency room when I could not obtain ankle treatment from my PCP; she took me to a pharmacy that gave me a covid shot when my PCP refused to do so; she found commercial toe spacers that prevented my toes from rubbing, instead of using wadded tissues that were not nearly as satisfactory, and which my PCP recommended.

In short, Cheryl provided me with more pain relief than my PCP ever did.

Going Public

For weeks after my PCP ran out on me, leaving me stranded in his office, I pondered what to do about him. I was not only tired of being thrown out of his office, and him running out on me, I was also dismayed because his continuous violations of the Hypocritic (sic) Oath left me without the medical treatment that I so desperately needed.

As a veteran of the Vietnam Conflict, I had gotten used to being called dirty names by civilian protesters. But there was a big difference between maltreatment and malpractice. According to the Hippocratic Oath, doctors held themselves to a higher code of ethics than that which was observed by nonpracticing citizens.

The Veterans Administration was supposedly honor bound to make medical treatment available to military veterans, especially to those who had been wounded in combat. Yet I was unable to obtain proper medical treatment from the PCP who had been assigned to me by the Wilkes-Barre VA Medical Center. I had already written thrice to the director of the medical center, begging for a change in doctors, but the director did not even take the time to acknowledge receipt of my complaint, much less do anything about it.

So where could I go from here? What was my next move when both my PCP and the hospital director refused to help me? Ultimately, instead of one move, I made several.

I started a letter campaign.

My first letter went to Michael Missal, the Director of Veterans Affairs in Washington, DC. After three months, my letter was returned to me unopened. It had been delivered, inspected, and X-rayed, but as far as I could determine it never reached the desk of Michael Missal or any of his subordinates. If the letter had been "inspected," then the Department of Veterans Affairs must have learned from my return address label that I was a veteran.

> Michael Missal   November 21, 2021
> Department of Veterans Affairs
> 810 Vermont Ave., NW, POB 1151
> Washington, DC 20420
>
> The enclosed letters should be self-explanatory, but I will add provenance for clarification.
>
> My elected representatives received only page number 1. I chose brevity in order to focus on the ultimate event which caused me to reach out to them for help. I did not want to overwhelm them with details at that time.
>
> The media received (and continues to receive) both page number 1 and page numbers 2-3. I wanted the media to have the full background events that led to my prayer for help.
>
> I did not bother to contact the Wilkes-Barre VA Medical Facility about this latest outburst because I tried that avenue before, and it did not work. At that time I thought that a diplomatic approach would achieve positive results while containing the situation in-house. But the Facility ignored my protest. Now I am in too much pain to care about "blowing the whistle" on my so-called caretakers and their dreadful lack of diligence; or about hurting people's feelings, especially those who ignored my original plea for help; or about painting the VA in its true light by rebuking the false image that it presents to the public.
>
> You now have all the information that is needed to initiate a full investigation into this matter, and to alleviate my personal situation.

I wasted no time in mailing a second copy to the same person and address. After another three months without a reply, I sent a third copy to the named recipient. I never received a reply. I surmised that the Director of Veterans Affairs had no interest in a wounded Vietnam veteran. Ultimately, I never received a reply to that letter either.

While I was waiting for a reply from the Department of Veterans Affairs, I sent a bevy of letters to newspapers and official representatives. Here is a summation of the results of my letter campaign:

Veterans Administration:
    Department of Veterans Affairs, Washington, DC
    3 letters, no replies, first letter returned unopened

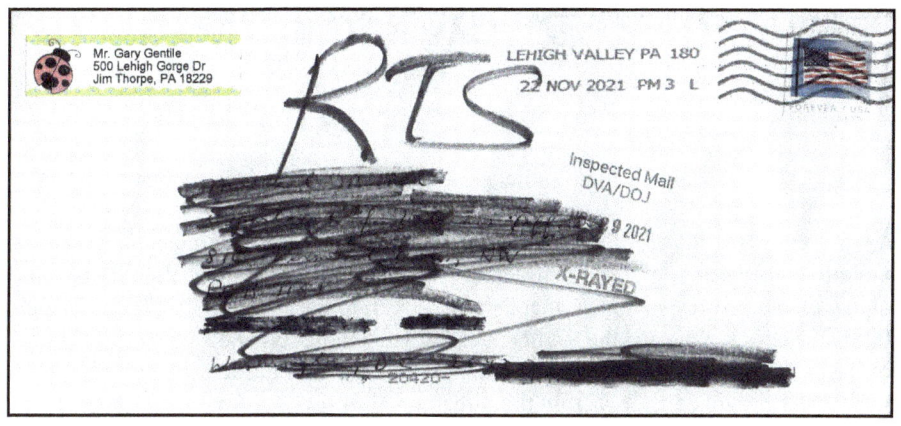

Director of the Wilkes-Barre VA Medical Center, Wilkes-Barre, Pennsylvania
5 letters, no replies
Director of Veterans Affairs, Jim Thorpe, Pennsylvania
2 letters, no replies

Local Pennsylvania newspapers:
Citizen's Voice	2 letters, no replies
Harrisburg Today	2 letters, no replies
Paxton Herald	2 letters, no replies
Philadelphia Inquirer	2 letters, no replies
Times Leader	2 letters, no replies

National newspapers:
Chicago Tribune	2 letters, no replies
Los Angeles Times	2 letters, no replies
New York Times	2 letters, no replies
Washington Post	2 letters, no replies

Representatives:
Senator Robert Casey   2 letters, no replies

Senator Doyle Heffley   3 letters, no replies, despite a face-to-face visit from my friend Jerry McAward, who knew Heffley personally, and who stressed to Heffley my difficulties with the VA. Heffley still did not reply. I expected more from Heffley because in his self-promotion brochure he claimed to be a staunch advocate for veterans. In my opinion, his stance as an advocate for veterans was a scam that was designed to garner votes but was totally lacking in substance.

Congressman Dan Meuser   2 letters, no replies

Senator Susan Wild   4 letters, no replies
She was another self-promoter who, in my opinion, used her familial connection (her husband was a veteran) as a way to trick people into believing that her adver-

tising as an advocate for veterans was real, instead of a scam that was intended to garner votes.

        Governor Tom Wolf   2 letters, no replies

        Senator John Yudichak   2 letters, no replies

        Senator Pat Toomey   1 letter, responded in less than a month via telephone. A staff member called to provide instructions about how to fill out an online privacy statement that I should return to the office so that Toomey could intervene between me and the VA hospital. I filled out the form and sent it to Toomey's office in Washington, DC. Toomey's letter to the director of the Wilkes-Barre VA Medical Center provoked a reply from the director.

Note that of the 44 letters that I sent, this is the only recipient who bothered to respond. It seemed to me that there was not much interest in helping a wounded soldier from a war that the country would rather forget.

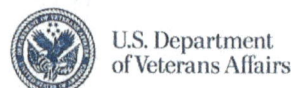

U.S. Department
of Veterans Affairs

Medical Center
1111 East End Boulevard
Wilkes-Barre, PA 18711

In Reply Refer to: 693/110
SSN 0747
GENTILE, John

The Honorable Patrick J. Toomey
United States Senator
1150 S. Cedar Crest Blvd., Suite 101
Allentown, PA 18103

RECEIVED
FEB 09 2022
Allentown

Dear Senator Toomey:

    Thank you for the opportunity to reply to your concerns regarding the healthcare provided to Mr. John Gentile at the Department of Veterans Affairs (VA) Medical Center, Wilkes-Barre, Pennsylvania.

    In response to the concerns noted in Mr. Gentile's recent correspondence, he was contacted by Lori A. Duda, Administrative Officer Primary Care, to further explore the specifics of his concerns and dissatisfaction he reported experiencing during recent exam appointments.

    We regret Mr. Gentile felt his appointment with Primary Care was unsatisfactory and we apologized for any inconvenience that may have resulted. Wilkes-Barre VA is dedicated to providing our Veterans with quality services. As a result of the events noted in his letter, a detailed discussion of his concerns has taken place.

    Mr. Gentile was made aware his Primary Care Provider, Dr. Atul Dalsania, has reviewed his requests and had placed orders for additional radiology testing, as well as orthopedic and pain management consultations which have, or will be subsequently scheduled. Mr. Gentile acknowledged understanding and agreement to this plan of care and expressed appreciation for assistance provided by staff.

    I want to assure you that at the Wilkes-Barre VA Medical Center, we believe that our Veterans are our nation's heroes. If you have additional questions regarding this issue, you may contact Ms. Lori A. Duda, Administrative Officer, at (570) 824-3721, Extension 24674.

                        Sincerely,

                        Russell E. Lloyd
                        Director

My letter to the director

I need help. I was badly wounded in combat. My ankle was damaged by an enemy grenade, and I received three bullet wounds: one shattered a femur, another passed through a lung and exited through a shoulder blade, the third was a flesh wound. I spent thirteen months recuperating in army hospitals. I have suffered chronic pain ever since. I was discharged with a disability rating of 60 %.

My level of pain has increased with age. I started to receive medication for pain in 2011. I am currently receiving treatment from the Wilkes-Barre Veterans Administration Hospital. I have been assigned to a doctor who treats my pain with disdain. Initially, he halved the amount of pain medication that was prescribed to me by my previous doctor. Now I need either a higher dosage or a more effective medication, neither of which my current doctor will prescribe.

Here is how my most recent visit went. The doctor spent five to six minutes going over my chart and viewing the results of my blood work. He listened to my heart for a minute. Then I told him that I had some issues that I needed to discuss with him. He looked at the clock and said to hurry. The time was three minutes till noon.

I showed him a problem that I was having with my unwounded foot, and asked what could be done about it because it was causing additional pain. He said that I needed an operation. When I asked him to schedule the operation, he looked at the clock, then said that I should wait until the problem gets worse. I certainly did not want the operation, but as it was necessary, I would rather have it before my condition got worse and I had to endure additional pain.

The doctor then looked at the clock and said that he had to go. I said that I needed to discuss my chronic pain issue because the pain was getting stronger. Much of the time I could not walk without a ski pole that I cut short to use as a cane or crutch. He started yelling at me and went into a tirade. Because he spoke so fast, and because he has such an indecipherable accent, I could not interpret everything he said. But I did hear him say that more pain medication was not good for me, because the pain was in my head.

The pain is certainly not in my head. X-rays showed how badly my ankle was damaged. When I put weight on that leg, I felt as if my ankle was being stabbed with an ice pick. After a neurological exam of my shattered femur, the neurologist told me that there was nothing that could be done except to treat the pain. An orthopedic doctor has recently given me a cortisone shot for displacement of and pain in my broken scapula. These are real pains in various parts of my body where I suffered debilitating wounds.

Like everyone else in the world, I am addicted to the absence of pain. My body is wracked with pains that needs treatment. These pains can be alleviated by proper medication, which this doctor is unwilling to prescribe. Pain medication is not necessarily bad; it is used by millions of Americans to alleviate pain and make life more comfortable and productive.

My pain is so bad that it sometimes wakes me at night. If I take the medication that the doctor has eked to me, then I run out of it before the end of the month when my prescription can be renewed. I work at home on a computer, but often the pain is so sharp that I cannot focus on my work.

I have never had a doctor yell at me before. Other doctors have listened to what I had to say as I described my symptoms, then prescribed suitable medication. Plus, I still had other issues to address. This doctor looked at the clock, quit his rant, and rushed out of the office, leaving me in the middle of an examination. I grabbed my ski pole and hobbled after him. I spotted him fifty feet away as he turned into another corridor. I caught up with him only because he stopped at the secretary's deck. Without speaking to me, he pointed to the secretary and departed without a backward glance. The secretary scheduled my next appointment – for a year from then!

All I got from the doctor was ten minutes of his time, most of which was taken with his telling me the results of my blood tests. He took one minute to listen to my heart. Then he yelled at me for three minutes because I mentioned chronic pain. He ignored my request for surgery which he himself recommended. Now he will not see me again for another year.

None of my issues was resolved. I am still suffering from chronic pain. I do not have the proper medicine to relieve that pain. He left me to suffer for another year, at which time the process will repeat itself – as it did this year.

More than a year ago I wrote to the Wilkes-Barre VA hospital and asked to be assigned to a different doctor. No one at the hospital has replied to my request, so I cannot rely on the Veterans Administration to help me. I need a doctor who is sympathetic to my condition, and who is less interested in lunch and more interested in the comfort and treatment of his patients. I have nowhere else to turn. Please intervene in my behalf.

I served my country. It is time for my country to serve me.

A Lick and a Promise

In response to Senator Pat Toomey's letter, the director of the Wilkes-Barre VA Medical Center promised to correct the abuse that I was currently receiving.

Noted in the director's letter to Toomey, an aide named Lori Duda would call to inform me that she had contacted the hospital's Chronic Pain Clinic, and that I would soon receive a call from someone at said clinic to make an appointment. Both calls were duly initiated.

This begs the question: why did my PCP not send me to the Chronic Pain Clinic years ago? He certainly knew that I was in chronic pain, because I managed to inform him of that fact on several occasions before he threw me out of his office or ran out on me. Yet he never mentioned that such a clinic existed in the very building in which he was purportedly practicing medicine and was supposedly caring for the welfare of his patients.

Paragraph 4 of the director's letter was written in such a misleading manner that it made it seem as if my PCP took the initiative to place orders for additional testing. Not true. It was *I* who, on my own volition, used the hospital memo system to *demand* a neurological examination of my leg as well as an MRI of my ankle. The only thing that my PCP did was to accept my demands instead of blocking them.

I neither "acknowledged understanding and agreement to this plan of care," nor "expressed appreciation for assistance provided by staff." I did everything on my own. I *created* "this plan of care," (except for the Chronic Pain Clinic, knowledge of which was maliciously withheld from me by my PCP). There was no one for whom I "expressed appreciation." In the absence of a caring and dedicated PCP, I was forced to do everything myself. The director made it seem as if the staff did something extraordinary for which they should receive appreciation. In fact, they were only doing their jobs after I put them in a position that forced them to do so.

When the clinic's secretary called to schedule the appointment, I gave her phone numbers for the Philadelphia VA hospital where my ankle surgery took place in 1985, and for the neurologists who examined me in Palmerton in 2011. I impressed upon her the facts that the Philly hospital had all my medical records, which could be forwarded to the Wilkes-Barre hospital; and that the neurologist who examined the results of the neurological test was now working in the Wilkes-Barre VA Medical Center, and had been working there for the past 10 years. The latter could be contacted through the interoffice communication system.

In the meantime, I had both the MRI of my ankle and the neurological test of my leg. I was happy to learn that due to technological advances in the testing equipment, the electrical bursts of the shock treatment were not only tolerable but were hardly noticeable. I had suffered far worse shocks when I worked in the electrical trade.

The findings of these tests were sent to my PCP. The result of the MRI was so alarming that the PCP called me at home in order to tell me the bad (and incriminating) news. He told me that the deterioration of the bones in my ankle was much greater than he ever would have imagined. (My words, not his.)

This was not news to me. I felt that deterioration every single day, every hour, every minute, with every step I took. It was the whole rationale for my asking the VA medical center for help. Help, I should add, that has been willingly and knowingly withheld from me.

The PCP left the issue hanging. But I knew right away what the facts implied: that had either he or the orthopedic doctor treated my condition when I first arrived at the hospital so many years ago, my ankle would not have reached such a horrible state of degeneration – which was still getting progressively worse.

Did the PCP now offer a solution to this progressively worsening problem? No.

Did he present a way in which to reduce the pain? No.

He just gave me the information and went on his merry way.

My PCP called me again at home a few days later with another alarming broadcast. It came as no surprise to me that the neurologist determined that the damage to my sciatic nerve could not be repaired, and that the only therapy available was to treat the pain. He had now told this to me twice: first in 2011 when I suffered the grand episode, and a few days earlier when he repeated his previous diagnosis.

The nerve damage was not getting any better, and there was no way to stop the nerve damage from getting worse.

Did the PCP now offer a solution to this progressively worsening problem? No.

Did he present a way in which to reduce the pain? No.

He just gave me the information and went on his merry way.

A few days later I sent him a memo in which I asked him to increase the dosage of tramadol. He reluctantly admitted that I could now have four pills per day instead of three. The increase in pain relief was slight.

NEUROLOGY CONSULTATION:-OUTPATIENT NEUROLOGY CONSULTATION.

REASON FOR CONSULTATION:-
Brief History: Patient status post gunshot wound in Vietnam, with damage to left sciatic nerve.
EMG study was done recently confirmed that. Patient requested to follow-up in Dr. Karim clinic, was seen by Dr. Karim in the community previously.

CHIEF COMPLAINTS:-
Brief History: Patient status post gunshot wound in Vietnam, with damage to left sciatic nerve.
EMG study was done recently confirmed that. Patient requested to follow-up in Dr. Karim clinic, was seen by Dr. Karim in the community previously.

HISTORY OF PRESENT ILLNESS:-
Patient is a 75-year-old white male with a past medical history significant for gunshot injury in the left thigh/left chest, osteoarthritis, hyperlipidemia, chronic pain syndrome. Back in July 14, 1967 while patient was in the services and deployed to Vietnam patient was hit in the left thigh area and also left chest area by 2 bullets by the enemy. The bullet in the left thigh area injured the left sciatic nerve while exiting the wound area. Subsequently over the years patient has been complaining of pain in the left buttock area radiating all the way down to the posterior aspect of the left thigh/left leg down to the

> left foot. Along with this he also has pain in the ball of the left ankle. He does have significant degenerative joint disease of the left ankle joint which is adding to this problem and pain. Recent EMG of left lower extremity revealed possible injury to the left sciatic nerve. Therefore clinically he does have left sciatic nerve injury. Since this is chronic pain he has already been referred to the chronic pain clinic. I have discussed the whole option of pain control with this patient and since there is no surgical options pain management is the only thing which is needed for this patient. He has already been started on Gralise which is slowly being titrated. Previously he was on other pain medications including oxycodone which I told patient was not a good idea. I do not know whether patient will benefit from injections in that particular area. I will defer that to the pain management team.

This image and the one on the previous page are screen shots from the VA email system. The neurologist made a mistake when he wrote "oxycodone." During our conversation I made no mention of oxycodone. I told him that my family doctor had prescribed hydrocodone. The neurologist must have misremembered.

Chronic Pain Clinic Buffoonery

Apparently there are two definitions for Chronic Pain Clinic. One might hope that it is a clinic which provides pain *relief*. The VA defines it differently, as a clinic that ignores a patient's pain symptoms by providing placebos. Who would have thought?

Come the day of the appointment, Cheryl accompanied me to the courtroom in which the trial was held. There were five people in the room, none of whom was a doctor.

The secretary who had called me to arrange the time for the meeting unabashedly announced that she had not gotten in touch with the neurologist, even though he worked in the present building; and had not bothered to contact the Philly VA hospital where all my medical records were readily available. This meant that my presentation of chronic pain would not be supported by medical evidence.

This was certainly an auspicious commencement for what I had hoped would be a prime opportunity to present my case to a hopefully impartial panel that was dedicated to aiding patients who were suffering from devastating chronic pain. I felt as if she was pooh-poohing my case as insignificant, and that I was not to be taken seriously. Instead of aiding my case she was deriding it at the outset.

Of the other four jurors in the room, one was a physician's assistant, one was a pharmacist, one was a psychologist, and the last one was a student. Oddly, the person who interceded the most was the pharmacist. The physician's assistant occasionally asked questions for a point of clarification. The psychologist kept quiet until after I completed the descriptions of my various lifelong pains and their worsening severity; then she asked a series of questions about my mental and emotional states. The student merely watched the proceedings. It seemed to me that his job was to learn how the other four people kept veterans from obtaining the pain relief that they needed.

As it turned out, none of the people took me seriously, even though Cheryl confirmed everything that I said, and added more detail from her personal observations.

The only good thing that I can say about my soliloquy was that at least no one yawned or fell asleep.

I did make one inconsequential mistake. As the psychologist rattled off a litany of questions, to which I kept responding "No," she asked me if I had trouble sleeping. I automatically said "No." Later that night, as I was preparing for bed, I realized that I should have told her about the increasing frequency of flashbacks, which prevented me from getting to sleep. I was taking a nightly dose of sleeping pills. In the long run, it didn't make any difference because that fact was not a tipping point on the result of the meeting.

Here is how I should have responded to her question. Decades ago, when I was scuba diving off the coast of Florida, I was stung by a Portuguese man-of-war. I immediately returned to the dive boat. The pain was so severe that I lost consciousness on the deck. After the boat returned to the marina, I was taken to a pharmacy where I was instructed to purchase Benadryl: an over-the-counter antihistamine that was commonly taken for the relief of allergic reactions. As I quickly learned, a side effect of Benadryl was drowsiness.

Fast forward a number of years. After my sciatic nerve "episode" in 2011, I started suffering from an increase in the number of flashbacks that I experienced as I tried to fall asleep at night. As I noted earlier in this book, the trigger for these flashbacks was pain. A throbbing leg reminded me of why I was in such pain: getting shot in Vietnam.

One night, while I was trying to get to sleep, I remembered the Portuguese man-of-war incident. I asked Cheryl to buy a box of Benadryl pills the next time she stopped at the Pharmacy. Two pills put me right to sleep. When I next visited my PCP, before he had time to throw me out the door, I mentioned this improvised sleep medication. He was in a rare mood because he prescribed a replacement called hydroxyzine. I worked like a charm and I've been taking it ever since.

Yet, sometimes the flashbacks were so strong that they overrode the medication. Plus, as my sciatic pain has increased in intensity and frequency due to the lack of adequate analgesics, my flashbacks have increased so that now I must take them every night.

This reminded me again about what one Army doctor said to another after examining me before my discharge, "He's going to have a tough time later on." (Or words to that effect.)

So, after an hour of pouring out my soul to a group of disinterested collaborators, they adjourned to an adjacent room in order to determine my ultimate fate with regard to chronic pain. The prejudiced jury returned in 3 to 4 minutes – perhaps the shortest deliberation in the history of criminal injustice. By ignoring all the facts that Cheryl and I presented, they agreed to provide me with a medication that contained a long and fancy-sounding multisyllabic chemical that meant nothing to me, but which I agreed to take on a trial basis.

Imagine my shock when it was delivered to my house via the United States Postal Service, only to learn that it was nothing more than an over-the-counter skin cream that I could have purchased at Walmart for 10 dollars plus tax.

Even a moron should know that sciatic pain cannot be cured by skin cream. If it could, a whole lot of chiropractors would have been put out of business a long time ago. Yet this team of VA medical personnel had somewhere in their training been hoodwinked into believing that ordinary skin cream could put an end to pain that resulted from a damaged sciatic nerve that was beyond repair.

I do not apologize for japing. It was well earned.

You Can't Push Rope

According to MedStar Health, "Injuries of the sciatic nerve can occur for a variety of reasons, including prolonged pressure, trauma, scarring, or other damage. They may be seen in cases of pelvis or femur fractures, *gunshot wounds*, poorly performed injections, tumors, complications from hip surgery, and specific positions during surgery." (Italics mine.)

As you can read, this description describes my symptoms perfectly.

Furthermore, "Depending on the severity of the lesion and symptoms, the pain management specialist may first recommend pain management medication and physical therapy. Patients with more serious symptoms will likely require surgery to repair the nerve."

Note that nowhere does MedStar Health mention skin lotion in any way, shape, or form. Here's why.

The pain from a damaged sciatic nerve may not be felt at the point of origin. A pinched nerve in the lower spine may be felt anywhere in the upper leg, lower leg, or foot. I've had pain in all these areas at the same time, and only in certain areas at other times. Presently I feel the most pain in the ball of my foot, while at the same time I feel numbness on the top of my foot and on the four small toes. Rubbing skin lotion on any of these locations did not relieve the pain that I felt at those locations because the nerve that caused the pain was damaged at the site of the bullet wound, or possibly in my buttock because of that other bullet wound, or both.

This is the reason that amputees sometimes feel "phantom pain": pain that was felt in a foot or leg that had been amputated. The pharmacist telling me to rub skin lotion on my foot was like telling an amputee to apply skin to the air where his foot used to be.

The VA neurologist told me specifically – on two occasions twelve years apart – that my left sciatic nerve was irreparably damaged and could not be repaired, and that the only way I could obtain relief was by treating the pain.

This begs the question: as the VA's own neurologist suggested treating the pain, why did the folks at the Chronic Pain Clinic not do what he recommended? After all, he knew more about my chronic pain issue than all five of those folks combined. The answer to this question is a simple one, but you will find it hard to believe.

They had not bothered to read either report!

How do I know this, you may ask. I know this because after I was sentenced to receiving nothing more than skin lotion for the relief of sciatic nerve pain, I had one face-to-face meeting with the pharmacist in the VA medical center, and one subsequent telephone conversation.

I asked the pharmacist directly if he or any of the others in attendance at my stakeless witch burning had read the report.

His answer was a simple, "No."

Worse yet, he did not promise to read the reports, or to use the information to alter his opinion about the type of medical treatment that I would receive. How do I know this? I know this because I asked him a direct question about whether I could expect to receive a stronger medication that would treat my level of pain.

He said, "No."

"No" seemed to be the only reply in his vocabulary. He had made his decision, and nothing was going to change it. New evidence was not allowed to be submitted. Case closed.

When I told him that the skin lotion was useless, he said that skin lotion was all I would get. However, he later relented and let me have three acetaminophen pills per day. Acetaminophen was the medicine that I used to take for headaches. It was an over-the-counter medicine that was slightly stronger than aspirin. Baby aspirin. Okay for headaches but useless for sciatic nerve pain.

Another question that I asked him at one of these conferences was, "Does the doctor in charge of the Chronic Pain Clinic even know that I exist?"

He said, "No."

There were two ways that I could interpret this answer. If he was telling the truth, then the doctor in charge of the Chronic Pain Clinic did not know that I existed, which consequently meant that he or she did not care enough about the patients who were assigned to him or her, to examine them in order to make certain that they were being treated properly. In other words, he or she had a job that was merely a sinecure or a no-show job.

Sinecure is defined as "an office, commission, or charge that requires no work yet provides compensation."

No-show job is defined as "a paid position that ostensibly requires the holder to perform duties, but for which no work, or even attendance, is actually expected. The awarding of no-show jobs is a form of political or corporate corruption."

This disorganization has left the patients to be handled by an unknowledgeable or non-caring or incompetent staff, or all of the above.

In other words, the Chronic Pain Clinic was a charade that looked good on paper and that allowed the VA to brag about the existence of such a clinic in case the VA was ever investigated about the efficiency of its management or the treatment of its patients. This scenario shows a clear case of dereliction of duty on the part of the hospital's director.

Shades of the scandal in the VA Health Care System in Phoenix, Arizona, where in 2014 some 40 veterans died while waiting for treatment, after which upper management personal awarded themselves bonuses for their non-existent efficiency. The VA hasn't changed much in the following decade, as this book has clearly shown.

On the other hand, if the pharmacist was lying, and there was no doctor in charge of the Chronic Pain Clinic, in which case the clinic was a mockery without adequate leadership. So who was in charge? Who oversaw the decisions that were made by the five individuals who presided over my case?

I did not know which of these interpretations was worse. For the forgotten Vietnam veteran, it didn't much matter because the outcome was the same: he remained forgotten and received little or no competent medical treatment.

As I have shown above, the five Chronic Pain Clinic people who moderated my case refused to obtain my medical history from the Philadelphia VA hospital, where my records were readily available. Plus, they refused to review the results of the MRI and the neurological examination: tests which I had demanded specifically for my meeting with the Clinic review panel. It seemed as if they, like my PCP, did not want to know anything about my medical history and the severity of my wounds.

Furthermore, this self-conceived quorum seem to have made a conscious decision not to believe what I told them about my wounds or medical history. If this kind of medical maltreatment was all that the hospital director could do for me, what else could I do?

When I worked in the electrical trade, we had a saying that goes like this: "You can't push rope." This means that when you push a length of conduit from one end, the entire length of conduit moves, but when you push a length of rope from one end, the rope merely bunches in the middle while the other end of the rope remains in place.

In other words, no useful work can be accomplished by workers who are dedicated to not doing their jobs.

The Chronic Pain Clinic was like rope. It could not be budged into doing work that it had purportedly been created to do. It was broken, and it seemed to me that no one wanted to fix it. The clinic was running out of control because it lacked a governor. It did me no good to push the clinic for help because it was just another length of rope.

Hippocratic Hypocrisy

I put another arrow into my bow. I wrote a letter of complaint to the American Medical Association. Three months later, I received a reply in which I was informed that the AMA "does not accept or process complaints against physicians, hospitals or medical centers. To file a formal complaint, please contact your state's medical licensure board."

As suggested, I then wrote to the Pennsylvania State Board of Medicine, and explained my situation. Two months later, I received an acknowledgment of receipt, in which I was told to "Promptly return any additional information to this office in writing."

The Board did not send me any information to return, so I wrote a new list of complaints and sent them to the Board.

A week and a half later, I received another letter from the Board in which I was informed, the "Normal processing time is 9-12 months."

Apparently, promptness was a one-way street.

The actual processing time turned out to be not a year, but three months shy of *two* years. In between, a representative of the Pennsylvania State Board of Medicine visited me at home in order to conduct one half of the investigation of my case against my PCP. The other half was a visit to the PCP for his side of the story.

The investigator was not only professional but helpful. After I gave him the gist of my complaint, and told him where the doctor worked, he informed us (Cheryl was in the room and prompted me when my memory lapsed) about a previous case in which the director of the Wilkes-Barre VA Medical Center had been so obstinate and contrary that the investigator had to serve him with a subpoena in order to obtain his cooperation. This didn't surprise me, but it should have warned me about how much trouble I was going to have with him. A lot of trouble.

I told the investigator everything about my PCP that I have already written in this book. There is no reason for me to repeat it. The investigator was so impressed by my case – and so astonished at the PCP's violent behavior – that he told me that he had never had a case in which the evidence against a doctor was so damning.

But, he was quick to add, he didn't make the decisions. Someone else did that. All he did was to present the evidence that I provided. Furthermore, I would not have the opportunity to face the pcp in court, to ask questions, to object, or even to plead my case in front of a jury of my peers. The Board was a one-sided system: the Board's side.

I could not even read a transcript of the PCP's testimony, and object to incorrect or misleading statements. Nor would I be allowed to file amendments as the PCP continued his un-Hippocratic behavior.

I was still nothing more than an annoying soldier from the Vietnam war: one that the VA in general and the VA hospital in particular would like to forget.

Vengeance is Mine, Saith the . . .

In response to the results of my MRI and neurological examination, my PCP begrudgingly prescribed one additional tramadol pill per day – not voluntarily, but only after I demanded the increase. He must have had second thoughts about it because he did a complete reversal by cutting me off tramadol completely, and without notifying me ahead of time. He did it on the sly.

I made my usual monthly request on the seventh day of the month. I began to get anxious after a week had passed without receiving the pills in the mail. They were not delivered the next day, nor the day after than, nor the day after that. That was when I sent an anxiety-filled reminder through the hospital email system.

The PCP did not answer. He never answered. But I received a memo from one of his nurses, who said that a follow-up memo that was sent to the pharmacy established that the PCP had not placed the order.

By careful hoarding, I had managed to build a two-week back-up supply for just such an occasion. But my "incaser" reserve was about to be consumed. I informed the nurse of my plight.

"It was just my luck" usually precedes a sentence that forewarns of dire circumstances, but this time it was just my luck that the doctor was out of the office that day. The nurses all knew about the disaccord that was ongoing between me and the PCP – and likely between other patients and the PCP – because they read all my memos first, then either forwarded them on their own recognizance to the appropriate recipient, or sent them to the PCP for execution (or discard).

I don't know the circumstances that occurred that day among the nurses and the substitute doctor, who to a certain extent had to rely on the nurses' advice for dealing with patients whose medical issues were unknown to him or her. I would not tell the tale if I did because it might result in one or more of the nurses being fired due to vindictiveness of my PCP. All I know for certain is the result.

The substitute doctor prescribed a full dose of six tramadol pills per day: enough to last until my next order date and then some. By the time the prescription was delivered to my house, I had only one tramadol pill remaining.

But wait! There's more.

The circumstances that I now have to relate are so devious and complex that I doubt that I can deliver the story perfectly straight. Indeed, immediately after the issue was resolved – not to my satisfaction – I had trouble remembering the precise order of events that led to the unacceptable conclusion. Due to the fact that most of the narrative unfolded over the telephone, the following confabulation is the best that I can do. Please bear with me. Keep in mind that although my PCP caused the problem, he did nothing to fix the problem. Nor did he ever apologize for his lack of affirmative action.

The Impossible Dream Becomes a Nightmare

Now that I had a new prescription from the substitute doctor, I had regenerated my back-up stash in case my PCP tried to play another trick on me. Before proceeding, my readers might want to know in the first place how I happened to have an overage of tramadol pills. The answer is simple, when I weaned myself off tramadol after the 2011 episode, I saved the leftovers to use as "incasers." Fortunately, over the next two years I did not need any incasers. When my VA PCP prescribed tramadol for the pain in my ankle, I swallowed the "incasers" first, before I started taking the newly prescribed pills.

Also, I still had the 11 hydrocodone pills. I didn't feel as if I needed them yet, so I continued to save them. Eventually, when I did need them several years later, I found that they were ineffective. The hydrocodone chemical must have separated into its constituent atoms and molecules.

Now to proceed. On the seventh of the following month, I signed in to myhealthvet on the VA hospital website, navigated to the page where I made my prescription requests, and ordered the current month's prescription of tramadol.

However, tramadol was blanked out so that I was unable to place my order. I sent a message to my PCP and explained the problem. One of the nurses intercepted the message, and responded to me via the hospital messaging system, stating that this time the issue was not with the PCP but with the pharmacy. The nurse had held a long conversation with the pharmacist but was unable to get him to fill the prescription. The issue was so difficult to explain that the nurse provided the name and phone number of the pharmacist and suggested that I speak with him directly, as he could explain the situation better than the nurse could transcribe it.

I called immediately. Over the course of this and two subsequent conversations, here was approximately how he described the problem. He would accept my tramadol prescriptions only every 30 days – not a minute over 29 days – but only after 30 days from the date on which the previous prescription was filled. Although I placed my request on the proper date, the PCP had not forwarded the prescription to the pharmacy when he was supposed to forward it. (As I learned, he never forwarded my prescription request.) The pharmacy did not receive the prescription request from the substitute doctor (who had been alerted to the problem by one of the nurses.) until the twentieth of the month, thus the twentieth of the month became my new order date.

You can easily understand how stupidly this system worked (or didn't work) in the real world. Suppose I neglected to place my tramadol order on the seventh of the month, but remembered to place my order on the following day. In that case, I would lose a day permanently, and the eighth would become my new ordering day. If this happened again, I would lose another day, and the ninth would become another new ordering day. Every month in which I was a day or two or three late on placing my order, meant that those days would be added to my previously lost days.

Worse than that, if the pharmacy failed to process my order on the day on which I ordered it, but processed the order on the following day, or the following two days, I would lose those days as well.

An intelligent ordering system would not accumulate lost days that could never be regained. If taken to the extreme, eventually I could end up lapping a month and be more than thirty days behind schedule. The system should be set to a monthly schedule so that no matter when in the month I posted a reminder to the pharmacy, the pharmacy would dispatch the prescription.

None of my other prescriptions were set to such a strict accounting system. I could order them whenever my stock got low, or whenever I anticipated that I might need more pills at a time when I might be away and not have access to my computer. In other words, I had a little leeway. But not a lot of leeway.

Now you can understand how the PCP wreaked havoc by taking advantage of the VA medical system. By not forwarding my monthly tramadol prescription to the pharmacy, I quickly ran out of this much-needed medication, and was left with no opportunity for recovery. Was his lack of action on my behalf an accidental event, a moment of forgetfullness, pure oversight, or a conscious attempt to keep me in pain. I think that his refusal to correct the situation or to apologize for creating the predicament indicates the appropriate answer. Admittedly, I am biased.

Why couldn't the pharmacy simply put my tramadol prescription on an automatic subscription, the way it does with some of my other monthly orders, instead of making me order tramadol manually? The answer was that the pharmacy functioned that way because that was the way the VA wanted the pharmacy to function. Does that make sense?

Just to be perfectly clear, did I mention that my PCP never intervened, never spoke with the pharmacy department, never helped to fix the problem that he created, never submitted a new prescription the way his substitute doctor did, and never apologized for all the trouble he had caused, but let the trouble continue? In short, once the system was corrupted, I was left out to hang.

The current system was designed in such a way that it was easy to corrupt by a doctor who wanted to take vengeance against his patients.

The only concession that the pharmacy made was to ship my tramadol by overnight express – not just this time but for all future orders for tramadol. This was important because forever more, quoth the raven, I would have only one tablet remaining when I received the new prescription.

However, the temporary PCP did not prescribe just enough tramadol pills to reach my next prescription date, he or she created a brand new prescription for a full month's supply. This thoughtfullness plus overnight delivery did not provide any leeway, but it did ensure that I would not run out of tramadol prematurely.

Full Name: GARY JOHN GENTILE
Patient ID: 185380747
Gender: Male
Date of Birth: 6/2/1946

Visit Date: 1/24/2022 10:08
Age: 75 Years
Examining Physician: Dr. Kroski:
Referring Physician: Dalsania
Height: 5 feet 11 inch
Weight: 160 lbs
History: SeeCPRS

Conclusion:

1. Abnormal electrodiagnostic examination.
2. There is electrodiagnostic evidence of a chronic left sciatic neuropathy with evidence of chronic nerve damage.

Speaking of Tramadol

As long as I am on the subject of tramadol, I will mention a couple of other issues that I did not know I had with my PCP until I reviewed my messages in the VA message board for inclusion in this book.

It turned out that after my meeting and subsequent phone conversation with the pharmacist who attended and took charge of my visit with the Chronic Pain Clinic, had second thoughts about my plight with respect to pain and quality of life. He condescended to suggest a partial or limited dosage of hydrocodone for use during what he termed "flare ups" of pain.

In order to keep me suffering, my PCP nixed his suggestion.

In a similar fashion, the neurologist who examined me, and the results of my neurological examination, stressed that I had "chronic nerve injury and there is not anything we can do to reverse that." The neurologist impressed upon me that in the VA medical system, he was not allowed to make prescriptions for his patients. Only the PCP could do that. Thus the PCP was a self-enforced barrier between the recommendations of doctors who knew more about my chronic pain situation than my PCP cared to know. As a result, my PCP was able to – and did – ignore those recommendations in order to keep me in chronic pain.

Keep in mind that this was the same neurologist who made the same recommendation twelve years earlier, at which time my family doctor took his advice. I eventually weaned myself off hydrocodone because my pain subsided to a point at which I no longer needed such a strong pain killer. Soon afterward, I weaned myself off tramadol. I even weaned myself off ibuprofen.

Now my damaged sciatic nerve has erupted, or "flared up," causing intense pain that must be treated by strong pain killers. But I was stuck with a PCP who would not let me have the pain killers that I needed.

I was also stuck with a hospital director – or is that dictator? – who supported a PCP who told a patient that he needed an operation, then had a tantrum and ran out of his office without scheduling the operation.

Welcome to my world of medical mistreatment. And likely the world of numerous Vietnam veterans, who have reached the age at which their wounds and disabilities were catching up with them, when they need medical care the most and received it the least.

At this point I should mention that Cheryl has several medical conditions that require different specialists. She also has a PCP who can make appointments with these specialists. In the civilian hospital system, each specialist can not only prescribe medicine, but once visited, can continue to work with patients on their own, without having to make appointments through a PCP. Thus each specialist is autonomous. This way, no PCP can block treatment or medication that is prescribed by a specialist.

Ankle Fusion

While I was dealing with the tramadol issue, I also had to deal with the orthopedic doctor. I was now suffering from two separate pain issues in my bad ankle. One issue resulted from post-traumatic arthritis which I felt above the ankle joint, while the other issue resulted from an undiagnosed condition which I felt below the ankle joint.

Keep in mind the fact that the reason I went to the VA hospital in the first place

```
1. mri left ankle
    Severe degenerative arthropathy with obliteration to the
        tibiotalar joint space with chronic depressed dome. Extensive
        synovitis, spurring, subchondral cyst throughout with extensive
        bone marrow edema within the distal tibia, fibula, and tail
        secondary to chronic repetitive trauma.
    Chronic sprains to the medial and lateral collateral ligaments.
    Chronic tendinopathy inframalleolar course of the peroneus
        longus/brevis as well as posterior tibial/flexor digitorum
        longus.
2. l/s spine xray
    Levoscoliosis with diffuse vacuum degenerative disease throughout
        entire lumbar spine. Posterior arthropathy L4-5 and L5-S1
        apophyseal joints.
```

was due to pain in my ankle. The first orthopedic doctor had only prescribed ibuprofen to reduce the swelling. But as the years passed, and the pain grew worse, no matter how much I complained about the increasing pain, neither doctor did anything about it. The PCP kept throwing me out of his office instead of sending me to the replacement orthopedic doctor. It was not until I demanded X-rays of my ankle that I met the replacement orthopedic doctor.

By that time it was too late. The replacement orthopedic doctor did nothing but increase the dosage of ibuprofen. The combined failure of all three doctors to take affirmative action allowed the damaged bones to deteriorate to the point at which the orthopedic doctor found that in his estimation, the only thing that could then be done was to fuse the ankle bones, because the pain was caused by the bones touching each other.

This surgical procedure required the implantation of screws to fasten the bones together. There was no guarantee that this operation would stop or reduce the pain. It could make the pain worse. Furthermore, the fused ankle joint would no longer move in any direction. The result was equivalent to wearing a ski boot fulltime, day and night.

The operation was permanent. There was no undoing it if it didn't work.

To me, this seemed like too much of a chance to take based on the lack of guaranteed success. I decided to get a second opinion, even if I had to pay for it myself.

I went to a local hospital that specialized in orthopedics. The chief orthopedic doctor ordered X-rays that were taken with my ankle bent in prescribed positions that would show the joint in various stretched and bent attitudes. I sat with the doctor as he examined the X-rays and asked various questions, largely about the history of the joint from the time the ankle had been damaged.

When I told him that the VA orthopedic doctor wanted to do an ankle fusion, he harumphed and replied, "An ankle fusion is the last thing I would advise." He told me that a number of other options were available to me before he would consider doing a fusion.

He wasted no time in prescribing a simple procedure called a "guided steroid injection." Then and there he made an appointment with the hospital's orthopedic team that would conduct the procedure at a different location several weeks later. In this procedure, because the bones were so close together, there was no space for an ordinary steroid injection; the surgeon could not be certain of inserting the needle in the precise location between the bones. Therefore, the needle was guided by either X-ray or ultrasound.

Because the VA orthopedic doctor obviously did not know that such a procedure existed, I sent a memo to the VA hospital in which I requested a referral for outside

> With regard to the ankle his option is going to be for ankle fusion. He has destroyed his ankle joint and his talus is completely flattened. All over his symptoms are tolerable as long as he uses brace and his medications. I explained to the patient that if his symptoms become intolerable his neck step would be for an ankle fusion.
>
> Currently do have an operative podiatrist at Wilkes-Barre VA who can perform ankle fusions. He should be referred to the operative podiatrist should he want to proceed with surgical intervention. In the meantime continue with his medications and use of his brace with no restriction on activity.
>
> Follow-up: Follow-up Ortho clinic as needed
>
> /es/ GEORGE RITZ
> Orthopaedic Surgeon
> Signed: 02/23/2022 13:52

The orthopedic doctor told me in person and wrote in his report that an ankle fusion was my only option.

care. Keep in mind that because of my 60 % disability rating, the VA was obligated to cover all my medical expenses when the VA was unable to provide a needed service. I provided the date and time of the procedure.

Also keep in mind that because I was now old enough to be insured by Medicare, the bulk of those expenses would be paid by the U.S. government no matter where I received the proper medical care. It mattered not whether the government paid for my medical expenses through the VA or through Medicare. The cost to the government was nearly the same.

Two days before the scheduled date for the guided steroid injection, I received a frantic phone call from the Wilkes-Barre VA Medical Center. The woman on the phone wanted to schedule two appointments for me: one to talk with a doctor the very next morning at 9:30, and the other to have a procedure performed. She was quite insistent that I accept her offerings immediately.

I was unaware that any appointment or procedure was on my VA calendar. So, the first question I asked was, "An procedure for what?"

Secretary: "You'll have to ask the doctor."

(The following dialogue is a condensation of our subsequent conversation.)

I hemmed and hawed at her lack of enlightenment. Finally, I said, "I have to work tomorrow."

Secretary, eagerly: "Okay, then I'll just cancel the appointment."

Me (hastily): "Do not cancel the appointments. Tell me what this procedure is for."

Secretary: "You'll have to ask the doctor."

Me: "I already have a procedure scheduled for the day after tomorrow. The VA hospital knows all about it because I contacted them for a referral. I want to know what procedure you're talking about."

Secretary: "You'll have to ask the doctor."

Me: "I'm asking *you*. It's an 85-mile trip for me." (That is roundtrip.)
Secretary: "I'll just cancel the appointments."
Me: "Do not cancel the appointment. Just postpone it until I learn what it's about." (Or words to that effect.)
Secretary: "You'll have to ask the doctor."
Me: "Tell me what the procedure is for."
Secretary: "I'll just cancel the appointments."
Me (hastily): "Do not cancel the appointments. I want to know what the procedure is for."
Secretary (belligerently trying to get me off the phone: "Alright, I'll just cancel the appointments."
Me (desperately because I didn't know what was going on and wanted to know more about it: "Do not cancel the appointments. If the doctor only wants to talk, ask him to call me tomorrow at 9:30. I'll have my phone with me."
Secretary: Silence.
Dial tone.
The secretary had disconnected without providing any information.

I immediately tried to call her, but the VA has this clever phone system in which all outgoing calls register the same number on the recipient's smartphone: 507-824-3521. When a person calls that number, he or she must listen to a multi-minute recorded message that is irrelevant to the purpose of the call, after which the caller is directed to press the 4-digit code of the person he or she is trying to reach.

The secretary did not give me either her name or the name of the doctor. She had effectively and, in my opinion, purposely disconnected so that I could not ascertain who had called or what the reason was for the call. I wrote "purposely" because by her words and aggressive demeanor, it sounded to me as if her real purpose in calling me was not to schedule a medical procedure, but to get me to cancel the "appointments," if in fact such appointments existed. The phone call made no sense to me.

Not until two years later did I learn the sinister truth about the call, when I reviewed the transcript of existing memos in the VA messaging system in preparation for writing this book. As you can read below, the call was designed to make it seem as if *I* canceled the appointments, when in fact *she* cancelled the appointments despite my repeated orders *not* to cancel the appointments (if such appointments truly existed).

Here is a transcript of the message that she sent to my PCP's nurse in response to my request to obtain a referral so that I would not have to pay for the guided steroid injection, a procedure that the orthopedic doctor did not offer to me as an option for reducing some of the pain in my ankle, after he told me that my only option was an ankle fusion:

Signed: 05/09/2022 08:19
Receipt Acknowledged By:
* AWAITING SIGNATURE * YEKEL,MAUREEN A
05/09/2022 ADDENDUM STATUS: COMPLETED
I spoke to veteran on two different occassions and offered an appt with Dr. Kroski; veteran declined appt. stating he was already scheduled for an appt. on the outside of the VA and was using his private insurance. Consult was d/c per his request. Thanks.

The secretary's version of the call is overwhelmed with lies and deletions:
She did not provide her name or station.
She called only once.
She did not offer an appointment with an named doctor; she *announced* an undisclosed appointment with an unnamed doctor.
She did not announce a single appointment; she announced two appointments, the second one for an undisclosed surgical procedure whose type she withheld.
I did not decline her offer; I reiterated four times *not* to cancel the undefined appointments.
I did not say anything about paying for a procedure with so-called "private insurance," as I did not have private insurance; I depended solely on the VA for my medical needs. Again, the appointment(s) were neither canceled nor declined "per my request." Her aggressive behavior was not represented in her distorted representation to my PCP's nurse.

She told more lies in a single paragraph than a politician could tell in a book. This begs the question: Why did she lie so many times to my PCP's nurse? What was her purpose?

It was obvious to me from the beginning that she *wanted* me to cancel or decline the appointments. That was why I grilled her about her purpose. (I have edited much of our conversation because I could not remember it all. But my readers should get the gist of what she said from this account.) I knew – or suspected with conviction – that she had an ulterior motive in trying to talk me out of accepting the appointments.

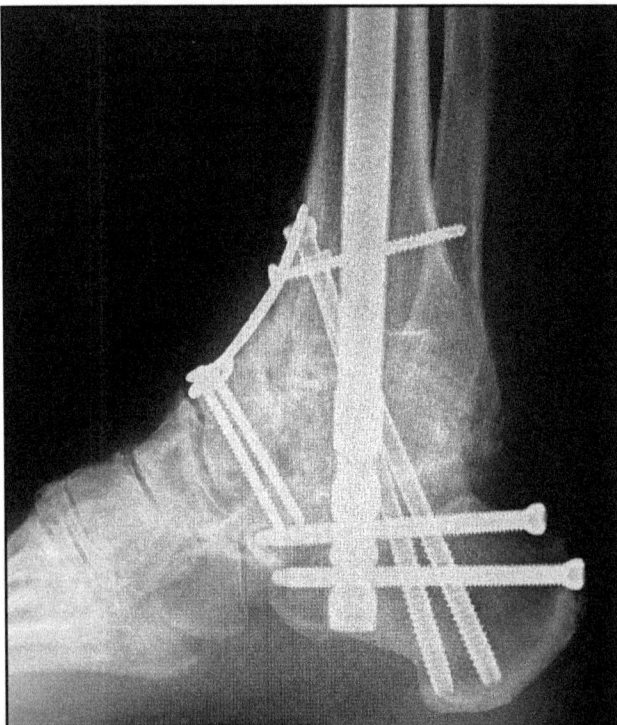

This is an x-ray of the ankle fusion of my friend Don DeMaria. The number, length, and position of the screws depend on the type of fusion that a patient's ankle damage requires. Sometimes plates of various sizes are employed. Don kindly sent this to me so I could see what I would be getting into if I have to make a decision about having my ankle fused. Thanks Don. It seems as if I have receive more and better medical advice from my friends and my other half than I have received from my VA doctors.

But what possible motive could a secretary have to harm me? What did she have to gain by lying to me. Or perhaps I should ask, who could have convinced her or forced her to lie to me, in order to get me to cancel two imaginary appointments? Was that person the doctor she mentioned in her message, or was it a person who was above her in the VA hierocracy; someone who had the authority to have her fired from her job? And what was the motive of that superior person in creating a fake phone call?

I do not know the answers to these questions, and I refuse to speculate about the scam. It is just another in a long line of inequities that I suffered at the hands of certain individuals within the Wilkes-Barre VA Medical Center.

Although I refuse to speculate about who was ultimately responsible for the creation of the phone call, I am more than willing to provide the *result* of the call: the VA hospital utilized the lies to deny my claim for reimbursement for the guided steroid injection, which I obtained from St. Lukes' hospital in place of the VA's offer to fuse my ankle.

Speaking of which . . .

Guided Steroid Injection

Although I was traveling during the day after the secretary's felonious phone call, I kept my phone with me, waiting for the VA doctor to "discuss" the medical issue. He or she never called during the appointed time – or at any time.

The following day I went to the St. Luke's hospital where the guided steroid injection was to take place. I had no idea what to expect.

The procedure was attended by two doctors and a technician. The doctors decided to conduct the procedure via the X-ray method instead of by Ultrasound. I made no input as I was basically a bystander, with no medical background knowledge about the procedure. I lay on a padded table throughout the procedure.

To explain the process, think of the difference between a still photograph and a movie. An X-ray is ordinarily perceived as a static picture, whereas in this case the X-ray image appeared to be moving as the doctors rolled the remote imaging device along my ankle. In fact, the device was moving and not the image of my ankle joint.

The doctors (one male and one female) were searching for a place in my ankle where the needle could fit between the adjacent bones. The technician's job was crucial because the X-ray image consisted of not just black and white images as the "roller" moved back and forth, but various shades of gray. She had to continuously alter the image as the roller passed over the different densities of bone versus flesh.

As the doctors studied the X-ray images, they drew lines on my skin with a black marker. This created a design in which, like a treasure map, X marked the spot. The female inserted the needle through the intersecting coordinates.

I felt only a pinprick. But as she pressed the syringe that forced the liquid steroid into my ankle, I felt the swelling as an increasing pain. This pain lasted no longer than a few seconds until it receded and the feeling in my ankle returned to normal.

The doctors knew about my medical history from the information on my chart. The male doctor left the room, the technician stowed her equipment, and the female doctor chatted with me. She noted that I had spent ten months in Valley Forge General Hospital, which was in the vicinity of where she was raised. The hospital was closed by that time, enabling her and her friends to play on the property. Her father had served in the Army but not in Vietnam.

After about five minutes, she told me to stand up. I slid off the table, placed my left foot on the floor ever so gently, then slowly put all my weight on the foot. Instead of feeling the stab of an icepick, I felt no pain. None. Nothing. Not a thing.

I was cured – and without the excruciatingly painful operation that I would have had to undergo if I had accepted the VA orthopedic doctor's ankle fusion; to say nothing of the months I would have had suffer – and be incapacitated – while the new scars healed.

It was a miracle!

The doctor told me that I could have another injection every three months. She also told me not to wait until the pain became unbearable, but to schedule another injection as soon as I felt the beginning of pain.

That was two years ago, and I haven't felt a bit of pain yet below my ankle.

I am forever grateful that non-VA hospitals have the tools to do the jobs that are required, and a dedicated staff who can provide such up-to-date medical service, to treat chronic pain without screaming in my ear and calling me a drug addict and running out of the office in the middle of an examination. Instead, they worked calmly and professionally, recognized my pain problem, and treated it properly.

Hail St. Luke's.

The Two-Front Battle

I have so far ignored the other battle that I was contesting while I was fighting mistreatment and lack of treatment from my PCP and the Chronic Pain Clinic. This other battle was on a different front. I have done this purposely so as not to lose the continuity between fronts. Imagine how confusing it would be to read a book about World War 2 in which the author alternated chapters between the Battle of the Atlantic and the Battle of the Pacific. As the United States did in World War 2, I was fighting in two theaters in which I was being squeezed between a pair of implacable enemies that shared a common alliance to defeat me by denying appropriate medical treatment and relief from pain.

Here goes.

The Ultimatum

The next time the VA scheduled an appointment for me with my PCP, I made a slight alteration in plans. Cheryl parked the car in the VA hospital parking lot. She stayed there while I checked into the laboratory where a nurse drew five vials of blood. She then escorted me to the rest room which she prepared for me to use. She handed me a small plastic jar with a screw top. She instructed me to urinate into the jar and screw the lid onto it, but not to flush the toilet or wash my hands until she had the opportunity to examine the rest room.

This was the standard VA procedure for testing a patient for illegal or unprescribed drugs. I had gone through this grind multiple times over the past ten years, and had never failed the test. The only part of the test procedure that I didn't like was the part that prevented me from drinking my morning coffee until after I completed the test, which was late in the morning.

My appointment with the PCP followed the blood and urine tests. Instead of going to the waiting room outside the PCP's office, I left the building, returned to the car, opened the unbreakable Stanley thermos bottle that I had owned ever since I worked as an electrician, and started drinking cup after cup of hot coffee.

Meanwhile, Cheryl drove to Steamtown, a National Historic Site that was located a few miles away in Wilkes-Barre. This was a railroad museum that contained a number of steam engines from yesteryear. We went on a guided tour of the various buildings where parts were manufactured and where steam engines were repaired. It was a fascinating place to visit.

Afterward, we went home where I still had time to do some work.

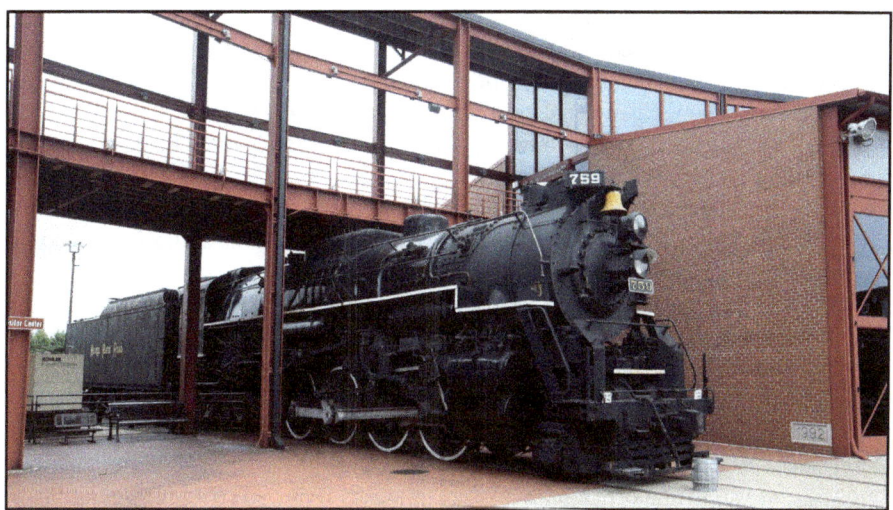

When I checked my email the following morning, I found a hostile memo from my PCP about missing the appointment. I didn't understand why his feathers were ruffled. Was he upset because I caused him to miss his opportunity to throw me out of his office? Or did I hurt his feelings because he couldn't scream at me and run out in the middle of an examination?

My reply was curt and to the point:

> Have you forgotten our previous exam? When I asked for help with the pain in my ankle, you threw a tantrum, screamed in my ear that I was a dope addict, then ran out of the office and never returned, leaving me alone in the middle of the exam. I swore that I would never let you humiliate me again. That is why I did not see you yesterday. I had my blood drawn and left a urine sample. In the nine years that I have been seeing you, you never once helped me with my bad ankle or damaged sciatic nerve.
>
> Since then, I visited a private hospital where a competent doctor performed a guided steroid injection which completely cured the stabbing pain in my ankle. From the hospital's doctor, I learned that *you* are responsible for allowing my ankle to deteriorate, by not treating me during the past nine years when a non-guided injection could have been performed. Now, thanks to you, my ankle is permanently ruined.
>
> Do not forget that twice during other exams, when I mentioned my ongoing

pain, you threw me out of the office. Worse yet, the hospital director condoned your childish behavior and mistreatment of me. That is why I had to seek help from a private hospital.

The Last Hurrah

Okay, maybe it wasn't curt. But it was to the point. Nor did I pull any punches. I told him like it was, and I didn't care if he didn't like what I wrote.

Of course, I knew that at least one of the nurses would read my memo before he or she forwarded it to the PCP. I was hoping for that, so they would know – if they didn't know already – how the PCP had been mistreating me throughout the years.

The PCP pulled one last trick on me: a trick that was not only an act of vengeance, but one that was surely against the Hippocratic oath, if not patently illegal. He threatened to cut off my medications if I did not see him in his office.

I had not anticipated such a dastardly action, but it certainly fitted his psychological profile. Not to worry; I had a backup plan, or an ace in the hole, or any other cliché that was appropriate for the situation. I was prepared to change VA hospitals. Neither the PCP nor the director of the Wilkes-Barre VA hospital had the authority to stop me from enlisting in the VA hospital in Allentown.

Before I made such a drastic move, I decided to try one other maneuver. I called the VA help line, and told the woman who answered that I wanted to change PCP's.

She said, "No problem. We do that all the time."

I was shocked! "You do?"

"Why do you want another doctor?"

I gave her a brief account about my PCP's tantrums that resulted in him twice throwing me out of the office, and his screaming fit followed by him running out of the office in the middle of an examination, and so on.

She replied (in effect), "I have a doctor who is very low-keyed. He should be just right for you."

In less than a minute, this woman solved a problem that I had been fighting for five years with the director of the hospital. It's amazing how things worked out sometimes. She immediately made an appointment for me visit her recommended doctor. Curiously, my new PCP asked why I wanted to switch PCP's. I gave him the same account. I also admitted how crazy this story must have sounded, but swore that it was true in every regard.

At the end of our meeting – which included a physical examination – he made it easy for me to obtain tramadol monthly without interference, by posting it on my pharmaceutical chart as an ordinary medicine like acetaminophen, so I could order it straight from the pharmacy instead of having to ask his permission every month. Now all I had to do was check the tramadol box and order it myself.

I could hardly believe that he could do this. He shrugged. I had to ask for renewals only every six months. This made me realize that my previous PCP had been keeping me on a short leash all these years by making me obtain his personal approval every month! He was dispensing pills the way a miser counted his money. It was his way of maintaining control over me.

The new doc let me have the same dose of tramadol – six per day – without comment.

Short Recap

If you will pardon the western cowboy expression, I jumped the gun a bit by ending the medical side of my battle with VA doctors, without explaining all that was happening concurrently with the hospital director and his staff: a different contentious argument but one that interacted with the incidents that I have already told. Here goes.

As I have previously suggested, due to the blatant lies that a secretary related to one of the VA doctors, it was my conclusion that the director and his minions were going out of their way to cause trouble for me.

After all, the director was not quite forthcoming in his letter to Senator Patrick Toomey when he took credit for making appointments that I had already made. This misinformation gave the impression that the director was taking my case seriously, when in fact he simply sloughed me off to a bunch of deadheads who called themselves the Chronic Pain Clinic, who lived up to their name by keeping me in chronic pain despite the recommendations of two in-house neurologists.

As I have already shown, the CPC did not bother to review the neurological report. And when I insisted that they do so after I learned that they had ignored it, and the pharmacist eventually took it upon himself to review the report and make the appropriate recommendation, my PCP consciously thwarted any attempt to prescribe the analgesics that would have alleviated my pain.

ASSESSMENT/PLANNING/IMPRESSION:-

#1. Injury to the left sciatic nerve status post bullet injury in 1967 while patient was in the services. — Chronic left sciatica/chronic pain syndrome.

RECOMMENDATIONS:-

#1. I have again explained to this patient that this was a chronic nerve injury and there is not anything we can do to reverse that at this point.
#2. Since this is chronic pain— this should be managed by the chronic pain management team.—I will defer management of pain to chronic pain management team.
#3. Advised healthy diet and daily exercises.
#4. Advised good sleep hygiene.
#5. Discharge patient from neurology clinic. Follow-up with primary care physician/pain management team.

Not so my new PCP. He took the bull by the horns and immediatelly prescribed hydrocodone after I gave him a copy of the recommendations that my previous PCP had buried.

So what good was a Chronic Pain Clinic if (1) it refused to call the Philly VA hospital to have my records forwarded; (2) if it refused to prescribe suitable pain killers as recommended by the hospital's neurologists, and (3), if a patient's PCP refused to acknowledge the CPC's)recommendations (assuming that it cared enough to make any?

The patient lost in either case. In short, VA medical treatment is a charade, and the wounded veteran remains untreated.

As you can see, both VA neurologists - the one who gave me the test and the one who interpreted the results - agreed that my damaged sciatic nerve could not be repaired, and therefore could be treated only with appropriate analgesics. Yet the CPC refused took their advice.

When I was in grade school, I had a book called *Doctor Dan the Bandage Man*. I could now get better treatment by rereading that book than I have gotten by putting myself in the hands of the Veterans Administration. At least Doctor Dan had a page full of real bandages that the reader could dispense. Certainly I exaggerate, but not by much.

The final irony is that I got kicked out of the Chronic Pain Clinic. It started like this . . .

No Service Available

Let me start this section by showing the conditions under which veterans are eligible for community care:

According to VA guidelines, "Drive times are calculated using geomapping software."

Yet when I tried to sign up for travel reimbursement at the Wilkes-Barre VA Medical Center, I was denied, despite the fact that drive time by the shortest route was an hour. (Several years later, time was reduced to 45 minutes after a new interchange was built on the Northeast Extension of the Pennsylvania Turnpike.) When I pointed this out to the man on the phone, he responded by disconnecting without a word. Such was the way the director allowed the hospital staff to operate.

As already noted, when the only option that the VA orthopedic doctor gave me for the relief of pain in my ankle was fusion, and I learned that I could obtain a guided steroid injection from a community hospital - a procedure that the VA could not provide - the director refused to reimburse me for my out-of-pocket expenses.

Stated differently, despite my disability rating of 60%, not only did the director of the Wilkes-Barre VA Medical Center force me to pay for medical treatment that the VA

---

1. A Veteran needs a service not available at any VA medical facility.
2. A Veteran lives in a U.S. state or territory without a full-service VA medical facility. Specifically, this would apply to Veterans living in Alaska, Hawaii, New Hampshire and the U.S. territories of Guam, American Samoa, the Northern Mariana Islands and the U.S. Virgin Islands.
3. A Veteran qualifies under the "grandfather" provision related to distance eligibility under the Veterans Choice Program.
4. VA cannot furnish care within certain designated access standards. The specific access standards are described below:

- Drive time to a specific VA medical facility

- Thirty-minute average drive time for primary care, mental health and noninstitutional extended care services.

hospital was unable to provide, but I had to pay for a simpler and more advanced treatment of which the VA orthopedic doctor had no knowledge.

Another deficiency of the VA hospital was the lack of a proper brace for the specific needs of my damaged ankle. Again, I had to go to a community hospital for an Arizona brace. To make this brace, a technician made a mold of my foot and lower leg, then built the brace around the mold.

Yet another deficiency was the substandard qualification for cataract surgery. The VA offered eye examinations that were limited to prescriptions for eyeglasses but not for contacts, and treatments for diseases of the eyes, including cataracts, but only if the condition was serious enough to threaten blindness.

I've had cataracts in one eye for several years, and I have been told by a community opthalmologist that my condition was serious. But the VA would not prescribe cataract surgery because I was not blind enough.

Whereas community opthalmologists prescribed cataract surgery for a patient whose vision was 20/30, the VA demanded a threshold of 20/40 for surgery. The only way in which I could see clearly was to close my right eye and look only with my left. This made driving an automobile somewhat difficult, especially at night when I saw double made worse by flares and the loss of binocular vision. The VA held no exceptions to its rule.

About the only way in which I was better off was due to the relaxation on the wearing of face masks in public buildings, as the threat of covid-19 faded. Because of my damaged lung, I could not breathe while wearing a face mask. That is, I could wear a mask for a few minutes, but I simply was unable to inhale enough oxygen to satisfy my need.

In a crowded room when no one was looking, I would pull the chin of the mask off my skin and take a number of deep breaths until I "caught up" on the deficit. Sometimes I left the room and caught my breath in the hallway.

In 2023, after both of us had gotten 4 vaccination shots, Cheryl visited her doctor because of a lingering cold that was in its fifth day. When she came home she told me

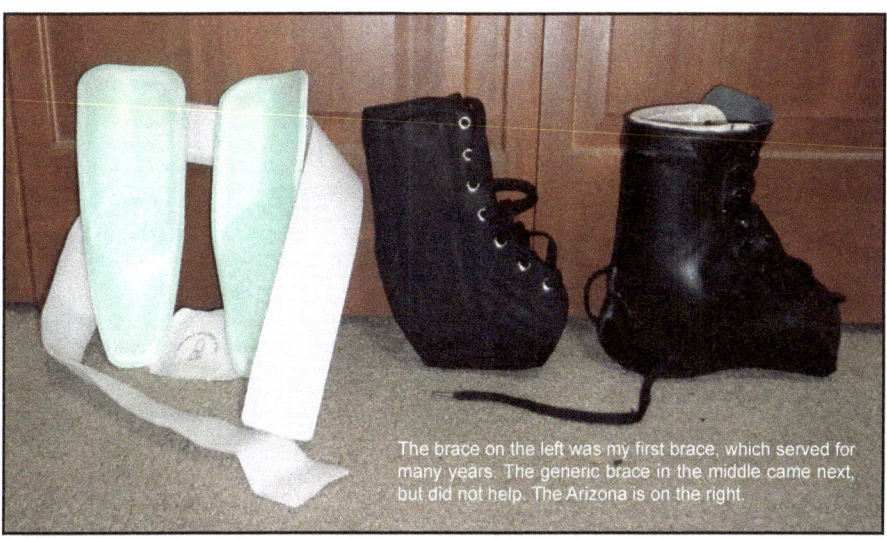

The brace on the left was my first brace, which served for many years. The generic brace in the middle came next, but did not help. The Arizona is on the right.

My letter to the director

Earlier this year I requested an EMG of my left femur, which had been shattered by an enemy bullet. I also requested an x-ray of my left ankle, which had been damaged by an enemy grenade. The purpose of these examinations was to support my assertion that the extreme chronic pain that I suffer was proven by valid testing procedures.

The neurologist informed me that there was no way to cure my permanently damaged sciatic nerve, and that the only remedy was to treat the pain.

Orthopedic Dr. ~ was giving me a steroid shot in my left shoulder blade – the result of an enemy bullet that had struck me in the chest, passed through my lung, and exited through the scapula – when I asked him if he could give me a steroid shot in my ankle as a way to treat the debilitating chronic pain. He examined the recent x-rays of my ankle and told me that the only remedy that might alleviate the pain was an ankle fusion.

As a result of Senator Patrick Toomey insistence, I was scheduled to meet with the pain clinic. This begs the question: why did my PCP not do this on his own, without being forced to do so? The primary reason I appealed to the VA ten years ago was because of pain in my ankle, which was constantly getting worse. Yet in all that time, my PCP did nothing to treat my pain. Worse yet, he was so incompetent that he not only refused to prescribe the pain medication that I was already taking, and that was having the most positive effect, but he reduced by half a substandard pain medication for which I also had a prescription.

I duly had a hearing with the pain clinic. If the clinic has a doctor in charge, he or she did not favor me with an appearance. My hearing was held by a pharmacist and four other individuals. The secretary failed to bring my medical records, despite the fact that I had told her in advance where to locate them. As I later ascertained, the arbiters of my case did not even bother to read the reports of the neurologists and the orthopedic doctor.

For an hour I testified about my various wounds, how I have suffered from them throughout my life, and how the pain from those wounds has increased dramatically with age: violent shooting pains that ran down my leg and felt as if my leg were on fire or being electrocuted; severe pain where the ankle bones rubbed against each other, which caused the feeling with every step that was similar to being stabbed with an icepick. For ten years Dr. ~ ignored my repeated requests for medical treatment.

As a result of this trial, the clinic judges recommended nothing more than over-the-counter skin lotion for my accumulated pains. When I complained that such placebos did nothing to alleviate my pain, the pharmacist told me that I was not going to get anything else. Such an action of surrender is not how a medical professional performs. If one treatment does not work, then another and stronger treatment must be tried – and another and another, until the patient obtains relief or is cured of his ailments.

I asked the pharmacist: "Don't you care about me? Don't you care about my suffering? Don't you care about my pain? Don't you care about my quality of life?" He did not respond, which in itself is an answer about how he feels about me as a patient.

In your letter to Senator Patrick Toomey, you wrote, "We believe that our Veterans are our nation's heroes." If I am your hero, why are you letting me be treated like shit?

As a result of your hospital's lackluster, reluctant, and absence of treatment, I decided to obtain another doctor's opinion about my ankle. I asked your hospital for a referral, but it was refused. I had to make my own appointments to the St. Luke's Hospital System. These orthopedic doctors recommended an ankle fusion solely as a last resort, and suggested alternative therapies that could alleviate my pain. These suggestions resulted in my having a guided steroid injection, whose existence Dr. ~ had not mentioned, apparently because he had no knowledge of such a procedure. I also obtained an ankle brace that outperforms the kind that your hospital provides.

From new x-rays that St. Luke's orthopedic doctors prescribed, I learned that my ankle has been deteriorating for years due to lack of treatment. You may recall from my previous correspondence that when I complained to my PCP about the pain in my ankle, he either did nothing, or he threw me out of his office (twice), or had a tantrum, screamed at me that I was a drug addict and that the pain was in my head, and walked out of his office and never returned, leaving me alone in his office. Yet despite this unprofessional behavior and lack of sympathy and performance on my behalf, he is still employed by the Wilkes-Barre VA Medical Center.

If my PCP had not been so incompetent, the first time I visited him he would have recommended a simple steroid injection. Instead, he allowed my damaged ankle to deteriorate more and more throughout the years, until the damage to the ankle bones is now irreparable.

Because I have a disability rating of 60%, the VA is obligated to cover all my medical expenses. I have enclosed the medical bills that Medicare did not fully cover so that the VA can compensate me for the overage that I had to pay on my own.

Part of my disability rating is based on pain and suffering. Because the VA, via the inaptly and ineptly named pain clinic, which has willfully and with malice aforethought, decided to make me continue to suffer, including extreme pain from a damaged sciatic nerve, I want you to submit paperwork to the Department of Veterans Affairs to increase my disability rating to 70%.

In compliance with bureaucratic transparency, you should write to Senator Patrick Toomey and tell him the truth about my situation: that the pain clinic is a sham, that I am still suffering from pain that the VA refuses to treat, and that the VA employs unqualified doctors and other medical personnel who care nothing about the well-being of their patients.

Keep in mind that I am supposedly one of your heroes. If that is true, I expect you to ensure that I am treated as such.

that she had tested positive for covid.

I said, "We've been sleeping together for five days and I haven't gotten it." I never did. That was proven by two subsequent tests.

Instead of sleeping in separate beds in different rooms, like two of our friends, we continued life as usual. I figured that if I hadn't gotten covid when Cheryl had it, at a time when we had mixed bodily fluids, then I was unlikely to get it under other circumstances.

The Director's Kiss-off Letter

As you can read, the director did not offer to do anything himself. In essence he told me to help myself. But I have already taken that route, and I was unable to get the VA to answer my requests, much less to aid in my distress. Now I wanted the director to use his position and authority to force the VA to take affirmative action. His answer proved that he did not care enough about his patients in general and me in particular to use his position to ensure that I obtained the treatment that I needed.

This letter was preceded by a phone call from one of the director's office workers. She started the conversation by telling me that I had been kicked out of the Chronic Pain Clinic. The act itself didn't matter to me because it hadn't done anything to treat my pain. But I did wonder who had the authority to have me kicked out of the clinic. And why.

Then she told me that her purpose in calling was to ensure that she understood what I had written in my letter to the director. She quoted a certain sentence, then asked if I had written it.

I did not have the letter in front of me because I was mountain biking in the woods. I dismounted and leaned my bike against a tree. I asked her if she had my letter in hand. After her acknowledgment, I said, "I think it's obvious that if you're reading from my letter, then I wrote it."

Unabashed, she read another sentence from my letter, then asked, "Did you write that?"

Her stupidity astonished me. How could she possibly not know that I had written that sentence if she was reading it from my letter?

"What don't you not understand about that sentence?"

"I just want to make sure that it's clear."

Reading and understanding are not the same thing. Yet never once did she ask for an explanation. She simply read a sentence, or part of a sentence, then asked if that was correct. This inanity continued five or six times before she announced that I would

---

There's an old construction joke about two nuns passing by a new building site where two workers were having an argument. One of the nuns said, "Do those men have to swear all the time?" The other nun said, "They're not swearing. They just call a spade a spade." The first nun replied. "No they don't. They call it a fucking shovel."

Having been a construction worker, I have heard more than my share of foul and filthy language. There's no doubt that it gets to the point in no uncertain terms. By the time I wrote the letter on the opposite page, I knew that the director was never going to help me in any way, shape, or form (to quote a cliche). So there was no sense in holding back my feelings about the inequities that I suffered in the hospital that he was responsible for "directing" - hence the title of his position. Therefore, I did not shirk from indicating how poor a job he was doing, and what I needed him to do in my behalf. I knew - or suspected with conviction - that he was not going to help me: no way, no how. I wanted to make him angry so I could publish his reply, in order to prove that he did not have the best interests of veterans at heart . He fell right into my trap. Here it is. Read on as I parse it.

The Director's Infamous Letter

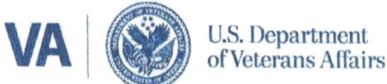

U.S. Department of Veterans Affairs

Medical Center
1111 East End Boulevard
Wilkes-Barre, PA 18711

In Reply Refer To: 693/110
SSN 0747
GENTILE, Gary J.

JUL 1 9 2022

Mr. Gary Gentile
500 Lehigh Gorge Dr.
Jim Thorpe, PA 18229

Dear Mr. Gentile:

Thank you for the opportunity to address your concerns regarding the healthcare provided to you at the Department of Veterans Affairs (VA) Medical Center, Primary Care Service, in Wilkes-Barre, Pennsylvania. We are honored to serve and provide care for our nation's Veterans.

In response to the concerns noted in your recent correspondence, you were contacted by Cassandra Sherrill, Program Support Assistant, Wilkes-Barre VA Medical Center. As discussed with Ms. Sherrill, you were last evaluated by your Primary Care Provider, Atul Dalsania, M.D., on October 29, 2020. It was recommended that a more current evaluation be conducted, to which you agreed, and an appointment has been scheduled on August 17, 2022, at 11:00 A.M. At this visit, Dr. Dalsania will evaluate your current symptoms and discuss recommendations on future treatment options.

Regarding your pain management treatment, a review of your care was performed by Dr. Thomas W. Hanlon, M.D. The review determined that the care provided was timely and appropriate for the treatment of chronic pain. It is recommended that you discuss your current symptoms with your Primary Care Provider during your upcoming appointment.

Regarding your request for reimbursement of the medical bills you have enclosed from St. Luke's University Health Network for your orthopedic care, you were notified on April 6, 2022, that community care was not approved by the Wilkes-Barre VA Medical Center, and therefore, these services would not be reimbursable.

In response to your request for service connection and disability rating increase, Ms. Sherrill instructed you to contact The Veterans Benefits Administration at,
I want to assure you that, at the Wilkes-Barre VA Medical Center, we believe that our Veterans are our nation's heroes. I encourage you to contact Ms. Cassandra Sherrill, Program Support Assistant, at 570 824-3521, extension 24253, to discuss your concerns.

Sincerely,

Russell E. Lloyd
Director

shortly receive a reply from the director.

Here were my thoughts about his replies:

Paragraph 1: The director used the same time-worn euphemistic word that all governmental administrators employed as a way to avoid the truth of a situation. To tell it like it was, he should have written the descriptive word "complaints" instead of the fuzzy and obfuscatory word "concerns." There's a big difference between a concern and a complaint.

He then followed this word with the sentence, "We are honored to serve and provide care for our nation's Veterans." Ten years passed before I obtained a Primary Care Provider who actually provided care for me. My initial PCP refused – yes, refused – to provide the care that I needed, and on at least one occasion took that care away from me.

The director's sentence was far from the truth as he emphasized in the succeeding paragraph, to which we now segue.

Paragraph 2: Due to my previous letters, the director was certainly aware that my first PCP would not provide the care that I needed, and that I wanted to be transferred to a different PCP. Yet he persisted in sticking me with a PCP whom the director knew had thrown me out of his office on two occasions, had thrown a tantrum and abandoned me in his office after he shouted at me and ran out of his office, and had persistently refused to prescribe the dosage of medicine that I needed. It was my firm suspicion that the director intentionally stuck me with that PCP because he wanted me to continue to be mistreated, and he knew that said PCP would continue to do so.

Paragraph 3: The director claimed that a doctor whom I had never seen, and who had never examined me, "determined that the care provided was timely and appropriate for the treatment of chronic pain." I am certain that the two neurologists who did examine me would beg to differ with said doctor, because they knew that skin cream would not suffice to treat chronic pain that was the result of a damaged sciatic nerve.

A third doctor agreed with them. (See page 175.) Yet the director ignored the findings of these experts in neurology in order to take the word of a doctor whose qualifications were not expressed; or should I say that the director's hand-picked doctor was chosen over the others because he was willing to provide the evaluation that the director wanted, in order to substantiate his claim that skin cream was all I needed for chronic neurological pain. As I could no longer be treated by the Chronic Pain Clinic, there was no one to stand against my PCP's mishandling of my true medical condition.

For ten years I tried to discuss my "current symptoms with [my] Primary Care Provider," but he consistently refused to listen, going as far as to twice throw me out of his office when I mentioned my pain, and once throwing a tantrum and leaving the office in a huff, and once failing to refill my tramadol prescription: all of which the director knew.

Even after my PCP read the neurologists' report, he refused to provide "timely and appropriate . . . treatment of chronic pain." In reality, he was not a Primary Care Provider; he was a Primary Care Preventer. To attempt to discuss this issue again with my PCP was an exercise in futility.

To go further, the director's review doctor had access only to those records of mine that were available at the Wilkes-Barre VA Medical Center. He did not have access to the vast number of background records that were located at the Philadelphia VA hospital. To make an analogy, if you were asked to add a sum of numbers, but were given only some of the numbers, could you give the correct answer?

Paragraph 4: I had a right to request reimbursement for community medical expenses because the VA orthopedic doctor told me that my only option for the relief of ankle pain was an ankle fusion, whereas a community hospital was able to conduct a guided steroid injection, which treatment was not offered to me by the VA orthopedic doctor.

To cover the fact that the guided steroid injection was not offered to me, a VA secretary - either on her own or because she was coerced into doing so under duress that was made by a VA administrative employee - concocted a fictitious story in which she claimed that I declined a VA medical service which she refused to describe, by a doctor she refused to name, to achieve a result that she refused to tell me.

She made me suspicious first by trying to rush me into making an blind appointment, then second by stating eagerly that she would cancel the blind appointment, then third by disconnecting in the middle of my sentence. None of these actions seemed ethical.

Paragraph 4: Notice that the director neglected to mention that the that orthopedic doctor gave me only one choice: an ankle fusion. He also neglected to mention that the Wilkes-Barre VA Medical Center did not have the capability – neither the staff nor the equipment – to perform a guided steroid injection: a far less invasive and a far more expedient procedure which completely cured my pain without leaving my ankle immobilized.

The director seemed not to care about the efficacy of the procedure, only about not having the VA pay for it. He would rather that I have a half-assed operation that would leave me more disabled than I already was, than to pay for me to have the proper procedure that I truly needed.

Paragraph 5: I have already told about my efforts to contact the central office of the VA, only to have it refuse to acknowledge receipt of my letters, much less deal with the issues at hand. That is why I needed the director to work on my behalf, to represent me in my dealings with the VA, which I thought fitted his job description. His selfish strategy was to tell me to stop bothering him and to make contact myself: a not very helpful effort on his part, as I have already tried that method and learned that the VA does not care about Vietnam veterans.

Paragraph 6: This is repetitive of his first letter, in which he used the same words, stating that he and the hospital that he misdirects believe that "our Veterans are our nation's heroes." He must also believe that the nation's heroes should be treated like shit, as that is the way he has consistently treated me.

The Last Straw

There is good news for doctors who have no patience with patients, who misuse their power to prescribe medicine, who love to make their patients suffer, and who patently abuse the Hippocratic Oath.

The Pennsylvania State Board of Medicine has used its authority to condone medical malfeasance and to support the unacceptable behavior of doctors who use their practice as a means to mistreat patients by throwing them out of the office, by screaming at them and calling them drug addicts, by running out of the office in the middle of an examination and never returning, by withholding much needed pain medication, and

Kiss-off Letter from the Pennsylvania State Board of Medicine

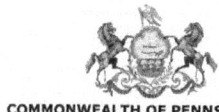

COMMONWEALTH OF PENNSYLVANIA
OFFICE OF GENERAL COUNSEL

Keith E. Bashore
Prosecuting Attorney

kbashore@pa.gov
Prosecution Division

January 11, 2024

Gary Gentile
500 Lehigh Gorge Drive
Jim Thorpe, PA 18229

  RE: Case No. 22-49-005876 (Atul O. Dalsania, MD)

Dear Mr. Gentile:

  The Prosecution Division of the Department of State's Office of Chief Counsel, on behalf of the Bureau of Professional and Occupational Affairs, has completed its inquiry into your complaint filed against Atul O. Dalsania, MD. Following review, this office has decided not to prosecute this case. Accordingly, this matter is now closed.

  Pursuant to section 907 of the Medical Care Availability and Reduction of Error (Mcare) Act, the act of March 20, 2002, P.L. 154, No. 13, *as amended,* 40 P.S. § 1303.907 and 63 Pa.C.S. § 3109, investigations by this office are confidential and privileged. Both Mcare and section 3109 prohibit this office from disclosing anything other than the final outcome of our investigation to you. Therefore, this office cannot provide you with a more detailed explanation of the evidence gathered during the investigation or the specific reasoning that led to this office's decision.

  While this office chose not to proceed further with your complaint, the very act of investigating a licensee can serve as a strong deterrent to professional misconduct. Additionally, the information you provided will be retained and can be referenced in the future to determine if there is a pattern of problems with this licensee.

  Thank you for taking the time to file the complaint.

         Sincerely,

         /s/ Keith E. Bashore
         Keith E. Bashore
         Prosecuting Attorney
         Commonwealth of Pennsylvania
         Department of State

KEB/keb

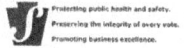

DEPARTMENT OF STATE / OFFICE OF CHIEF COUNSEL / PROSECUTION DIVISION
2601 NORTH 3RD STREET / P.O. BOX 69521 / HARRISBURG, PA 17106-9521
PHONE: 717-783-7200 / FAX: 717-787-0251 / WWW.DOS.PA.GOV

Protecting public health and safety.
Preserving the integrity of every vote.
Promoting business excellence.

---

by doing to me everything else that I have described in this book.

  It is a sad state of affairs when mistreated patients are further mistreated by government agencies that were created to protect the public from harm and abuse. Keep in mind that in a democracy, the sole purpose of government is to protect its citizens. In my case, the government chose not to protect me from authoritarian perversion, but left me to wallow in the hands of federal torturers. Worse, the Veterans Administration is a hopelessly corrupt and inadequate institution to treat and care for what is supposed to be "the nation's heroes."

Not that I think of myself as a hero. I am simply one of a large cadre of Vietnam veterans who has suffered, and is still suffering, from the vicious wounds of combat. As such, I expected my country to treat me more fairly than it has allowed its minions to treat me.

> The major recommendations from Part Two concern the VA hospitals. There we suggested that as health insurance programs are developed on the national level, the VA system be phased out in favor of a program of insurance credits graded according to the level of service-connected disability and number of years since military discharge. We made this proposal for many reasons, three of which are particularly important. First, an insurance system would provide veterans—particularly young veterans who may not be enthralled with the character of VA hospitals—with a wider choice as to where they can receive free medical care. Second, it is our belief that the nature of the VA as a system essentially of chronic care facilities on the periphery of American medicine cannot be altered by any statutory reforms. Third, if the VA remains an independent hospital system, it will make regional coordination among health services that much more difficult. There will be unnecessary duplication of facilities and equipment, discontinuities of care, artificial barriers that prevent patients from getting to the institution that can best handle their problems (as in the case of spinal cord injury). All these considerations militate against the maintenance of a separate system of veterans' health services—which, as we have pointed out, deviates from all other veterans' programs in that it involves a separate *institutional system*, not just separate financing, as in the GI Bill.
>
> The theory of the VA hospital system is that its principal task is to care for all service-connected medical problems. Second, because the nation owes a special debt to wartime veterans, it treats their most serious nonservice-connected conditions (i.e., those which require hospitalization) on occasions when they cannot afford treatment themselves. The trouble with this reasoning is that it leaves VA patients half in the system and half outside. This makes no sense medically or economically. The proposal for insurance credits, on the other hand, would allow veterans to receive all their medical care from one institution, if they so wished. This would be consistent with the new emphasis on health maintenance organizations. The proposal preserves—or rather, restores—the proper role of veterans' benefits. It provides permanent aid for those with permanent service-connected disabilities and readjustment assistance for those who are not disabled.

As For the Future

At this stage in my trials and tribulations with the VA, I am breathing easier than I have been for the past 10 years. My ankle is mostly pain free, and I know where to go to obtain relief when my symptoms return - not to the VA but to St. Luke's. I now have a PCP who cares about me and my health, and who I am certain will treat any unforseen forthcoming symptoms as well as is medically possible.

As for actual breathing, meaning inhaling and exhaling, I am still limited with how hard I can work myself without getting out of breath. Covid was a difficult time for me whenever I had to enter a building where masks were required, because I could not get enough air through the fabric to satisfy my need. When no one was looking, I turned my face toward the floor, lifted the bottom of the mask, and hyperventilated. This trick enabled me to catch my breath and store some oxygen for the next several minutes.

Ever since I started having issues with my PCP, I have kept my 800+ Facebook friends informed about my ongoing issues with the VA. I will continue to keep my Facebook friends informed about the VA's improprieties.

One issue which has yet to be resolved concerns optometry. My assigned optometrist has continued to perform beyond the call of duty. When she retired, my next scheduled visit was postponed for several months; then *that* visit was postponed for several more months; then *that* visit was postponed for an additional 7 months. I have yet to see her replacement. Instead of semi-annual visits, a year and a half will have passed before my worsening cataracts will be examined . . . unless yet another appointment gets postponed.

The Discarded Army

The quote on the facing page is from a book called *The Discarded Army: Veterans After Vietnam* (The Nader Report on Vietnam Veterans and the Veterans Administration), by Paul Starr. It is found on page 266, in Part 4: Conclusion. The book was published in 1973. Unfortunately, this invaluable report was ignored by the American Congress that authorized the investigation. One of the primary thrusts of the book was the senseless duplication of veteran hospitals. The book argued that instead of building an entire and redundant system of hospitals, which served only veterans, it would be more economical to simply allow veterans to use community hospitals whose veteran services would be paid by allocations from the Veterans Administration.

In other words, instead of a veteran being forced to go to a hospital that was located an hour away from his or her home, that veteran could go to a local hospital, after which the bill would be sent to the Veterans Administration. What could be simpler?

Better yet, being a private entity, I assure you that a community hospital would quickly fire a doctor who mistreated patients and who withheld medication from them the way my original PCP did to me. Nor would a community hospital suffer a director who allowed the hospital patients to be mistreated in any manner, the way I was.

Nor would a community hospital stand for a doctor who submitted a false report about a patient that said doctor never examined; nor let a secretary make a fake phone call and then lie about the contents of the call. Nor, as happened in the Phoenix, Arizona VA hospital, would it let patients die instead of treating them for a life-threatening condition.

The VA hospital system must be abolished.

Addendum

I had an "interesting" experience while exploring the Greater Hazleton Rails to Trails. I had just reached a gate that separated the Great Dreck Trail from the dirt road on which I was riding. I dismounted and sat on the ground to mark a waypoint on my GPS unit. As I lay the unit on my lap, my peripheral vision detected an object partly covered by my left leg: a hand grenade!

I had thrown enough of them in combat to recognize it immediately as an M2 fragmentation grenade. I used to carry six of them clipped to the front suspender straps of my pistol belt: three on each strap.

The grenade was mostly buried in the dirt. I could see only half of the exposed hemisphere and fuse cap, but not the arming lever or pull ring. Although I sat as still as a statue, goose bumps coursed along my spine. I stared at the grenade ... and stared. And kept staring.

A pain developed in my chest and slowly grew worse. When the pain became unbearable, I realized that I was not breathing. I did not gasp. Slowly, without moving the position of my body, I inhaled a deep gulp of air. After a few seconds, I commenced to breathe almost normally.

The loose flap of my pants leg was covering some of the grenade. Carefully, even delicately, I fingered the loose fold and lifted it off the grenade. Now I could see that my leg was not actually resting on the grenade but was perched on the ground adjacent to it. My combat training and experience warned me not to jump away. If the grenade had been planted as a booby trap, pressing the earth could cause it to detonate. Instead, I gradually rolled away from the grenade, onto my stomach, and up to my knees.

Now I examined the grenade closely. I was afraid to touch it but I didn't want to leave it for some hapless biker to step on. I recalled the patrol in which I dug my hand through grains in a rice crib, and pulled out a wire contraption that was an anti-personnel mine in the making: a fuse without the explosive charge.

After considerable study of the present situation, I used my fingers to gently rub away the dirt on both sides of the "device." The top of the grenade was tilted down and buried. Gradually I exposed more and more of the grenade until I could see the entire hemisphere and most of the fuse cap. Oddly, the fuse cap appeared to be light brownish in color instead of silvery (as in a new grenade) or reddish (if the fuse cap were rusted). I presumed that the arming lever and pull ring were facing down and were still hidden. As I swiped more dirt away from the fuse cap, it grew in length until it extended longer than it should have been.

I sighed with both relief and frustration. I tapped the body of the grenade with my fingernail. Then I stuck my finger under the fuse cap and jerked the device out of the ground. The "grenade" was made of plastic, and instead of a fuse cap the top opening was plugged with rolled cardboard. It was a child's toy! Nonetheless, it scared to hell out of me. My experiences in combat in Vietnam continue to haunt me.

This incident reminded me of watching the movie *Planet of the Apes* in 1968, shortly after my discharge from the Army. There is a scene in which an ape turned his rifle directly toward the camera – and the hero – and fired. I jumped in my seat as the muzzle blast reminded me of the time that enemy soldier shot me in the chest.

I never know when another backflash will occur. Vietnam is always in my subconscious mind, ready to erupt at a moment's notice.

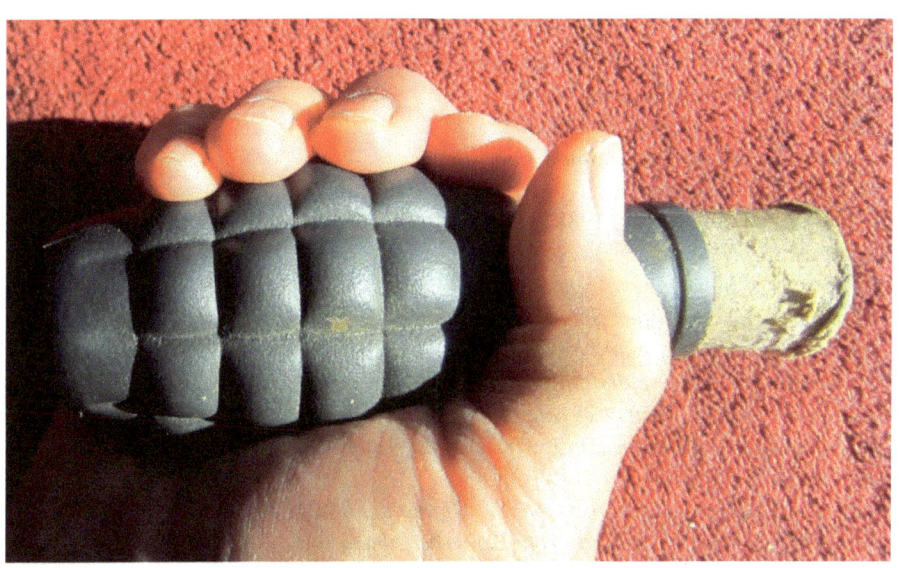

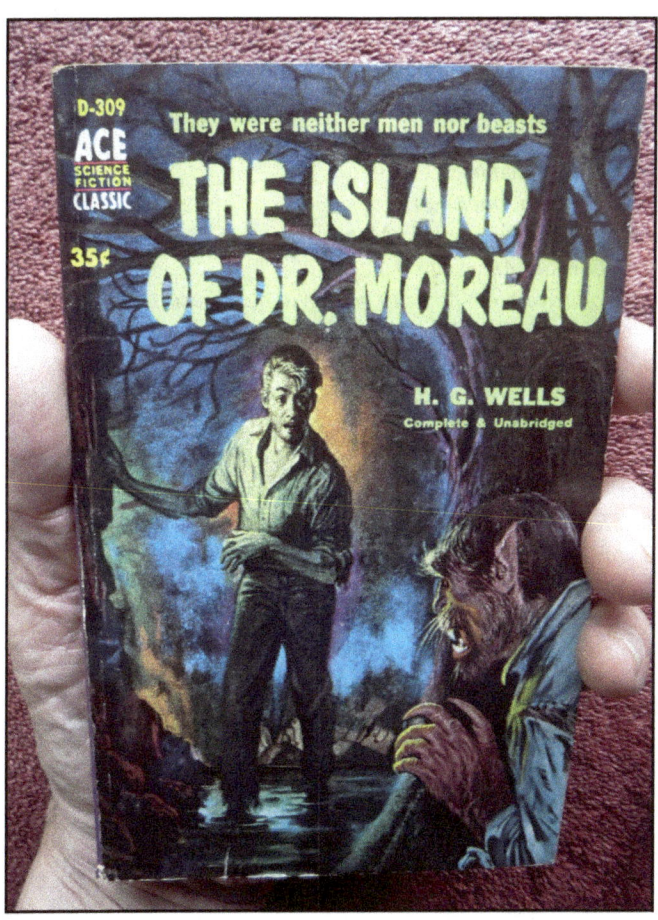

The Popular Dive Guide Series

Shipwrecks of Maine and New Hampshire
Shipwrecks of Massachusetts: North
Shipwrecks of Massachusetts: South
Shipwrecks of Rhode Island and Connecticut
Shipwrecks of New York
Shipwrecks of New Jersey (1988)
Shipwrecks of New Jersey: North
Shipwrecks of New Jersey: Central
Shipwrecks of New Jersey: South
Shipwrecks of Delaware and Maryland (1990 Edition)
Shipwrecks of Delaware and Maryland (2002 Edition)
Shipwrecks of the Chesapeake Bay in Maryland Waters
Shipwrecks of the Chesapeake Bay in Virginia Waters
Shipwrecks of Virginia
Shipwrecks of North Carolina: from the Diamond Shoals North
Shipwrecks of North Carolina: from Hatteras Inlet South
Shipwrecks of South Carolina and Georgia

Shipwreck and Nautical History

Andrea Doria: Dive to an Era
Deep, Dark, and Dangerous: Adventures and Reflections on the Andrea Doria
Great Lakes Shipwrecks: a Photographic Odyssey
The Great Navy Wreck Scam
The Fuhrer's U-boats in American Waters
Ironclad Legacy: Battles of the USS Monitor
The Kaiser's U-boats in American Waters
The Lusitania Controversies: Atrocity of War and a Wreck-Diving History
The Lusitania Controversies: Dangerous Descents into Shipwrecks and Law
The Nautical Cyclopedia
NOAA's Ark: the Rise of the Fourth Reich
Paukenschlag, Hardegen, and the SS Octavian
Shadow Divers Exposed: the Real Saga of the U-869
Shipwreck Heresies
The Shipwreck Research Handbook
Shipwreck Sagas
Stolen Heritage: the Grand Theft of the Hamilton and Scourge
Track of the Gray Wolf
The $25 Dollar Wreck of the Robert J. Walker
U-111 Exposed
Underwater Reflections
USS San Diego: the Last Armored Cruiser
Wreck Diving Adventures

Dive Training
Primary Wreck Diving Guide
Advanced Wreck Diving Guide
The Advanced Wreck Diving Handbook
Ultimate Wreck Diving Guide
The Technical Diving Handbook

Nonfiction
The Absurdity Principle
The House of Pain
Lehigh Gorge Trail Guide
Lehigh River Paddling Guide
Wilderness Canoeing

Science Fiction
A Different Universe
A Different Dimension
A Different Continuum
Entropy (a novel of conceptual breakthrough)
A Journey to the Center of the Earth
The Mold
Return to Mars
Second Coming
Silent Autumn
Subaqueous
Tesla and the Lemurian Gate
The Time Dragons Trilogy
   A Time for Dragons
   Dragons Past
   No Future for Dragons

Sci-Fi Action/Adventure Novels
Memory Lane
Mind Set
The Peking Papers

Supernatural Horror Novel   *The Lurking: Curse of the Jersey Devil*

Vietnam Novel   *Lonely Conflict*

Videotape or DVD   *The Battle for the USS Monitor*

Visit the GGP website for availability of titles:
http://www.ggentile.com

Lonely Conflict is Gary Gentile's gutsy, hard-bitten drama of America clashing with itself. It is not a stereotypic war novel. Although it focuses on Vietnam, it is first and foremost a work of literature, with strong emphasis placed on character development. The story centers on a group of teenagers who are each affected by the war in different ways. The narrative follows Anthony Giovanni: a college student who is drafted between semesters. While his friends remain at home in South Philadelphia, Tony is trained in jungle warfare and sent into combat in Vietnam.

Through Tony's eyes, the reader sees America at its lowest ebb: from campus demonstrations to trainee humiliation to an insensitive military machine that was totally lacking in compassion for the men who were forced to fight a war that was not of their choosing. Tony's friends provide divergent viewpoints on American involvement.

Even though *Lonely Conflict* is a work of fiction, the scenes depicted in the book represent actual events. The author experienced many of the incidents firsthand; others he witnessed, some he heard from the participants. No matter how absurd or preposterous they may seem, the depicted situations actually occurred in one form or another.

In this respect, *Lonely Conflict* personifies historical fiction. The author did not create or originate any of the plots or subplots. Rather, he compiled the storyline from his own experiences in the Army and in Vietnam, along with events which he knew to have occurred, and arranged the narrative in a sequence that presented scenes in such a way as to maximize the dramatic appeal. Each scene is therefore a combination of various situations that he parsed, rearranged, merged, or blended in order to create a cohesive whole, and to achieve a semblance of allegory.

The characters are composites or extrapolations of real people. The author recreated the dialogue, but based the words, thoughts, ideas, opinions, and dialect on those of people he actually met. His purpose in this regard was to convey the polemics that ran rampant during those tempestuous times, when the United States was embroiled in, and torn apart by, the Vietnam conflict. The characters symbolize controversial attitudes.

The purpose of this novel is to exemplify the turmoil of the Vietnam era for present and future generations. In one way or another, every American citizen, no matter how tangentially, was affected by the political appeal to arms. Particularly affected were those men who fought in the war, those draft-age males who avoided the war, those dissidents who actively protested the war, and those fortunate youths who - due to physical disqualification, sexual discrimination, or pure luck of the draw - managed to escape the war. Never in American history have such a large percentage of citizens demonstrated against a war.

The manner in which Americans reacted to the war was a testament to the evil of conscription, which violated the Constitutional creed by enslaving American citizens to fight in a foreign country for freedoms which Americans themselves did not possess.

Lonely Conflict is broken into five parts, which include shocking but true depictions of basic training and jungle warfare school that preceded the horror of combat that the author saw first hand.

At 380,000 words, this one book is equivalent to five books in length. After reading this volume, you will have great respect for those involuntary soldiers who were forced to fight a war that should never have been fought.

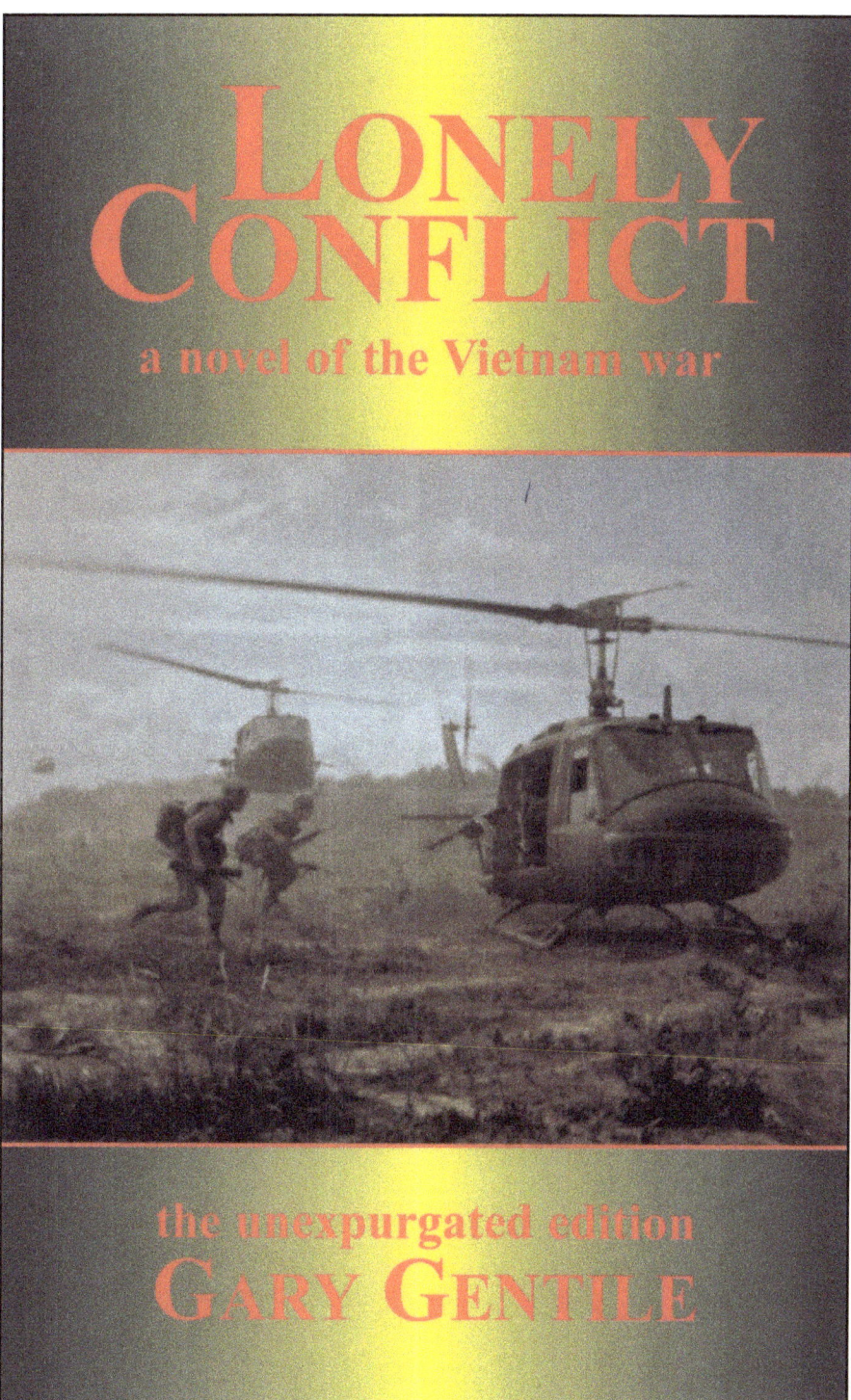

www.ingramcontent.com/pod-product-compliance
Lightning Source LLC
Chambersburg PA
CBHW071201160426
43196CB00011B/2148